20

W9-CHK-167

third edition

APPLETON & LANGE'S
REVIEW
for the usmle step 2

Carlyle H. Chan, MD, FAPA
Department of Psychiatry & Mental Health Science
Medical College of Wisconsin
Milwaukee, Wisconsin

Appleton & Lange Reviews/McGraw-Hill
Health Professions Division

New York   St. Louis   San Francisco   Auckland   Bogotá   Caracas   Lisbon   London
Madrid   Mexico City   Milan   Montreal   New Delhi   San Juan
Singapore   Sydney   Tokyo   Toronto

McGraw-Hill

A Division of The **McGraw·Hill** *Companies*

Appleton & Lange's Review for the USMLE Step 2, Third Edition

1234567890 CCICCI 99

ISBN 0-8385-0341-1

Notice

Medicine is an ever-changing science. As new research and clinical experience broaden our knowledge, changes in treatment and drug therapy are required. The author and the publisher of this work have checked with sources believed to be reliable in their efforts to provide information that is complete and generally in accord with the standards accepted at the time of publication. However, in view of the possibility of human error or changes in medical sciences, neither the author nor the publisher nor any other party who has been involved in the preparation or publication of this work warrants that the information contained herein is in every respect accurate or complete, and they are not responsible for any errors or omissions or for the results obtained from use of such information. Readers are encouraged to confirm the information contained herein with other sources. For example and in particular, readers are advised to check the product information sheet included in the package of each drug they plan to administer to be certain that the information contained in this book is accurate and that changes have not been made in the recommended dose or in the contraindications for administration. This recommendation is of particular importance in connection with new or infrequently used drugs.

This book was set in Palatino by Rainbow Graphics, LLC.
The editor was Patricia Casey.
The production supervisors were Frank Del Vecchio and Robert R. Laffler.
The cover designer was Elizabeth Schmitz.

Courier Printing was printer and binder.

This book is printed on acid-free paper.

Cataloging-in-Publication Data for this title is on file at the Library of Congress.

Contents

Contributors

Tilahun Adera, PhD
Associate Professor of Epidemiology
Department of Preventive Medicine and
    Community Health
Medical College of Virginia Campus
Virginia Commonwealth University
Richmond, Virginia

James Aiman, MD
Professor of Obstetrics and Gynecology
Director of Reproductive Endocrinology
Medical College of Wisconsin
Milwaukee, Wisconsin

C. M. G. Buttery, MD, MPH
Professor of Public Health
Department of Preventive Medicine and
    Community Health
Medical College of Virginia Campus
Virginia Commonwealth University
Richmond, Virginia

Elizabeth A. Caspary, MD
Assistant Professor of Psychiatry
Medical College of Wisconsin
Milwaukee, Wisconsin

Carlyle H. Chan, MD, FAPA
Professor of Psychiatry
Vice Chair for Education and Informatics
Department of Psychiatry & Mental Health Science
Medical College of Wisconsin
Milwaukee, Wisconsin

Rebekah Wang Cheng, MD
Professor of Medicine
Division of General Internal Medicine
Department of Internal Medicine
Medical College of Wisconsin
Milwaukee, Wisconsin

Patricia Lye, MD, MS
Assistant Professor of Pediatrics
Department of Pediatrics
Medical College of Wisconsin
Milwaukee, Wisconsin

W. R. Nelson, MD, MPH
Associate Clinical Professor of Public Health
Department of Preventive Medicine and
    Community Health
Medical College of Virginia Campus
Virginia Commonwealth University
Richmond, Virginia

Phillip N. Redlich, MD, PhD
Associate Professor of Surgery
Department of Surgery
Medical College of Wisconsin
Milwaukee, Wisconsin

Andrea Winthrop, MD, FRCS
Assistant Professor of Surgery
Division of Pediatric Surgery
Department of Surgery
Medical College of Wisconsin
Children's Hospital of Wisconsin
Milwaukee, Wisconsin

Preface

Taking the USMLE Step 2 can be an anxiety-provoking exercise. Extensive clinical exposure plus comprehensive study, including rehearsing the examination process, can aid in the preparation. The questions in this review were constructed according to the parameters set forth by the National Board of Medical Examiners. All of the subjects, types of questions, and techniques that will be encountered on the USMLE Step 2 have been updated and presented in this book. In addition to the questions in the various clinical disciplines, two practice exams covering all the clinical areas are provided at the end. Finally, we increased the number of color photos and the number of illustrations from the previous edition.

The author team is composed of experienced educators and clinicians, most of whom have been either medical student clerkship directors or medical student education directors for their respective specialties.

We believe this book will provide you with a valuable tool to assess your readiness to take the exam. We hope you will find the questions, explanations, and format to be of assistance to you in your review. Good luck!

Carlyle H. Chan, MD

Review Preparation Guide

This book is designed for those preparing for the United States Medical Licensing Examination (USMLE) Step 2. It provides a comprehensive review, with 1,200 clinical science multiple-choice questions and referenced, paragraph-length explanations of each answer. In addition, the last section of the book consists of two integrated practice tests for self-assessment purposes.

This introduction provides information on question types, question-answering strategies, specifics on the USMLE Step 2, and various ways to use this review.

THE UNITED STATES MEDICAL LICENSING EXAMINATION STEP 2

The USMLE Step 2 is currently a 2-day examination consisting of approximately 800 questions testing your knowledge in the clinical sciences. It contains multiple-choice questions organized within three dimensions: (1) System, (2) Process, and (3) Organizational Level. Although each dimension is weighted, the projected percentage for each is subject to change from exam to exam. The application materials illustrate the percentage breakout and offer a detailed content outline to aid you in your review.

ORGANIZATION OF THIS BOOK

This book is organized to cover sequentially each of the clinical science areas specified by the National Board of Medical Examiners (NBME). There are six sections, one for each of the clinical sciences, and an integrated practice test section at the end of the review. The sections are as follows:

1. **Obstetrics and Gynecology** (including biology of reproduction; fetus, placenta, and newborn; primary care of the OB/GYN patient; normal and abnormal clinical obstetrics; clinical gynecology)
2. **Pediatrics** (focusing on pediatric content and tasks and competencies)
3. **Internal Medicine** (including infectious disease, immunology, and allergy; diseases of the respiratory, cardiovascular, hematopoietic, gastrointestinal, renal, musculoskeletal, nervous, and integumentary systems; nutritional, metabolic, endocrine, oncologic, and fluid and electrolyte disorders; clinical pharmacology; legal medicine)
4. **Surgery** (including the general topics of physiology, anesthesiology, wounds, neoplasms, and forensic medicine; specific surgical treatment of the various body systems)
5. **Psychiatry** (including theories; social, community, and family relationships; assessment techniques; psychopathology; interventions; ethical and legal aspects of psychiatry)
6. **Preventive Medicine** (including biostatistics, epidemiology, disease control, provision of health services, and ethical and legal aspects of medicine)
7. **Practice Tests** (includes 300 questions from all six clinical sciences presented in an integrated format)

Each section is authored by an experienced teacher in the discipline. However, you will find that the author covers material of a general nature which is appropriate for Step 2. As a result, the basic concepts of clinical pathophysiology are covered. As in the examination itself, topics which might be classified as general or internal medicine are included in each section.

Each of the seven chapters is organized in the following order:

1. Questions
2. Answers and Explanations
3. References
4. Subspecialty List

These sections and how you might use them are discussed below.

Question Format

The style and presentation of the questions have been fully revised to conform with the USMLE. This will enable readers to familiarize themselves with the types of questions to be expected and practice answering questions in each format. Following the answer to each question, a reference refers the reader to a particular and easily available text for further reference and reading.

Each of the seven basic science chapters contains multiple-choice questions (or "items"). Most of these are one best answer—single item questions, some are one best answer—matching sets, and some are comparison—matching set questions. In some cases, a group of two or three questions may be related to one situation. In addition, some questions have illustrations (graphs, x-rays, tables, or line drawings) that require understanding and interpretation. Moreover, each question may be categorized at one of three levels of difficulty depending on the level of skill needed to answer it: rote memory, a clear understanding of the problem, or both understanding and judgment. Since the USMLE seems to prefer questions requiring judgment and critical thinking, we have attempted to emphasize these questions. Finally, some of the questions are stated in the negative. In such instances, we have printed the negative word in capital letters (eg, "All of the following are correct EX-

CEPT," "Which of the following choices is NOT correct," and "Which of the following is LEAST correct").

One Best Answer—Single-Item Question. The majority of the questions are posed in the A-type, or "one best answer—single item" format. This is the most popular question format in most exams. It generally consists of a brief statement, followed by five options of which only ONE is entirely correct. The options on the USMLE are lettered A, B, C, D, and E. Although the format for this question type is straightforward, these questions can be difficult because some of the distractors may be partially right. The instructions you will see for this type of question will generally appear as below:

DIRECTIONS: Each of the numbered items or incomplete statements in this section is followed by answers or by completions of the statement. Select the ONE lettered answer or completion that is BEST in each case.

The following is an example of this question type:

1. An obese 21-year-old woman complains of increased growth of coarse hair on her lip, chin, chest, and abdomen. She also notes menstrual irregularity with periods of amenorrhea. The most likely cause is

    (A) polycystic ovary disease
    (B) an ovarian tumor
    (C) an adrenal tumor
    (D) Cushing's disease
    (E) familial hirsutism

In the question above, the key word is "most." Although ovarian tumors, adrenal tumors, and Cushing's disease are causes of hirsutism (described in the stem of the question), polycystic ovary disease is a much more common cause. Familial hirsutism is not associated with the menstrual irregularities mentioned. Thus, the most likely cause of the manifestations described can only be "(A) polycystic ovary disease."

One Best Answer—Matching Set Questions. This format presents lettered options followed by several items related to a common topic. The directions you will generally see for this type of question are as follows:

DIRECTIONS (Questions 2 through 4): Each set of matching questions in this section consists of a list of 4 to 26 lettered options followed by several numbered items. For each item, select the ONE best lettered option that is most closely associated with it. Each lettered heading may be selected once, more than once, or not at all.

Below is an example of this type of question:

For each adverse drug reaction listed below, select the antibiotic with which it is most closely associated.

(A) tetracycline
(B) chloramphenicol
(C) clindamycin
(D) cefotaxime
(E) gentamicin

2. Bone marrow suppression

3. Pseudomembranous enterocolitis

4. Acute fatty necrosis of liver

Note that unlike the single-item questions, the choices in the matching sets *precede* the actual questions. However, as with the single-item questions, only one choice can be correct for a given question.

Extended One Best Answer—Matching/Choosing Questions. The USMLE Step 2 uses a new type of matching question that is similar to the one above, but can contain up to 26 lettered options followed by several items. The directions you will see for this type of question will generally read the same as the ones listed for the best answer—matching sets since this is another version of the same question. An example of this type of question is:

(A) sarcoidosis
(B) tuberculosis
(C) histoplasmosis
(D) coccidioidomycosis
(E) amyloidosis
(F) bacterial pneumonia
(G) mesothelioma

(H) carcinoma

(I) fibrosing alveolitis

(J) silicosis

627. A right lower lobectomy specimen contains a solitary 1.2-cm-diameter solid nodule. The center of the nodule is fibrous. The periphery has granulomatous inflammation. With special stains, multiple 2- to 5-μm budding yeasts are evident within the nodule. Acid-fast stains are negative.

628. A left upper lobectomy specimen is received containing a 4.6-cm nodule with central cystic degeneration. Microscopically, the nodule is composed of anaplastic squamous cells. Similar abnormal cells are seen in a concomitant biopsy of a hilar lymph node.

629. After a long history of multiple myeloma, a 67-year-old male is noted to have abundant acellular eosinophilic deposits around the pulmonary microvasculature at autopsy. A Congo red special stain demonstrates apple green birefringence.

630. A large pleural-based lesion is found on chest x-ray of an asbestos worker. Electron microscopy of the biopsy shows abundant long microvilli.

Note that, like other matching sets, the lettered options are listed first.

STRATEGIES FOR ANSWERING EXTENDED ONE BEST ANSWER—MATCHING/CHOOSING QUESTIONS

1. Read the lettered options through first.
2. Work with one item at a time.
3. Read the item through, then go back to the options and consider each choice individually.
4. As with the other question types, if the choice is partially correct, tentatively consider it to be incorrect.
5. Consider the remaining choices and select the answer.
6. Fill in the appropriate circle on the answer sheet.
7. Remember to make a selection for each item.
8. Again, the test allows for 50 seconds per item.

Answers, Explanations, and References

In each of the sections of this book, the question sections are followed by a section containing the answers, explanations, and references to the questions. This section (1) tells you the answer to each question; (2) gives you an explanation/review of why the answer is correct, background information on the subject matter, and why the other answers are incorrect; and (3) tells you where you can find more in-depth information on the subject matter in other books and/or journals. We encourage you to use this section as a basis for further study and understanding.

If you choose the correct answer to a question, you can then read the explanation (1) for reinforcement and (2) to add to your knowledge about the subject matter (remember that the explanations usually tell not only why the answer is correct, but also why the other choices are incorrect). **If you choose the wrong answer** to a question, you can read the explanation for a learning/reviewing discussion of the material in the question. Furthermore, you can note the reference cited (eg, "Last, pp 478–484"), look up the full source in the bibliography at the end of the section (eg, "Last JM, Wallace RB, Barrett-Connor E. *Maxcy-Rosenau-Last Public Health and Preventive Medicine.* 13th ed. Norwalk, CT: Appleton & Lange; 1992."), and refer to the pages cited for a more in-depth discussion.

Subspecialty Lists

At the end of each section of this book is a subspecialty list for each subject area. These subspecialty lists will help point out your areas of relative weakness, and thus help you focus your review.

For example, by checking off your incorrect answers on, say, the preventive medicine list, you may find that a pattern develops in that you are incorrect on most or all of the biostatistics questions. In this case, you could note the references (in the explanation section) for your incorrect answers and read those sources. You might also want to purchase a biostatistics text or review book to do a much more in-depth review. We think that you will find these subspecialty lists very helpful, and we urge you to use them.

Practice Tests

The 126-question practice tests at the end of the book consist of approximately 20 questions from each of the six clinical sciences. The questions are grouped according to question type (one best answer—single item, one best answer—matching sets, and comparison/matching sets, with the subject areas integrated. This format mimics the actual exam and enables you to test your skill at answering questions in all of the clinical sciences under simulated examination conditions.

The practice test section is organized in the same format as the six earlier sections: questions, answers and explanations, references, and subspecialty lists (which, here, will also list the major subject heading).

HOW TO USE THIS BOOK

There are two logical ways to get the most value from this book. We will call them Plan A and Plan B.

In **Plan A,** you go straight to the practice tests and complete them. After taking the practice tests, you check your answers and then tick off the ones you got wrong on the subspecialty lists on pages 312–313 and 360–361. The *number* of questions you got wrong will be a good indicator of your initial knowledge state, and the *types* of questions you got wrong will help point you in the right direction for further preparation and review. At this point, you can use the first six sections of the book, with the lists and discussions, to help you improve your areas of relative weakness.

In **Plan B,** you go through the clinical science sections (from OB/GYN to preventive medicine), checking off your answers, and then compare your choices with the answers and discussions in the book. Once you've completed this process, you can take the practice tests, check your answers as described above, and see how well prepared you are at this point. If you still have a major weakness, it should be apparent in time for you to take remedial action.

In Plan A, by taking the practice tests first, you get quick feedback regarding your initial areas of strength and weakness. You may find that you know all of the material very well, indicating that perhaps only a cursory review of the six clinical science sections is necessary. This, of course, would be good to know early on in your exam preparation. On the other hand, you may find that you have many areas of weakness (say, for example, in all of pediatrics and psychiatry and in some of the subspecialties of preventive medicine). In this case, you could then focus on these areas in your review—not just with this book, but also with text-

books of pediatrics and psychiatry.

It is, however, unlikely that you will not do some studying prior to taking the USMLE Step 2 (especially since you have this book). Therefore, it may be more realistic to take the practice tests *after* you have reviewed the six clinical science sections (as in Plan B). This, of course, will probably give you a more realistic test-type situation since very few of us just sit down to a test without studying. In this case, you will have done some reviewing (from superficial to in-depth), and your practice tests will reflect this studying time. If, after reviewing the six clinical science sections and taking the practice tests, your scores still indicate some weaknesses, you can then go back into the clinical science sections and supplement your review with your texts.

SPECIFIC INFORMATION ON THE STEP 2 EXAMINATION

The official source of all information with respect to the United States Medical Licensing Examination Step 2 is the National Board of Medical Examiners (NBME), 3930 Chestnut Street, Philadelphia, PA 19104. Established in 1915, the NBME is a voluntary, nonprofit, independent organization whose sole function is the design, implementation, distribution, and processing of a vast bank of question items, certifying examinations, and evaluative services in the professional medical field.

In order to sit for the Step 2 examination, a person must be either an officially enrolled medical student or a graduate of an accredited medical school. It is not necessary to complete any particular year of medical school to be a candidate for Step 2. Neither is it required to take Step 1 before Step 2.

In applying for Step 2, you must use forms supplied by NBME. Remember that registration closes *10 weeks* before the scheduled examination date. Some United States and Canadian medical schools require their students to take Step 2 even if they are noncandidates. Such students can register as noncandidates at the request of their school. A person who takes Step 2 as a noncandidate can later change to candidate status, and after payment of a fee, receive certification credit.

Scoring

You will receive two scores after completing Step 2. According to the information booklet provided by the National Board of Medical Examiners, a minimum score of 176 is recommended to pass Step 1, and 167 is recommended to pass Step 2. These two scores (from the three-digit scale) equate to a score of 75 on the two-digit scale. Keep in mind that the passing score for all three steps is determined on your proficiency of the examination content. Although the number of correct items to obtain these passing scores may change, the percentage of correct responses necessary to achieve them will fall between 55 and 65 percent.

Remember, there is no deduction for wrong answers, so even if you are unsure, you should answer every question.

Physical Conditions

The NBME is very concerned that all their exams be administered under uniform conditions in the numerous centers that are used. Except for several No. 2 pencils and an eraser, you are not permitted to bring anything (books, notes, calculators, etc) into the test room. All examinees receive the same questions at the same session. However, the questions are printed in different sequences in several different booklets, and the booklets are randomly distributed. In addition, examinees are moved to different seats at least once during the test. And, of course, each test is policed by at least one proctor. The object of these maneuvers is to frustrate cheating or even the temptation to cheat.

Standard Abbreviations

ACTH: adrenocorticotropic hormone
ADH: antidiuretic hormone
ADP: adenosine diphosphate
AFP: α-fetoprotein
AMP: adenosine monophosphate
ATP: adenosine triphosphate
ATPase: adenosine triphosphatase

bid: 2 times a day
BP: blood pressure
BUN: blood urea nitrogen

CT: computed tomography
CBC: complete blood count
CCU: coronary care unit
CNS: central nervous system
CPK: creatine phosphokinase
CSF: cerebrospinal fluid

DNA: deoxyribonucleic acid
DNase: deoxyribonuclease

ECG: electrocardiogram
EDTA: ethylenediaminetetraacetate
EEG: electroencephalogram
ER: emergency room

FSH: follicle-stimulating hormone

GI: gastrointestinal
GU: genitourinary

Hb: hemoglobin
hCG: human chorionic gonadotropin
Hct: hematocrit

IgA, etc: immunoglobulin A, etc
IM: intramuscular(ly)
IQ: intelligence quotient
IU: international unit
IV: intravenous(ly)

KUB: kidney, ureter, and bladder

LDH: lactic dehydrogenase
LH: luteinizing hormone
LSD: lysergic acid diethylamide

mRNA: messenger RNA

PO: oral(ly)
PRN: as needed

RBC: red blood cell
RNA: ribonucleic acid
RNase: ribonuclease
rRNA: ribosomal RNA

SC: subcutaneous(ly)
SGOT: serum glutamic oxaloacetic transaminase
SGPT: serum glutamic pyruvic transaminase

TB: tuberculosis
tRNA: transfer RNA
TSH: thyroid-stimulating hormone

WBC: white blood cell

CHAPTER 1

Obstetrics and Gynecology
Questions

James Aiman, MD

DIRECTIONS (Questions 1 through 108): Each of the numbered items or incomplete statements in this section is followed by answers or completions of the statement. Select the ONE lettered answer or completion that is BEST in each case.

1. A 27-year-old woman has used oral contraceptives (OCs) without problems for 5 years. However, she just read an article about complications of OCs in a popular women's magazine and asks you about the risks and hazards of taking OCs. You inform her that

   (A) the risk of developing ovarian cancer is increased
   (B) the risk of developing pelvic inflammatory disease (PID) is increased
   (C) the risk of developing endometrial cancer is decreased
   (D) the risk of bearing a child with major congenital anomalies is increased if taken while pregnant
   (E) the risk of ectopic pregnancy is increased

Questions 2 Through 4

The mother of a 3-year-old girl brings her daughter to see you because the girl developed breasts 6 months ago. The girl has had no vaginal bleeding and there is no pubic hair. She takes no medication.

2. The most appropriate next diagnostic step is

   (A) an ultrasound of the pelvis
   (B) a pelvic exam under general anesthesia
   (C) computed tomography (CT) scan of her head
   (D) a serum estradiol concentration
   (E) a serum follicle-stimulating hormone (FSH) concentration

3. The tests you ordered on this girl were normal for a prepubertal girl. The most likely diagnosis is

   (A) ingestion of the mother's oral contraceptive pills
   (B) a granulosa cell tumor
   (C) 21-hydroxylase deficiency
   (D) polycystic ovary syndrome
   (E) premature thelarche

4. Your management of this girl is

   (A) pituitary suppression with a gonadotropin-releasing hormone (GnRH) agonist
   (B) laparoscopy
   (C) assurance that the condition is benign and self-limiting
   (D) corticosteroid suppression of adrenal function
   (E) breast biopsy

5. After an appropriate diagnostic evaluation, a 59-year-old woman with postmenopausal bleeding had a total abdominal hysterectomy and bilateral salpingo-oophorectomy. The pathologic diagnosis is adenocarcinoma of the endometrium. An endometrial adenocarcinoma that is confined to the uterus and extends more than 50% through the myometrium is stage

(A) IC
(B) IIA
(C) IIB
(D) IIIA
(E) IVA

6. A 39-year-old woman at 16 weeks' gestation complains of headaches, blurred vision, and epigastric pain. Her blood pressure is now 156/104. Her uterine fundus is palpable 22 cm above her symphysis pubis. Fetal heart tones could not be heard with a handheld Doppler. She has 3+ proteinuria. The most likely diagnosis is

(A) anencephaly
(B) twin gestation
(C) maternal renal disease
(D) hydatidiform mole
(E) gestational diabetes mellitus

7. A 23-year-old woman develops painful vulvar vesicles that contain intranuclear inclusions on cytological examination. She is 22 weeks pregnant. Which of the following statements about genital herpes is correct?

(A) Herpes simplex viral shedding and the duration of symptoms are shortened by acyclovir.
(B) Herpes cultures from the cervix should be obtained weekly beginning at 36 weeks' gestation.
(C) An active genital herpetic lesion any time after 20 weeks' gestation requires a cesarean section.
(D) Intrauterine infection with herpes is common after 20 weeks in women with primary herpes.

(E) Pitocin induction of labor should be started within 4 hours after ruptured amniotic membranes in a woman at term with active genital herpes.

8. A 63-year-old woman has a raised, red lesion on her right labia majora. Several lymph nodes are palpable in the right inguinal region. A biopsy of the vulvar lesions is reported as malignant. The most common type of vulvar malignancy is

(A) sarcoma
(B) melanoma
(C) squamous cell carcinoma
(D) adenocarcinoma
(E) basal cell carcinoma

Questions 9 Through 11

A 48-year-old woman had a biopsy of a friable, bleeding lesion on her cervix. She had not had a pelvic exam or Papanicolaou (Pap) smear for about 12 years. The biopsy is reported as invasive squamous cell carcinoma of the cervix. On bimanual examination, there is induration to the side wall of her pelvis.

9. The stage of her cervical cancer is

(A) IA
(B) IB
(C) IIB
(D) IIIB
(E) IV

10. To complete the staging of her cancer according to International Federation of Gynecology and Obstetrics (FIGO) standards, she should have a

(A) lymphangiogram
(B) pelvic venogram
(C) cystoscopy
(D) magnetic resonance imaging (MRI) scan of her abdomen
(E) laparoscopy

✓ 11. Most deaths from cervical cancer occur as a consequence of

    (A) liver failure from metastatic disease

    (B) uremia and pyelonephritis

    (C) infection

    (D) uncontrollable hemorrhage

    (E) intestinal obstruction

✓ 12. A 35-year-old G_3P_3 woman has been experiencing bilateral breast pain for the past year. Breast examination and mammography are normal. Conservative measures have failed. The medication most likely to bring relief would be

    (A) clomiphene

    (B) stilbestrol

    (C) danazol

    (D) bromocriptine

    (E) medroxyprogesterone

13. Which of the following conditions would a gynecologist be most likely to treat with the use of dilator therapy?

    (A) dysmenorrhea

    (B) vaginismus

    (C) dyspareunia

    (D) primary anorgasmia

    (E) secondary anorgasmia

14. At a follow-up routine prenatal visit, the uterine fundus of a healthy 23-year-old pregnant woman is palpated halfway between her symphysis pubis and umbilicus. The test most appropriate at this stage of her pregnancy is _16 wk_

    (A) serum human immunodeficiency virus (HIV) titer

    (B) glucose tolerance test

    (C) amniocentesis

    (D) maternal serum alpha-fetoprotein (MSAFP)

    (E) cervical culture for group B streptococcus

✓ 15. Acute left ventricular failure may be associated with the use of the antineoplastic agent

    (A) cisplatin

    (B) cyclophosphamide

    (C) bleomycin

    (D) vincristine

    (E) doxorubicin /adriamycin

✓ 16. A 13-year-old girl had growth of breast buds at age 11 years, followed by the appearance of pubic hair between the ages of $11^1/_2$ and 12 years. The next pubertal event likely to occur is

    (A) beginning of accelerated growth

    (B) menarche

    (C) Tanner stage 5 breast development

    (D) maximal growth rate

    (E) Tanner stage 5 pubic hair

17. A 32-year-old G_2P_1 woman is now 13 weeks pregnant. Her first pregnancy was uncomplicated, and she delivered vaginally at 39 weeks' gestation 9 years ago. She has a history of rheumatic heart disease. She currently denies dyspnea, dizziness upon standing, or syncope with exertion. Which of the following is most helpful in determining the functional capacity of this patient during pregnancy?

    (A) an electrocardiogram

    (B) elevated diaphragms and an enlarged cardiac silhouette on chest film

    (C) pedal edema

    (D) an S_3 heart sound

    (E) the presence or absence of symptoms

✓ 18. Labor and vaginal delivery occur successfully in a 29-year-old woman after administration of Pitocin for 9 hours. Spontaneous onset of labor at term is the result of

    (A) cortisol production in the amniotic cavity

    (B) prostaglandin release from the fetal membranes

    (C) prolactin produced in the decidua

    (D) fetal pituitary secretion of oxytocin from the neurohypophysis

    (E) events that are currently uncertain

19. Extramedullary hematopoiesis is very common in the human fetus. At 8 months' gestation, the most important site of hematopoiesis is the

    (A) yolk sac
    (B) spleen
    (C) bone marrow
    (D) liver
    (E) lymph nodes

Questions 20 and 21

A 27-year-old woman with amenorrhea of 6 months' duration relates a 4-month growth of thick, black hair on her face, chest, and abdomen. She takes no medications with androgenic effects. Her family history is negative for hirsutism. The hirsutism is confirmed by your examination. Her pelvic exam is normal other than a mild male pubic hair pattern.

20. The most appropriate next step in her evaluation is a

    (A) serum prolactin concentration
    (B) 24-hour urine for 17-ketosteroid excretion
    (C) serum dehydroepiandrosterone sulfate (DHEAS) concentration
    (D) CT scan of the pituitary sella
    (E) pelvic ultrasound

21. Your evaluation of this hirsute, amenorrheic woman is normal except for a significantly increased serum DHEAS concentration. Additional history discloses that her menses have always been somewhat irregular since menarche at age 10 years. She has a 23-year-old sister with irregular menstrual intervals and hirsutism to a lesser degree. This patient has a blood pressure of 96/64. The most likely diagnosis is

    (A) polycystic ovary syndrome
    (B) 21-hydroxylase deficiency
    (C) 11-hydroxylase deficiency
    (D) 17-hydroxylase deficiency
    (E) Sertoli–Leydig cell tumor

22. A 31-year-old pregnant woman 6 to 7 weeks from her last menses comes to the emergency department of your hospital complaining of lower abdominal pain for 3 hours. The pain is diffuse in the lower abdomen but worse on the right side. Her serum human chorionic gonadotropin (hCG) concentration is 4600 mIU/mL. The strongest evidence that she has a tubal ectopic pregnancy is

    (A) absence of an extrauterine sac on ultrasonography
    (B) absence of blood on culdocentesis
    (C) absence of a mass on bimanual examination
    (D) absence of an intrauterine sac on ultrasonography
    (E) her hCG concentration

23. A 22-year-old primiparous woman is in premature labor at 30 weeks' gestation. Despite administration of tocolytic agents, it appears that she will deliver soon. Pulmonary maturity might be enhanced by the administration of

    (A) magnesium sulfate
    (B) betamethasone
    (C) hydroxyprogesterone
    (D) chloroprocaine
    (E) digitalis

24. A 28-year-old woman with 28-day menstrual cycles is attempting to conceive and is considering the use of a home ovulation predictor kit to time intercourse at ovulation. She asks you what day of her menstrual cycle her luteinizing hormone (LH) peak is most likely to occur. You tell her day

    (A) 12
    (B) 14
    (C) 18
    (D) 20
    (E) 27

25. A 48-year-old woman with five children complains of urinary incontinence with coughing and stair climbing. She likely has genuine stress urinary incontinence if loss of urine

    (A) is secondary to involuntary bladder contractions

    (B) is associated with a strong desire to void immediately

    (C) occurs in relation to anxiety or depression

    (D) occurs when intravesical pressure exceeds maximal urethral pressure

    (E) is due to increased intravesical pressure associated with bladder distension

26. An 18-year-old nullipara has suddenly stopped menstruating. She recently lost 8.6 kg when she started long-distance running. The laboratory test most consistent with her cause of secondary amenorrhea is

    (A) a serum prolactin level of 86 ng/mL (normal < 20)

    (B) a serum LH level of 48 mIU/mL (normal 6 to 35)

    (C) a serum estradiol level of 128 pg/mL (normal 40 to 300)

    (D) a serum FSH level of 3 mIU/mL (normal 5 to 18)

    (E) a serum testosterone level of 156 ng/dL (normal 40 to 110)

27. A 22-year-old woman with cystic fibrosis is engaged to be married and asks you about childbearing. You should advise her that

    (A) an amniocentesis should be done to detect fetal cystic fibrosis

    (B) pregnancy is contraindicated because maternal mortality is significantly increased

    (C) her children have a 25% chance of having cystic fibrosis

    (D) pregnancy and delivery are usually successful with special care and precautions

    (E) she should use nasal oxygen throughout pregnancy to minimize fetal hypoxemia

28. On the first pelvic examination of an 18-year-old nulligravida, a 3-cm paravaginal cyst is found. This likely represents remnants of the

    (A) wolffian duct   Gardner cyst

    (B) müllerian duct

    (C) urogenital sinus

    (D) metanephric duct

    (E) squamocolumnar junction

29. Mrs. Smith has just had twins and wonders if there is any way to determine whether the twins are identical. You tell her that

    (A) close examination of the placenta can often provide this answer

    (B) there is no way to tell unless one is a girl and one a boy

    (C) only matching of human lymphocyte antigens could determine this with certainty

    (D) identical twins occur only once in about 80 births of twins

    (E) it is unlikely because the birth weights differed by more than 200 g

30. The average female has her maximum number of oocytes at

    (A) 6 weeks' gestation

    (B) 20 weeks' gestation

    (C) 36 weeks' gestation

    (D) 1 year after birth

    (E) puberty

31. A patient with postpartum endometritis does not seem to be responding to her regimen of ampicillin and gentamicin. Important gynecologic pathogens not well covered by this therapy include

    (A) *Pseudomonas* species

    (B) enterococci

    (C) staphylococci

    (D) *Bacteroides fragilis*

    (E) *Proteus mirabilis*

32. The etiologic agent in condyloma lata is

    (A) human papillomavirus
    (B) *Hemophilus ducreyi*
    (C) herpesvirus, type 2
    (D) *Treponema pallidum*
    (E) *Neisseria gonorrhoeae*

33. A 24-year-old nullipara is being evaluated for infertility. A diagnostic laparoscopy shows a double uterus. The next method of assessment would most likely be

    (A) a postcoital test
    (B) a karyotype
    (C) an intravenous pyelogram (IVP)
    (D) a luteal-phase progesterone concentration
    (E) a hysterosalpingogram

34. A 58-year-old $G_6P_4Ab_2$ diabetic woman who weighs 122.6 kg (270 lb) has her first episode of vaginal bleeding in 5 years. Her physician performs an outpatient operative hysteroscopy and dilatation and curettage (D&C) with a preoperative diagnosis of

    (A) endometrial cancer because of her high parity
    (B) endometrial cancer because of her obesity
    (C) cervical cancer because of her age
    (D) cervical cancer because of her diabetes
    (E) ovarian cancer because of her obesity

35. A pregnant woman is being followed by a nephrologist for chronic glomerulonephritis. Which of the following findings is normal at 28 weeks' gestation?

    (A) blood pressure of 132/86
    (B) blood urea nitrogen (BUN) of 21 mg/100 mL
    (C) serum creatinine of 1.1 mg/100 mL
    (D) glomerular filtration rate of 100 mL/min
    (E) glycosuria with a plasma glucose of 130 mg/100 mL

36. A 25-year-old woman has a positive cervical culture for *Neisseria gonorrhoeae*. She has had

at least two positive cultures for gonorrhea treated in the past. She is afebrile and has no symptoms. The incidence of penicillin-resistant gonorrhea in some areas of the United States is currently as great as 10%. Because of this, the recommended treatment for gonorrhea includes

    (A) 125 mg intramuscular ceftriaxone as a single dose
    (B) 1 g spectinomycin
    (C) 2 g ampicillin orally as a single dose
    (D) 2 g intramuscular cefoxitin
    (E) 2 g metronidazole as a single dose

37. Of the following methods of assessing fetal well-being, the one with the greatest specificity (ie, the test is normal when the infant is normal) is

    (A) nonstress tests (NSTs)
    (B) oxytocin challenge tests
    (C) urinary estriol determinations
    (D) fetal movement counting
    (E) fetal biophysical profile

38. In the past 10 years, the major advance in the treatment of diabetic pregnancy has been

    (A) the ability to detect major anomalies by ultrasonography and provide therapeutic abortion
    (B) home monitoring of blood glucose by the patient
    (C) the advent and use of respiratory stimulants like betamethasone
    (D) the ability of pediatric surgeons to save infants born with congenital heart defects
    (E) the administration of glucagon to the infants of diabetic mothers

Questions 39 and 40

39. The diagnosis of septic pelvic thrombophlebitis is best made by

    (A) venography
    (B) ^{131}I tagging studies
    (C) clinical response to clindamycin

(D) clinical response to heparin

(E) MRI of the pelvis

40. Once a diagnosis of septic pelvic thrombophlebitis is made, affected patients should be managed by

(A) intravenous (IV) antibiotics and heparin for at least 7 days

(B) IV heparin alone for at least 7 days

(C) warfarin (Coumadin) administration and continuation of IV antibiotic therapy

(D) ovarian vein ligation and antibiotic therapy

(E) total abdominal hysterectomy and bilateral salpingo-oophorectomy

41. A 27-year-old woman has carcinoma in situ of the cervix. By colposcopy, the squamocolumnar junction is completely visible and the lesion does not extend into the endocervical canal. The most appropriate treatment for this woman is

(A) cryosurgery

(B) loop electroexcision procedure (LEEP)

(C) total hysterectomy

(D) radical hysterectomy

(E) local radiation therapy

42. A 16-year-old girl is brought to see you by a social worker. She has run away from home several times in the past 6 months. Her school grades have dropped noticeably. She has been arrested twice in the last month for shoplifting. She appears healthy and intelligent. The most plausible explanation for her behavior is

(A) boredom with school

(B) cocaine abuse

(C) incest

(D) depression

(E) peer pressure

Questions 43 and 44

You see a 23-year-old woman in the emergency department because she states that she was raped 3 hours ago.

43. Which of the following history or physical findings are sufficient to document a diagnosis of rape on her record?

(A) bruises on her torso

(B) acid phosphatase from a pool of vaginal fluid

(C) nonmotile sperm in the vagina

(D) motile sperm in the cervical mucus

(E) none of the above permit a diagnosis of rape

44. Your examination of this woman includes a search for sperm. Sperm remain motile the longest

(A) in the oropharynx

(B) in the rectum

(C) in the vagina

(D) in the endocervix

(E) on the vulva

45. A 19-year-old primigravid woman at 39 weeks' gestation is in active labor and her cervix is 4 cm dilated, 90% effaced. Her amniotic membranes have been ruptured for 4 hours. Contractions are strong at 2- to 3-minute intervals and of 60- to 70-second duration. For the past 30 minutes, repetitive variable decelerations of the fetal heart rate have occurred. They have lasted 60 to 90 seconds, and the fetal heart rate has dropped as low as 60 beats per minute. You explain that there is a risk that the baby will become hypoxic and recommend a cesarean section. She refuses. You should

(A) obtain permission for the cesarean section from her mother

(B) perform a cesarean section as an emergency

(C) obtain a court order permitting a cesarean section

(D) counsel her carefully about the fetal risks but accede to her wishes

(E) assign her care to another obstetrician

46. A 35-year-old primigravid woman with a history of cyclic menses at 28- to 30-day intervals began her last menses on August 18. A home pregnancy test was positive on September 20. At her first prenatal visit, she asks you what the duration of pregnancy is and what her due date is. You tell her that the average number of days from the onset of menses to delivery is

   (A) 250
   (B) 260
   (C) 270
   (D) 280
   (E) 290

47. The earliest you would expect to hear the fetal heart with a fetal stethoscope (unamplified) is at a gestational age of

   (A) 10 weeks
   (B) 12 weeks
   (C) 14 weeks
   (D) 16 weeks
   (E) 20 weeks
   (F) 26 weeks

Questions 48 and 49

A 44-year-old woman had a normal Pap smear 3 years ago. She has had intermenstrual and postcoital spotting intermittently for the past 6 months. The pelvic exam is normal.

48. The most appropriate test to perform is

   (A) an endometrial biopsy
   (B) an endocervical curettage
   (C) a conization of the cervix
   (D) a Pap smear
   (E) a hysteroscopy

49. All tests performed on the woman were normal. She returns one year later for her annual gynecologic exam. On speculum exam, she has a visible 7-mm lesion on her cervix that bleeds on contact. The most appropriate procedure is

   (A) colposcopy
   (B) cervical biopsy
   (C) Pap smear
   (D) conization of the cervix
   (E) vaginal hysterectomy

50. A 24-year-old woman lost her previous two pregnancies at approximately 20 weeks' gestation, without having noted any contractions. She is currently at 15 weeks' gestation and denies having uterine contractions. Her cervix is undilated and uneffaced. Treatment should consist of

   (A) bedrest
   (B) terbutaline
   (C) hydroxyprogesterone
   (D) diethylstilbestrol (DES)
   (E) a cervical cerclage

51. A 24-year-old woman with a previous infant with anencephaly is receiving genetic counseling at 16 weeks' gestation. She should be counseled that the approximate risk for recurrence of an open neural tube defect (NTD) is

   (A) 0.1%
   (B) 2%
   (C) 10%
   (D) 25%
   (E) 50%

52. A 69-year-old woman with diabetes mellitus complains of urinary incontinence. Her diabetes is well controlled with oral hypoglycemic agents. She has no complaints other than the wetness. The test most likely to demonstrate the cause is

   (A) urinalysis
   (B) urine culture and sensitivity
   (C) intravesical instillation of methylene blue
   (D) the Q-tip test
   (E) measurement of residual urine volume

53. A 48-year-old G_5P_5 woman has genuine stress incontinence. Kegel exercises have not helped, and her incontinence is gradually worsening. Her urethrovesical junction is prolapsed into the vagina, and her urethral closure pressure is normal. The procedure most likely to cure her incontinence is

(A) retropubic urethropexy
(B) anterior colporrhaphy
(C) suburethral sling procedure
(D) needle suspension of paraurethral tissue
(E) paraurethral collagen injections

54. On a routine annual examination, a 43-year-old woman is found to have a 2-cm mass in the lateral aspect of her right breast. The most appropriate next step is

(A) repeat the breast exam after her next menses
(B) mammography
(C) aspirate the mass with a 23-gauge needle and syringe
(D) open biopsy
(E) segmental resection

55. A 37-year-old pregnant woman has a genetic amniocentesis at 16 weeks' gestation. A concurrent ultrasound shows normal fetal anatomy. Her prenatal course has been unremarkable. Her prenatal labs include a B-negative blood type, a negative rubella antibody titer, a negative hepatitis B surface antigen, and a hematocrit of 31%. Which of the following is most appropriate for this woman?

(A) rubella immunization at the time of the amniocentesis
(B) a serologic test for the presence of hepatitis B surface antibody
(C) a follow-up ultrasound in 1 week to assess for intra-amniotic bleeding
(D) administration of Rh immune globulin at the time of the amniocentesis
(E) chorionic villus biopsy at the time of the amniocentesis

Questions 56 Through 58

A 23-year-old pregnant woman at 5 postmenstrual weeks took Coumadin until about 3 days after her menses was due. She has monthly menses. A home pregnancy test was positive on the day she took Coumadin. She is concerned that the Coumadin will cause birth defects.

56. You tell her that the conceptus is most susceptible to teratogenesis

(A) between menses and ovulation
(B) from ovulation to implantation
(C) between implantation and the day of expected menses
(D) between the day of expected menses and 12 postmenstrual weeks
(E) during the second and third trimesters

57. Your advice to this woman is to

(A) abort the pregnancy because the fetus is likely to have birth defects
(B) have an ultrasound in 1 to 2 weeks to search for fetal anomalies
(C) have a genetic amniocentesis at 16 postmenstrual weeks
(D) begin prenatal care because the probability of birth defects is low
(E) take 10 mg vitamin K to reverse the effects of Coumadin

58. The most common birth defect associated with Coumadin is

(A) nasal hypoplasia
(B) transposition of the great vessels
(C) spina bifida
(D) anencephaly
(E) achondroplasia

59. A 19-year-old primigravida at term has been completely dilated for $2^1/_2$ hours. The vertex is at +2 to +3 station, and the position is occiput posterior. She complains of exhaustion and is unable to push effectively to expel the fetus. She has an anthropoid pelvis. The most appropriate management to deliver the fetus is

(A) immediate low transverse cesarean section

(B) immediate classical cesarean section

(C) apply forceps and delivery the baby as an occiput posterior

(D) apply Kielland forceps to rotate the baby to occiput anterior

(E) cut a generous episiotomy to make her pushing more effective

Questions 60 and 61

A 22-year-old woman whose last pregnancy was terminated by salpingostomy for removal of a tubal pregnancy is attempting to conceive.

60. The average number of ovulatory cycles to achieve a pregnancy by normally fertile couples is

(A) 1

(B) 3

(C) 6

(D) 8

(E) 10

61. This woman is aware that her chances of another tubal pregnancy are increased. What is the earliest that a serum β-hCG will be positive?

(A) 4 days after fertilization

(B) during the week before the expected date of menses

(C) on the day of the expected menses

(D) 1 week after the missed menses

(E) 2 weeks after the missed menses

Questions 62 and 63

A 46-year-old G_3P_3 woman has had postcoital spotting for 6 months. On pelvic examination, she has a fungating, exophytic lesion arising from her vagina that is approximately 2 cm in diameter. Biopsy of this lesion is interpreted as invasive squamous cell carcinoma of the cervix. There is no evidence of extension of the cancer onto the vagina. The parametria are not indurated by bimanual examination. CT scan of her pelvis and abdomen discloses enlarged para-aortic lymph nodes and metastatic lesions in the parenchyma of her liver.

62. The FIGO stage of her cancer is

(A) IA

(B) IB

(C) IIA

(D) IIIB

(E) IVB

63. This woman's childbearing is complete. She is a healthy woman who is close to ideal body weight, exercises regularly, and does not smoke. Appropriate treatment of this woman is

(A) total abdominal hysterectomy and bilateral salpingo-oophorectomy (TAH-BSO)

(B) radical hysterectomy with pelvic and para-aortic lymph node dissection

(C) pelvic exenteration

(D) multiagent chemotherapy

(E) combined brachytherapy and external radiation therapy

64. A 32-year-old registered nurse has her second prenatal visit at 9 postmenstrual weeks. Her 7-year-old son was recently exposed to mumps. Her prenatal lab results are reviewed. She is rubella nonimmune. Her hepatitis B surface antigen is negative, but her hepatitis B surface antibody is positive. She has not had a tetanus toxoid injection for at least 10 years, and she cannot recall whether she has received a polio vaccine. Which of the following injectable vaccines is contraindicated during pregnancy?

(A) tetanus

(B) poliomyelitis

(C) rubella

(D) influenza

(E) rabies

65. A pregnant woman has been taking phenytoin (Dilantin) for a seizure disorder. She is concerned that the drug will cause fetal abnormalities. Which of the following defects is the most common anomaly associated with phenytoin?

(A) atrial septal defect

(B) ventricular septal defect

(C) cleft lip/palate

(D) spina bifida

(E) hydrocephalus

66. When counseling pregnant women about the dangers of drug use during pregnancy, they should be told that the rate of spontaneous major malformations in newborns is

(A) less than 1%

(B) 2 to 4%

(C) 6 to 8%

(D) 10 to 12%

(E) more than 12%

Questions 67 and 68

A 34-year-old woman just delivered a 4100-g boy after a 15-hour labor, including a 2^1/$_2$-hour second stage. During the repair of a midline episiotomy, there is a marked increase in the amount of vaginal bleeding.

67. Of the following, the most common cause of immediate postpartum hemorrhage is

(A) retained placental fragments

(B) uterine atony

(C) cervical laceration

(D) vaginal laceration

(E) disseminated intravascular coagulation

68. Immediate management of the probable cause of this postpartum hemorrhage is

(A) massage and compression of the uterine fundus

(B) intravenous administration of 20 units of oxytocin

(C) intramuscular administration of 0.2 mg methylergonovine

(D) insertion of a gauze pack into the uterine cavity

(E) hypogastric artery ligation

Questions 69 Through 73

A 55-year-old woman has a bloody discharge from her left breast. A mammogram discloses a cluster of microcalcifications 3 cm beneath her left nipple.

69. The next step in her evaluation is

(A) cytologic evaluation of the nipple discharge

(B) fine-needle aspiration under radiologic guidance

(C) CT of the breast and axillary nodes

(D) open biopsy of the left breast

(E) segmental mastectomy

70. The principal advantage of a fine-needle aspiration of a breast mass is that it

(A) reassures the patient if it is negative

(B) reduces the number of open breast biopsies

(C) differentiates between noninvasive and invasive cancer

(D) replaces the need for subsequent mammography

(E) helps to determine the extent of in situ breast carcinoma

71. The factor associated with the greatest lifetime risk for developing breast cancer is

(A) obesity

(B) early menarche

(C) late menopause

(D) postmenopausal hormone replacement longer than 10 years

(E) having a mother with a history of breast cancer

72. If the woman has breast cancer, the most common type is

    (A) inflammatory carcinoma
    (B) lobular carcinoma in situ
    (C) lobular infiltrating carcinoma
    (D) infiltrating ductal carcinoma
    (E) ductal carcinoma in situ

73. The best predictor of breast cancer that has spread outside the breast is

    (A) an initial tumor larger than 2 cm in diameter
    (B) the absence of estrogen receptors
    (C) the presence of progesterone receptors
    (D) a high mitotic index
    (E) a low thymidine labeling index

74. A 39-year-old woman known to have fibrocystic disease of the breast complains of persistent fullness and pain in both breasts. The most effective drug to relieve her symptoms is

    (A) tamoxifen
    (B) bromocriptine
    (C) medroxyprogesterone acetate
    (D) danazol
    (E) hydrochlorothiazide

75. A couple consults you because each has neurofibromatosis and wish to know what their reproductive possibilities are. You should tell them that

    (A) the disease is lethal and results in spontaneous abortion of homozygous fetuses
    (B) 25% of the females will be affected
    (C) 50% of all offspring will be homozygous for the abnormal gene
    (D) 75% of all offspring will have the disease
    (E) 100% of the offspring will either have the disease or be carriers

76. A 26-year-old woman complains of a vaginal discharge causing burning and itching of the perineum. The pH of the discharge is 4.5. The most likely cause of her discharge is

    (A) monilial vaginitis
    (B) trichomonas vaginitis
    (C) chlamydial cervicitis
    (D) gonococcal cervicitis
    (E) bacterial vaginosis

Questions 77 and 78

77. A wet smear of a vaginal discharge is illustrated in Figure 1–1. The cause of the discharge is

    (A) monilial vaginitis
    (B) trichomonas vaginitis
    (C) *Chlamydia trachomatis*
    (D) *Neisseria gonorrhoeae*
    (E) bacterial vaginosis

78. The most appropriate treatment for the discharge illustrated in Figure 1–1 is

    (A) clindamycin
    (B) erythromycin

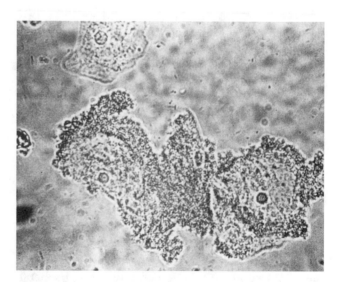

Figure 1–1. Vaginal epithelial cells studded with bacteria on their surface.

(C) metronidazole

(D) miconazole

(E) doxycycline

79. A 37-year-old man and his wife seek help for their 5-year history of primary infertility. Her infertility investigation is normal. However, the husband has an ejaculate volume of 0.4 mL and there are no sperm in the ejaculate. A qualitative test for fructose in the semen is negative. The probable diagnosis is

(A) germ cell aplasia

(B) bilateral occlusion of the vasa deferentia

(C) 17α-hydroxylase deficiency

(D) congenital absence of the vasa deferentia

(E) Klinefelter syndrome

80. According to the World Health Organization (WHO), the minimal sperm concentration associated with normal fertility is

(A) 1 million/mL

(B) 10 million/mL

(C) 20 million/mL

(D) 60 million/mL

(E) 100 million/mL

81. The duration of spermatogenesis, the formation of mature spermatozoa released into the epididymis from spermatogonia, is approximately

(A) 33 days

(B) 53 days

(C) 73 days

(D) 93 days

(E) 120 days

82. Once spermatozoa are released into the epididymis, the approximate time required for the sperm to appear in the ejaculate is

(A) 3 hours

(B) 7 days

(C) 21 days

(D) 28 days

(E) 60 days

Questions 83 Through 85

A 19-year-old pregnant woman at 38 weeks' gestation comes to labor and delivery with profuse vaginal bleeding and abdominal pain of sudden onset.

83. The most likely diagnosis is

(A) bloody show

(B) vaginal laceration from coitus

(C) cervicitis

(D) placenta previa

(E) placental abruption

84. If the patient has a placental abruption, which of the following is the most common risk factor?

(A) maternal age

(B) high parity

(C) abdominal trauma

(D) maternal hypertension

(E) cocaine abuse

85. This patient has an external fetal monitor placed. Uterine tone appears to be increased and there are occasional variable decelerations of the fetal heart to 90 beats per minute. The most appropriate management is

(A) tocolysis with a β-receptor agonist

(B) pitocin induction of labor

(C) continued monitoring of mother and baby

(D) amniotomy

(E) cesarean section

Questions 86 Through 88

A 58-year-old woman with stage IIB squamous cell carcinoma of the cervix is receiving radiation therapy.

86. The phase in which a cell is most sensitive to ionizing radiation is

(A) mitosis

(B) ribonucleic acid (RNA) synthesis

(C) deoxyribonucleic acid (DNA) synthesis

(D) protein synthesis

(E) the resting phase

87. This woman is to receive external radiation therapy. The usual dose to treat invasive cervical cancer is

(A) 500 to 1000 cGy
(B) 1500 to 2000 cGy
(C) 4500 to 5000 cGy
(D) 7500 to 8000 cGy
(E) 9500 to 10,000 cGy

88. The earliest complication of radiation therapy is

(A) diarrhea
(B) hemorrhagic cystitis
(C) vaginal stenosis
(D) ureteral fibrosis
(E) rectovaginal fistula

89. A 45-year-old woman has bilateral breast pain that is most severe premenstrually. On palpation, there is excessive nodularity, tenderness, and cystic areas that diminish in size after menses. The most likely diagnosis is

(A) fibrocystic disease
(B) fibroadenomas
(C) intraductal papilloma
(D) breast cancer
(E) engorgement due to increased prolactin

90. Which feature of fibrocystic disease of the breast is associated with the greatest risk of developing breast cancer?

(A) number of nodules
(B) serous nipple discharge
(C) size of the dominant mass
(D) presence of epithelial hyperplasia
(E) presence of a palpable axillary node

91. A 35-year-old woman at 30 weeks' gestation discovers a lump in her left breast. Examination reveals a 2 × 3 × 3-cm, firm nodule in the upper outer quadrant. The next step in the management of this patient is

(A) observation until after delivery
(B) thermography
(C) application of hot packs
(D) needle aspiration
(E) needle biopsy

92. A 2-cm carcinoma of the breast is diagnosed by an excisional biopsy in a 36-year-old woman at 14 weeks' gestation. The axillary nodes are negative. The best management of this patient is to

(A) terminate the pregnancy immediately
(B) terminate the pregnancy at 16 weeks' gestation with intra-amniotic saline
(C) induce labor at 34 weeks' gestation, then give chemotherapy
(D) terminate the pregnancy at 36 weeks' gestation by cesarean delivery
(E) allow the pregnancy to proceed to term and manage it expectantly

Questions 93 and 94

A woman at 31 weeks' gestation complains of feeling dizzy and lightheaded when she lies on her back. The diagnosis is probably the supine hypotensive syndrome.

93. This results in

(A) a decreased fetal heart rate
(B) an increased frequency of uterine contractions
(C) a decreased tolerance to pain
(D) a decreased effect of epidural analgesia
(E) an increased risk of placental abruption

94. During this woman's labor, the nurse describes the presenting part as engaged when the woman is 6 cm dilated. The most accurate definition of engagement in a woman with a vertex presentation is

(A) the vertex has passed through the pelvic inlet
(B) the vertex reaches the pelvic floor
(C) the biparietal diameter has passed through the pelvic inlet
(D) the biparietal diameter has reached the pelvic floor
(E) the vertex is at +1 station

95. An Rh-negative woman is pregnant. In which of the following circumstances is the administration of anti-D immune globulin unnecessary?

   (A) threatened abortion and first-trimester bleeding
   (B) genetic amniocentesis at 16 weeks' gestation
   (C) at 28 weeks
   (D) at 40 weeks with the onset of labor
   (E) after delivery of an Rh-positive fetus

96. Regarding the administration of anti-D immune globulin, which of the following statements is true?

   (A) Administration of anti-D immune globulin in the second trimester of pregnancy has not been shown to decrease the incidence of Rh sensitization.
   (B) It is a form of passive immunization.
   (C) It has a high association with HIV.
   (D) To be effective, it must be delivered within 24 hours after birth.
   (E) Once administered in one pregnancy, it does not need to be given in subsequent pregnancies.

Questions 97 Through 99

A 19-year-old primigravida is at 39 weeks' gestation. Her prenatal course had been normal since her first visit at 9 weeks' gestation. Her blood pressure is now 144/96. She has 2+ proteinuria. Her patellar reflexes are hyperactive.

97. The most likely diagnosis is

   (A) acute glomerulonephritis
   (B) essential hypertension
   (C) pheochromocytoma
   (D) preeclampsia
   (E) polycystic kidneys

98. The treatment of this patient would be

   (A) bedrest
   (B) oral magnesium sulfate

   (C) a thiazide diuretic
   (D) propranolol
   (E) induction of labor

99. Magnesium sulfate may be the preferred treatment in this patient if she is not at least at 37 weeks' gestation and there is no evidence of fetal distress. The purpose of magnesium sulfate is

   (A) tocolysis to prevent preterm labor
   (B) decrease her blood pressure into the normal range
   (C) reduce the risk of eclampsia
   (D) increase uteroplacental blood flow
   (E) prevent fetal hypertension

Questions 100 and 101

A 39-year-old multiparous woman has a retained placenta 60 minutes after the vaginal birth of a 3650-g healthy boy. There was no episiotomy and no lacerations of her perineum, vagina, or cervix. She now has profuse vaginal bleeding and her blood pressure is 80/50 with a pulse rate of 120 per minute. Her uterine fundus is firm.

100. The probable etiology of her postpartum hemorrhage is

   (A) cervical laceration
   (B) uterine atony
   (C) Couvelaire uterus
   (D) acute thrombocytopenia
   (E) placenta accreta

101. The most appropriate treatment of this patient is

   (A) transfusion with whole blood
   (B) uterine packing
   (C) supracervical hysterectomy
   (D) hypogastric artery ligation
   (E) intravenous administration of methylergonovine

102. Ligation of the hypogastric (internal iliac) artery effectively controls intractable pelvic hemorrhage because

(A) there is no collateral circulation to the uterus

(B) uterine blood flow is stopped

(C) arterial pulse pressure to the uterus is reduced

(D) clotting in uterine capillaries is enhanced

(E) blood flow is shunted to the ovarian veins

Questions 103 Through 105

A 53-year-old woman with five adult children complains of losing urine shortly after coughing or jumping. She occasionally loses urine while lying in bed if she happens to cough vigorously. She is unable to stop the urine once it has begun to flow.

103. The most likely diagnosis is

(A) genuine stress incontinence

(B) a vesicovaginal fistula

(C) a urethrovaginal fistula

(D) an atonic bladder

(E) detrusor dyssynergia

104. The test or procedure most likely to confirm the cause of this woman's incontinence is

(A) a urine culture

(B) a Q-tip test

(C) urethroscopy

(D) urethrocystometry

(E) an IVP

105. The treatment of choice for this woman's urinary incontinence is

(A) a course of nitrofurantoin

(B) a selective serotonin reuptake inhibitor (SSRI)

(C) oxybutynin chloride (Ditropan)

(D) vaginal hysterectomy and anterior colporrhaphy

(E) a Marshall–Marchetti–Krantz urethropexy

Questions 106 Through 108

A 14-year-old girl complains of monthly pelvic pain for the past 6 months. She has never menstruated. Breast development began at the age of $11^1/_2$ years, and pubic hair first appeared about the age of 12 years. Accelerated linear growth occurred about 1 year ago. On examination, there are no palpable abdominal masses, although the suprapubic region is tender to deep palpation. The external genitalia are normal, but there is no vaginal orifice. There is an outward bulge between the labia minora and a slight bluish tinge in this area. On rectal exam, there is a soft mass palpated anterior to the lower rectum. A uterus is palpated and feels somewhat enlarged and tender for a nulligravid adolescent.

106. The diagnosis is

(A) vaginal agenesis

(B) androgen insensitivity

(C) labial adhesions

(D) imperforate hymen

(E) transverse vaginal septum

107. The embryologic explanation for this girl's abnormality is

(A) failure of formation of the müllerian ducts

(B) failure of formation of the mesonephric ducts

(C) failure of formation of the urogenital sinus

(D) failure of canalization of the urogenital sinus

(E) failure of formation of the metanephric ducts

108. Treatment of this patient would be

(A) McIndoe vaginoplasty

(B) hysterectomy

(C) laparoscopy

(D) hymenotomy

(E) gonadectomy

DIRECTIONS (Questions 109 through 121): Each set of matching questions in this section consists of a list of 5 to 11 lettered options followed by several numbered items. For each item, select the indicated best lettered options that are most closely associated with it. Each lettered heading may be selected once, more than once, or not at all.

Questions 109 Through 113

Match the structure(s) with the phrase that best describes its anatomic location.

(A) cardinal ligament
(B) infundibulopelvic ligament
(C) ovarian ligament
(D) round ligament
(E) uterosacral ligament

109. Attaches to the cervix at the level of the internal os (select two) *a, e cardinal / uterosacral*

110. Attaches to the uterine fundus (select two) *c d round / ovarian*

111. Passes out of the pelvis with an attachment in the labia majora (select one) *d round*

112. Contains the ovarian artery and vein (select one) *b infundibulopelvic*

113. There are no vascular structures contained within (select two) *e ovarian / uterosacral C*

Questions 114 Through 121

For each of the following ovarian cancers, select the clinical and microscopic feature(s) most commonly associated.

(A) Call–Exner bodies *= granulosa cell*
(B) cords of lymphocytic infiltration *dysgerm*
(C) epithelium resembling endocervix *mucin*
(D) epithelium resembling endometrium *endo CA*
(E) epithelium resembling fallopian tube *serous*
(F) hormonally active *dys, granulosa*
(G) presence of neurectoderm *imm. terat*
(H) propensity for late recurrence *granulosa*
(I) psammoma bodies *= serous cystadem*
(J) Schiller–Duval bodies *= E.S.T*
(K) sensitive to radiation *dysg*

114. Serous cystadenoma (select two) *e, i*

115. Mucinous cystadenoma (select one) *C like endocervix*

116. Endometrial adenocarcinoma (select one) *D like endometrium*

117. Dysgerminoma (select three) *K B, F*

118. Endodermal sinus tumor (select one) *J*

119. Immature teratoma (select one) *G*

120. Granulosa cell tumor (select three) *f A, F, H*

121. Sertoli–Leydig cell tumor (select one) *f F*

Answers and Explanations

1. **(C)** The incidence of ovarian cancer in OC users is 50% less than that found in nonusers. The incidence of PID is also decreased by 50% in OC users. The risk of endometrial cancer is decreased by 50% after 1 year of OC use and the protective effect appears to persist after stopping the OC. In well-controlled studies, there is no increase in the risk of having a child with a major malformation, cardiac malformation, or limb abnormality. The risk of ectopic pregnancy is reduced by 90%, perhaps because the risk of any pregnancy approaches zero when the OC is taken correctly. *(Speroff et al, pp 715–763)*

2. **(D)** Breast development in an infant or young child is the consequence of increased estrogen secretion, exposure to exogenous estrogens, or increased response of breast tissue to normal, prepubertal amounts of estrogen. After excluding exposure to exogenous estrogens (eg, OCs, estrogen creams, etc), increased response to estrogen is more common than increased estrogen secretion from the ovaries or adrenal glands when breast development is the only sign of precocious puberty. The uterus and adnexa can be palpated abdominally in prepubertal girls if they are pathologically enlarged. For this reason, an estrogen-secreting ovarian tumor (granulosa cell is the most common type) is usually palpable and an ultrasound is unnecessary. For the same reason, a pelvic exam under anesthesia is not necessary, especially if the serum estradiol concentration is normal. Computed tomography of the head and a serum FSH concentration are unnecessary if breast development is the only sign of pre-cocious puberty and the serum estradiol concentration is normal in the prepubertal range. *(Yen and Jaffe, pp 537–538)*

3. **(E)** Premature thelarche is a disorder that probably occurs as a consequence of increased sensitivity of breast tissue to the low levels of circulating estradiol in prepubertal girls. The disorder occurs most commonly before the age of 3 years. The estradiol concentration may be normal in young girls ingesting estrogen if the serum estrogen concentration is not obtained at the time the estrogen is ingested. A negative medication history is helpful to exclude this possibility. The absence of a palpable lower abdominal mass and a prepubertal concentration of estradiol exclude a granulosa cell tumor. Adrenal 21-hydroxylase deficiency and polycystic ovary syndrome are function disorders that require the stimulation of adrenocorticotropic hormone (ACTH) and pituitary gonadotropins (FSH and LH) respectively to become clinically apparent. Both disorders do not appear until after the onset of puberty. Moreover, both are associated with androgen excess and masculinization, not estrogen excess and precocious breast development. *(Yen and Jaffe, pp 537–538)*

4. **(C)** Premature thelarche is a benign, self-limited disorder that does not progress. Breast development may actually regress, though the regression may not be complete. The girl and her parents should be assured that the events of puberty will be normal at a normal age. Examination of the girl should be repeated at 3- to 6-month intervals for

about 1 year to be certain that additional pubertal events do not occur (such as growth of pubic hair, accelerated linear growth, and vaginal bleeding). Since pituitary and adrenal function are normal for a prepubertal girl, therapy with a GnRH agonist (Lupron, Synarel, etc) or a corticosteroid is ineffective and inappropriate. While breast cancer is a rare possibility in prepubertal girls, the presence of bilateral breast buds effectively excludes this diagnosis. A breast biopsy may destroy breast anlage, and these girls will not have breast development at puberty. *(Yen and Jaffe, pp 537–538)*

5. **(A)** In general, gynecologic cancers confined to the organ of origin are stage I. Thus, this patient has a stage I cancer. In 1988, FIGO revised the staging of endometrial cancer from a clinical staging to surgical staging. Cancer limited to the endometrium is stage IA. Myometrial invasion less than 50% is stage IB, and myometrial invasion more than 50% but not involving the serosa is stage IC. *(Mishell et al, p 876)*

6. **(D)** The onset of preeclampsia before the 20th week of pregnancy is clinically seen only with a hydatidiform mole. Advanced maternal age, uterine size greater than gestational weeks, and the absence of a fetal heartbeat are added features to suggest gestational trophoblastic disease. Hydramnios, which can be associated with anencephaly and other fetal developmental abnormalities, also predisposes to preeclampsia, but its onset does not occur before 24 weeks. Renal disease, diabetes mellitus, and chronic hypertension also increase the likelihood of pre-eclampsia, but not before 24 weeks of pregnancy. The incidence of preeclampsia is increased in twin gestation, but again its onset is not before 24 weeks. *(Cunningham et al, p 680)*

7. **(A)** Acyclovir shortens the period of viral shedding and decreases the severity of symptoms during primary attacks of herpes. Weekly cultures are unreliable to exclude active herpes lesions in pregnancy and are not recommended to base the decision to per-

form a cesarean section. A cesarean section should be performed if a woman develops an active genital lesion at term. However, genital herpetic lesions before 36 weeks do not necessitate a cesarean section because there is no evidence that vertical transmission to the fetus is increased until the pregnancy is within 2 to 4 weeks of delivery. Intrauterine infections via transplacental or transmembrane transmission of the herpesvirus is rare. Most infections of the infant occur after passage through an infected birth canal. A cesarean section should be performed at term if the amniotic membranes rupture in a woman with an active herpetic lesion in the genital area. The cesarean section should be performed immediately, even if the membranes have been ruptured more than 4 to 6 hours. *(Creasy and Resnik, pp 666–668; Sweet and Gibbs, pp 119–128)*

8. **(C)** Squamous cell carcinoma is the most common malignancy of the vulva, accounting for approximately 85% of all vulvar cancers. Melanoma accounts for about 5%, sarcoma 2%, basal cell carcinoma 1 to 2%, and adenocarcinoma less than 1%. The average age of patients with vulvar cancer is 60 to 70 years. Any gross lesion visible in the genital tract should be biopsied to make a diagnosis. Such tests as colposcopy, cytology, and wet smear are only screening tests. *(DiSaia and Creasman, p 203)*

9. **(D)** Cancer of the cervix that has not invaded cervical stroma is stage 0, carcinoma in situ. Cancer that has invaded the cervical stroma but has not spread beyond the cervix is stage I. Involvement of the upper vagina or parametria (but not to the pelvic sidewall) is stage II. Stage III is involvement of the lower third of the vagina (IIIA) or parametria to the pelvic side wall (IIIB). Extension outside the reproductive tract is stage IV. *(DiSaia and Creasman, p 64)*

10. **(C)** The intent of staging is to judge the results of various treatments and to compare treatment results worldwide. Because advanced procedures such as venography, lymphangiography, MRI scans, and laparoscopy

are not universally available, staging of cervical cancer remains primarily clinical. Such tests as cystoscopy, proctosigmoidoscopy, barium enema, intravenous pyelography (IVP), and plain radiographs of the abdomen and chest are permitted. (*DiSaia and Creasman, pp 65–66*)

11. **(B)** Most deaths from cervical cancer occur as a consequence of local spread within the pelvis. Uremia is caused by compression of the ureters by tumor, producing hydronephrosis and pyelonephritis—the cause of death in about 60% of patients with cervical cancer. Infection is the second most common cause of death, accounting for about 30%. Another 5% of patients die from uncontrollable hemorrhage. About 30% of patients who die from cervical cancer have metastatic disease in the liver, lungs, or spleen at autopsy, but these lesions rarely are a direct cause of death. (*Scott et al, p 916*)

12. **(C)** Breast discomfort is a problem premenstrually for many women. Simple palliative measures include administration of vitamin E, 600 units daily, and limiting methylxanthines by eliminating coffee and other caffeine-containing substances, although the mechanism of action is not well understood. Danazol (Danocrine), in doses of 200 to 400 mg daily, is often effective in relieving breast pain. Clomiphene can have estrogenic side effects, and stilbestrol, a synthetic estrogen, can stimulate breast tissue. Many women receiving progesterone note breast discomfort secondary to fluid retention. Although bromocriptine lowers prolactin levels, it does not seem to relieve mastalgia because most women have normal prolactin levels. (*Speroff et al, pp 560–561*)

13. **(B)** Vaginismus is the painful, involuntary spasm of the musculature of the pelvis and lower third of the vagina. It will respond to properly administered dilator therapy. Dyspareunia may be associated with dysmenorrhea and may result from painful scarring of the external genitalia, vaginal infection, fibroids, endometriosis, or ovarian cysts. These all require specific therapies other than dil-

 atation. Anorgasmia usually requires extensive counseling to discover and treat the underlying causes, although organic causes such as neurologic disorders, diabetes, or drug abuse must be investigated. (*Mishell et al, pp 181–182*)

14. **(D)** The fundal height corresponds to 16 gestational weeks. Between 15 and 20 weeks, screening for open neural tube defects should be offered. In addition to MSAFP, the American College of Obstetricians and Gynecologists recommends hCG and unconjugated estriol to screen for Down syndrome and trisomy 18 as well. MSAFP is a screening test only; an abnormal result must be evaluated further by ultrasonography to identify the presence or absence of open neural tube defects or abdominal wall defects. In skilled hands, an ultrasound reduces the risk of such an anomaly by 95%. If the diagnosis is still uncertain, the woman should be offered amniocentesis for measurement of alpha-fetoprotein and acetylcholinesterase activity (increased in neural tube defects). While testing for HIV can be done any time, it is most appropriate at the first prenatal visit because earlier onset of prophylaxis with acquired immune deficiency syndrome (AIDS) drugs reduces the risk of transmission to the fetus significantly. Routine culture for group B streptococcus (GBS) is not recommended because of the high recurrence rate after treatment and the low attack rate to the fetus. Amniocentesis is not a screening procedure and is reserved for those women with a specific indication, such as elevated MSAFP, low MSAFP (risk of Down syndrome), advanced maternal age, and others. A glucose tolerance test may be appropriate if there is a clinical indication for diabetes mellitus: previous macrosomic infant or stillbirth, strong family history of diabetes mellitus, persistent glycosuria, previous gestational diabetes, or elevated random serum glucose concentration. (*Cunningham et al, pp 232–233, 921–927, 1305–1307*)

15. **(E)** Doxorubicin (Adriamycin) is an antibiotic used in the treatment of adenocarcinoma of the female genital tract (uterus, fallopian tube, and ovary), as well as uterine sarcomas,

ovarian cancer, and other tumors. Dosages must be reduced in patients with impaired liver function. The drug should not be given to women with significant heart disease. Patients should be monitored for electrocardiographic abnormalities and signs of heart failure. Acute left ventricular failure occurs more frequently with patients who have received a total dose in excess of 550 mg/m^2. (*DiSaia and Creasman, pp 519–523*)

16. **(D)** The mean age of onset of any pubertal event is approximately 11 years, beginning with the appearance of breast buds. Pubic hair appears approximately 6 months later, and this is followed by the peak height velocity (greatest rate of linear growth per unit time). Six to 12 months later, menstrual bleeding begins. Increased rate of growth begins early in the pubertal process. The sequence of pubertal events and the approximate age of appearance of each event is sufficiently predictable that significant variation in age of onset or sequence should lead to an evaluation of a cause of abnormal puberty. (*Speroff et al, pp 365–370*)

17. **(E)** There is no clinically applicable test for accurately measuring functional capacity of the heart. The most helpful guide to functional status is the mother's symptoms or the lack of symptoms. Enlargement of the heart and elevation of the diaphragm on a chest x-ray in pregnancy are normal findings. Pedal edema in mild degrees is also a very common finding. An S$_3$ in pregnancy is an abnormal finding and indicates cardiac disease but is not in and of itself predictive of functional status. (*Cunningham et al, pp 1083–1085*)

18. **(E)** Although many mechanisms involving the fetal pituitary axis, placental membranes, decidual secretions, and fetal–placental interaction have been investigated, no mechanism has been established for the initiation of labor in humans. Cortisol mechanisms probably initiate labor in sheep, and sheep generally are the experimental animals used to study human parturition. It has, however, been shown that this mechanism does not incite labor in humans. Women who are pregnant

with an anencephalic fetus often do not begin labor until after 42 weeks, but they do begin spontaneous labor even in the absence of a fetal pituitary gland. The most current thinking is that a fetal–placental–uterine interaction initiates labor. It is uncertain exactly how the pieces fit in this puzzle. (There is a comprehensive and complex review of the physiologic and biochemical processes of human parturition in Cunningham et al.) (*Cunningham et al, pp 273–313; Scott et al, pp 534–539*)

yolk sac → liver → bone marrow

19. **(C)** The first site of hematopoiesis in the fetus is the yolk sac. Between 12 and 24 weeks' gestation, the fetal liver makes the largest contribution. After 28 weeks, the fetal bone marrow is the most important site. An important learning point from this question is to read the questions carefully—this question asked for the site of hematopoiesis, not extramedullary hematopoiesis at term. (*Cunningham et al, p 166*)

20. **(C)** Hirsutism occurs when a woman is exposed to increased amounts of biologically active androgens, or when hair follicles are extrasensitive to normal amounts of androgens. Women with regular menstrual intervals usually have familial hirsutism, and it usually begins at or soon after puberty. Hirsutism associated with menstrual disturbances usually means exposure to increased amounts of androgens, either endogenous secretion from the ovaries or adrenal glands or ingestion of a drug with androgenic effects. The amenorrhea suggests increased androgen exposure, while the negative drug history suggests an endogenous source. Testosterone may arise from the ovaries, the adrenal glands, and from extraglandular formation. A serum testosterone concentration is not helpful to distinguish which source of androgen is responsible for hirsutism. Furthermore, the serum testosterone level is often misleadingly low because increased production rates of testosterone stimulate an increase in the rate of removal (the metabolic clearance rate) of testosterone from the circulation. The degree of hirsutism is the best gauge of the amount of excessive androgen production. Most virilizing ovarian tumors

are palpable in young women, and a pelvic ultrasound is useful only when the bimanual exam is inadequate. Elevated prolactin levels may cause amenorrhea but do not cause hirsutism. There is no use for measurement of urinary androgen (17-ketosteroid or 17-ketogenic steroid) excretion in modern gynecology. The best next step is to measure a serum DHEAS concentration, because it is elevated in adrenal disorders and normal or only slightly elevated in ovarian causes of hirsutism. *(Speroff et al, pp 486–490)*

21. **(B)** A history of irregular menses from menarche suggests a functional disorder, such as polycystic ovary syndrome or attenuated adrenal hyperplasia due to an inherited enzyme deficiency. The absence of a unilateral ovarian mass on pelvic exam, the positive family history, and the early menarche favor a diagnosis of attenuated adrenal hyperplasia over that of a virilizing ovarian tumor. Women with 17-hydroxylase deficiency or 11-hydroxylase deficiency are hypertensive. Women with 17-hydroxylase deficiency are also sexually infantile, not hirsute, because they are unable to produce androgens or estrogens in normal amounts. Women with 21-hydroxylase deficiency may have salt wasting and hypotension if the enzyme deficiency is sufficiently severe. *(Speroff et al, pp 494–498)*

22. **(D)** At serum hCG concentrations above the discriminatory zone (usually about 2000 mIU/mL), transvaginal sonography should reveal an intrauterine pregnancy. The absence of such a finding suggests either an extrauterine pregnancy or a spontaneous abortion. Higher levels of hCG are necessary before an extrauterine gestational sac may be seen by sonography. At each week of gestation, hCG concentrations normally vary by a large amount. For this reason, a single measurement is not helpful, although serial measurements to determine whether the hCG fails to double in 48 hours is helpful to suggest a failing pregnancy (ectopic or intrauterine). Nonclotting blood obtained from the cul-de-sac by a culdocentesis may be the result of a ruptured ectopic pregnancy or a ruptured ovarian cyst. An adnexal mass is palpated in only 50% of women with an ectopic pregnancy. *(Mishell et al, pp 444–452)*

23. **(B)** The only agents currently recognized to enhance production of fetal pulmonary surfactant are glucocorticoids. There is good evidence that pulmonary immaturity is reduced by 50% when corticosteroids are given to mothers at a gestational age less than 31 weeks. Also, there is evidence that neonatal death is decreased by about 50% with corticosteroid therapy, and other major infant morbidity is reduced as well (intraventricular hemorrhage, necrotizing enterocolitis). To achieve these benefits, delivery must be delayed 48 hours. Of the agents listed, magnesium sulfate can prevent eclamptic seizures and may inhibit uterine contractions. The other agents have no role in the treatment of fetal lung immaturity. *(Creasy and Resnik, pp 432–434)*

24. **(B)** The LH surge classically triggers ovulation 14 days before the onset of the subsequent menstrual period. Subtract 14 days from the typical cycle length to estimate the cycle day of the LH surge and ovulation. It is pertinent to remind this woman that her probability of conceiving in each cycle is no higher than 15 to 20%, even with intercourse timed to the preovulatory LH surge. *(Speroff et al, p 191)*

25. **(D)** Genuine stress incontinence occurs when there is immediate involuntary loss of urine with increased intravesical pressure greater than maximal urethral pressure in the absence of detrusor contractions. These women can usually stop the flow of urine by voluntary contraction of the muscles that close the urethra. Loss of urine with a strong desire to void immediately suggests urge incontinence, often occurring as a result of detrusor contractions. Loss of urine associated with seemingly unrelated conditions should raise the suspicion of a drug-associated incontinence. Maximal bladder distension and greatly increased bladder capacity suggest a diagnosis of an atonic bladder with overflow incontinence. *(Mishell et al, p 569)*

26. (D) Women with amenorrhea owing to weight loss and stress have decreased hypothalamic secretion of GnRH, and secondarily decreased serum levels of FSH and LH. As a consequence, serum estradiol levels will be low. While women with weight loss amenorrhea may have mild hirsutism, it is probably the result of a decreased estrogen secretion and decreased estrogen:androgen ratio, rather than an increase in serum testosterone levels. *(Speroff et al, pp 435–441)*

27. (D) With improved care, women with cystic fibrosis now survive into the reproductive age and are capable of carrying a pregnancy successfully. No special precautions such as prolonged hospitalization, oxygen supplementation, bedrest, or others are necessary. Likewise, there is no need for routine cesarean section or other labor modifications, except ensuring adequate hydration and normal serum electrolytes. An amniocentesis is unnecessary. There is no constituent of amniotic fluid that is diagnostic of cystic fibrosis. Also, the fetus is at risk for cystic fibrosis only if the father is a carrier. If not, the fetus will be a carrier only. Chorionic villus biopsy can be done to determine whether the fetus has cystic fibrosis if the father carries one of the 150 alleles for cystic fibrosis or the couple had a previously affected child. *(Creasy and Resnik, pp 54–56, 896–897)*

28. (A) Gartner's duct cysts are formed from the remnants of the wolffian (or mesonephric) duct. In the absence of testosterone in the developing embryo, this tissue will regress. These cysts are usually asymptomatic and benign. Embryonic müllerian tissue becomes the fallopian tubes, uterus, and upper vagina. The urogenital sinus develops into the lower portion of the vagina. The metanephric duct becomes the ureter and lower collecting system of the kidney. The squamocolumnar junction is the anatomic border between the endocervical columnar and ectocervical squamous epithelium. *(Scott et al, pp 876–877)*

29. (C) Different-sex twins must be dizygous. Prenatal ultrasound can detect monochorionic, monoamnionic twins, and these must

be monozygous. For same-sex twins, careful examination of the amnionic membranes after birth can reveal monozygous twins if the placental membranes are monochorionic. Dichorionic membranes can occur with either monozygous or dizygous twins. Ultimately, assessment of DNA polymorphism is the best way to determine twin zygosity. *(Creasy and Resnik, pp 586–587)*

30. (B) The ovary at 6 weeks' gestation is relatively undifferentiated. By 20 weeks' gestation, after rapid division of oogonia and entrance into the first meiotic division, there are 4 to 6 million oocytes. By birth, half are lost. The oocytes remain in the prophase of the first meiotic division until puberty, when the first meiotic division is completed. At puberty, both ovaries contain approximately 300,000 oocytes. *(Speroff et al, pp 95–104)*

31. (D) Most gram-positive aerobes are sensitive to a penicillin derivative such as ampicillin. Ampicillin and gentamicin are particularly synergistic for the treatment of enterococci. Gentamicin will usually attack the gram-negative rods, including most *Pseudomonas* species. It is also effective against *Staphylococcus aureus*, although *S aureus* is very rarely a significant gynecologic pathogen. The combination of ampicillin and gentamicin will not, however, eradicate infections with *Bacteroides fragilis*, and another antibiotic must be administered if that is a suspected pathogen. Clindamycin, metronidazole, or a third-generation cephalosporin is a good option. *(Creasy and Resnik, pp 646–651)*

32. (D) The lesions of condyloma lata are large, raised, flattened, and grayish-white, and are characteristic of secondary syphilis. Human papillomavirus infection causes condyloma acuminatum, which characteristically occurs in clusters and may be large and cauliflower-like, or small and asymptomatic. The other infectious agents listed do not cause condylomatous eruptions. *(Mishell et al, pp 609–623)*

33. (C) Approximately 30% of women with a uterine anomaly will have a urinary tract anomaly. Likewise, there is an increased likelihood of a genital tract anomaly in women with a urinary tract anomaly. Most women with uterine anomalies have no difficulty conceiving and carrying a pregnancy to term. However, a uterine anomaly may be present in as many as 25% of women with repeated spontaneous abortions and preterm labor and delivery. An infertility investigation is appropriate only if the couple has not achieved a conception after 1 year of intercourse without contraception. (*Speroff et al, pp 127–130*)

34. **(B)** Obesity, advanced age, and hepatic disease are associated with an increased risk of endometrial adenocarcinoma. While postmenopausal bleeding is most commonly due to atrophic changes in the genital tract, cancer must be considered. Cervical cytology and examination of endometrial histology are absolutely indicated. The risk of endometrial cancer is increased approximately threefold in diabetic women, and obese women have a three- to fourfold increased risk. High parity is a risk factor for cervical cancer; low parity is a risk factor for ovarian and endometrial cancer. Postmenopausal bleeding is a sign of ovarian cancer only if the malignancy secretes estrogen to stimulate the endometrium. An office endometrial biopsy has a sensitivity of about 90%. If postmenopausal bleeding persists, a D&C with hysteroscopy should be done. A D&C alone samples about 50% of the endometrium. For this reason, many gynecologists are performing a hysteroscopy and directed endometrial biopsy in addition to a D&C. (*DiSaia and Creasman, pp 134–142*)

35. **(D)** Blood pressure tends to drop slightly in normal pregnancy. This woman's blood pressure of 132/86 is definitely higher than would be expected and suggests the possibility of chronic hypertension. Since the glomerular filtration rate (GFR) in pregnancy increases normally by as much as 50% to a peak of approximately 160 mL/min, serum creatinine and BUN should be less than 0.9 mg/100 mL and 13 mg/100 mL, respectively. The observed values in this patient are elevated for pregnancy. The renal threshold for

glucose normally decreases in pregnancy. Therefore, glycosuria does not always mean diabetes in pregnancy. Several plasma glucose measurements should be obtained in pregnant women with glycosuria to correlate urinary and plasma glucose levels. (*Cunningham et al, pp 211–212*)

36. **(A)** The current treatment guideline from the Centers for Disease Control and Prevention for uncomplicated gonococcal infections is cefixime, 400 mg orally; ceftriaxone, 125 mg IM; ciproflaxacin, 500 mg orally; or ofloxacin, 400 mg orally. Each is given as a single dose. To the chosen drug is added azithromycin, 1 g orally, or doxycycline, 100 mg orally twice daily for 7 days. The second drug is added to treat *Chlamydia trachomatis*, which is present in a significant percentage of women with gonorrhea. Sexual partners should be treated at the same time. (*MMWR, pp 67–70*)

37. **(E)** A sequence of antepartum fetal assessment tests seems to be emerging in clinical practice. Basic screening with fetal movement counts by the mother is followed by nonstress testing if the fetal movement count is low or the pregnancy is high risk. If the NST is nonreactive (ie, three or fewer 10- to 15-beat/minute fetal heart rate accelerations with fetal movement within 30 minutes), then a contraction stress test (CST) is performed. If the contraction stress test is suspicious or positive for fetal heart rate decelerations, many obstetricians will proceed with a biophysical profile. The biophysical profile assesses fetal breathing movements, gross body movements, fetal tone, reactivity of the fetal heart rate, and amniotic fluid volume. The biophysical profile is reported to have a lower false abnormal rate than an NST or a CST. (*Creasy and Resnik, pp 322–325*)

38. **(B)** Improved control of diabetes prenatally and during pregnancy has dramatically changed the management of diabetes. Diabetic patients using blood glucose monitors at home four times daily yields better glucose control than frequent monitoring of urinary glucose or less frequent plasma glucose determinations. Rigid diabetic control with diet

and insulin adjustments if needed has decreased the incidence of congenital anomalies, preterm birth, uteroplacental insufficiency, and the sudden death of the fetus associated with late diabetic pregnancy. *(Creasy and Resnik, pp 934–971)*

39. **(E)** The diagnosis of septic pelvic thrombophlebitis should be considered in women suspected of having a pelvic infection, but who fail to respond to broad-spectrum antibiotics and continue having spiking fevers after 3 to 4 days. A pelvic abscess or infected hematoma should be excluded by a pelvic exam or an imaging study. While women with septic pelvic thrombophlebitis typically respond rapidly to anticoagulant doses of heparin, an MRI of the pelvis is the most definitive test. Venography and a ^{131}I-fibrinogen scan are cumbersome and imprecise. A 48-hour course of heparin therapy should render patients with septic pelvic thrombophlebitis completely afebrile. *(Cunningham et al, pp 556–558)*

40. **(A)** Septic pelvic thrombophlebitis is believed to occur in some women as a complication of bacterial endomyometritis. The range of organisms causing endomyometritis should be considered in the choice of antibiotics. Broad-spectrum and usually multiple antibiotics should be given. In the absence of a pelvic abscess, heparin in full anticoagulant doses should be added and the combination of antibiotics and anticoagulant continued until the woman is afebrile for at least 24 to 48 hours. Coumadin will not be effective in blocking the inflammatory response in affected patients. *(Scott et al, p 468)*

41. **(B)** Cryosurgery and electrocautery have the advantage of being office procedures and therefore treatments with relatively low cost. However, cryosurgery has at least two drawbacks: lack of tissue for histologic exam and the possibility that recurrences will not be detected by cytology or colposcopy. The latter problem occurs because the cryosurgery can cause the formation of a new squamocolumnar junction that grows over persistent or recurrent dysplastic cells. Any type of hysterectomy will effectively eradicate the lesion but is too much therapy for the problem. Local radiation is inappropriate for cervical cancer in situ but is usually the principal mode of therapy for stage II or greater invasive cervical cancer. The LEEP procedure has several advantages. A tissue specimen can be examined to be certain that the margins are disease free. The procedure can be done in the office with a paracervical anesthetic block. The procedure does not decrease the value of future cervical cytology or colposcopy. *(DiSaia and Creasman, pp 23–29)*

42. **(C)** Incest should be suspected in a child or adolescent with behavioral changes, anger, guilt, lying, stealing, school failure, running away, and sleep disturbances. The physician should ask appropriate questions, such as, "Were you physically or sexually abused?" The question must be asked in a nonjudgmental manner. In many states, physicians have a legal requirement to report suspected abuse to Child Protective Services. An estimated 336,000 children are sexually abused each year in the United States. As many as 15 to 25% of all women and 12% of all men may have been victims of incest. The sexual abuse is committed by a family member in approximately 80% of instances. The other choices may describe some of her problems, but only incest encompasses all her problems. *(Mishell et al, pp 202–203)*

43. **(E)** Each of the first four choices may be present in a woman who was raped. However, rape is a legal statement rather than a medical term. You should record your findings in the medical record and record a diagnosis of "alleged sexual assault." *(Mishell et al, pp 200–201)*

44. **(D)** Sperm maintain viability and motility for 48 to 72 hours in the cervical mucus if the woman is preovulatory. The duration of sperm motility in cervical mucus is shorter at other times in a woman's menstrual cycle. Sperm become nonmotile within several hours in the other sites. Thus, the presence of motile sperm in the vagina is evidence of recent intravaginal ejaculation. Motile sperm in

cervical mucus may be from the assailant or from a prior consensual act of intercourse. For this reason, documentation of sperm in the posterior vaginal fornix is more important than sperm within cervical mucus when evaluating a victim of sexual assault. (*Mishell et al, pp 200–201*)

45. **(D)** In many states, a pregnant woman under the age of 21 years is considered an emancipated minor and is the only person who may make legal decisions pertaining to the pregnancy. Though an immediate cesarean section is indicated because of the severe fetal heart rate decelerations, to perform it without her permission violates the ethical principle of autonomy. This is a principle that states that human beings should have their wishes respected as autonomous persons if they are capable of self-determination. Obtaining a court order may fulfill the ethical principle of beneficence, a physician acting to do no harm and to help the patient. In this situation, the ethical (moral) decision is complicated by a conflict between beneficence and autonomy. However, proceeding with a cesarean section exposes the obstetrician to a legal charge of battery. Assigning her care to another physician is a standard and accepted solution when there is a moral conflict between patient and physician. However, this is not an acceptable option in an emergency situation. The obstetrician is at risk for abandonment. Though not a satisfying choice, the choice most ethically sound is to counsel her carefully, but eventually accede to her wishes. Placing her in the lateral position, giving her oxygen by mask, and providing adequate intravenous hydration should be instituted to minimize the risk of fetal hypoxia. (*Scott et al, pp 1063–1071*)

46. **(D)** The mean duration of human pregnancy is 266 days from conception. To this is added 14 days for the interval between the onset of the last menses and the conception date. Thus, it is important to ascertain the range of days for each woman's menstrual cycles. The more variable a woman's menstrual cycles are, the less certain is the estimated due date calculated from the last menstrual period (LMP).

The standard deviation of pregnancy duration is ± 17 days. Thus, 95% of human pregnancies will deliver between 263 and 297 days after the onset of the LMP. (*Cunningham et al, p 229*)

47. **(E)** While ultrasonography can detect a fetal heartbeat as early as 5 to 6 postmenstrual weeks, detection of the fetal heart with a handheld Doppler is not possible before 10 to 12 weeks. The fetal heartbeat is detectable in 80% of pregnant women by 20 weeks, and in 100% by 22 weeks of pregnancy. Patient size, the hearing acuity of the examiner, and the persistence of the examiner affect when the fetal heartbeat is first audible with a stethoscope. (*Cunningham et al, p 232*)

48. **(D)** Postcoital spotting and intermenstrual spotting in a woman with cyclic menses is suggestive of a cervical abnormality, rather than an endometrial hormonal abnormality. In the absence of a visible lesion, a Pap smear that includes cells from both the ectocervix and endocervix is the preferred method of evaluation, especially when the woman has no history of cervical pathology or a normal Pap smear in the recent past. Endometrial biopsy and hysteroscopy assess the endometrium, not the cervix. A conization of the cervix should be reserved for women with documented cervical neoplasia when determination of the extent of the lesion is necessary. An endocervical curettage is usually reserved for women with unsatisfactory Pap smears and persistent abnormal bleeding. (*Mishell et al, pp 141–142*)

49. **(B)** Pap smear and colposcopy are screening tests appropriate when there is no visible cervical pathology. In the presence of a lesion, pathologic evaluation is necessary to make a diagnosis. An office cervical biopsy is the procedure of choice to establish the diagnosis. If the diagnosis from the biopsy is cancer, a conization of the cervix is indicated to determine the extent of the disease—surface spread as well as depth of stromal invasion. (*Mishell et al, pp 141, 822–825*)

50. **(E)** The patient described in the question has a classic history of an incompetent cervix: ex-

pulsion of a fetus without labor. It is believed to be caused by previous cervical trauma, DES exposure, or, most commonly, a congenital defect in cervical stroma. In the absence of preterm labor, there is no indication for terbutaline or other tocolytic agents. DES is contraindicated in pregnancy, but was used in the past to treat repeated pregnancy loss. Hydroxyprogesterone is a progestational compound that is being used by some hospitals for patients in premature labor, but its use is controversial. Bedrest is occasionally encouraged by some practitioners for patients with a history of premature deliveries. The probability of a successful pregnancy after a cervical cerclage increases from 20% to approximately 80%. It is crucial to eliminate the possibility of preterm labor before placing a cerclage. (*Mishell et al, pp 410–411*)

51. **(B)** NTDs and other single organ system defects are transmitted via polygenic/multifactorial inheritance. The recurrence risk for any NTD is approximately 2% after having one affected child. The recurrence risk is also 2% if one parent has an NTD. The risk is 0.5 to 1% if the mother's sister or brother has a child with an NTD, but is lower if the father's brother or sister has a child with an NTD. (*Creasy and Resnik, p 78*)

52. **(E)** The combination of aging and diabetes suggests the likelihood of a neurologic defect in the bladder, resulting in overflow incontinence. This occurs when the detrusor muscle becomes hypotonic or atonic. Such women complain of voiding small amounts but still having the feeling of a full bladder. In addition, these women are incontinent of small amounts of urine and are unable to stop the flow. This helps to distinguish those with overflow incontinence from those with genuine stress incontinence; the latter are able to increase urethral pressure enough to stop urine flow. Cystitis commonly causes urgency and increased urinary frequency, but not incontinence. A urinalysis and urine culture are not likely to be revealing in this patient. Instillation of methylene blue into the bladder after placement of a vaginal tampon should be done when a vesicovaginal fis-

tula is suspected. This occurs most often following gynecologic surgery and should be suspected in women complaining of constant urine leakage. The Q-tip test is useful to demonstrate posterior urethral rotation found in women with genuine stress incontinence. (*Mishell et al, p 592*)

53. **(A)** In a patient with genuine stress incontinence, a retropubic approach offers the best long-term cure of the incontinence. The Burch procedure and the Marshall–Marchetti–Krantz procedure are the most common retropubic procedures. With an anterior colporrhaphy, plication sutures are placed at the urethrovesical junction (UVJ) in an effort to support and elevate it. Long-term results are not as good as a retropubic urethropexy or a suburethral sling. A suburethral sling procedure is used when urethral closing pressure is low, less than 20 cm H_2O. A needle suspension procedure is most often done when there is associated genital prolapse with potential incontinence. Collagen injections at the UVJ have been attempted to partially obstruct the urethra. Incontinent patients who may benefit the most from collagen injections are those with intrinsic sphincter deficiency and a fixed bladder neck. (*Scott et al, pp 856–865*)

54. **(C)** The presence of a dominant mass requires immediate evaluation. Insertion of a 23- to 25-gauge needle attached to a syringe will resolve whether the mass is cystic or solid. If clear or cloudy fluid is aspirated and the mass disappears, the woman should have a repeat breast exam in one month. If the mass remains after aspiration, if the fluid is bloody, or if there is a residual mass on a follow-up visit in one month, an open biopsy should be done. Mammography is a screening tool, not a diagnostic tool. It cannot replace aspiration and biopsy in the presence of a dominant mass. A segmental resection is a therapeutic option for a circumscribed carcinoma, but is not an appropriate diagnostic tool. (*Scott et al, pp 703–709*)

55. **(D)** Rh immune globulin should always be administered to an Rh-negative pregnant

woman who sustains any trauma or has any type of invasive procedure, such as an amniocentesis. Detectable fetomaternal hemorrhage occurs in 6% of women having an amniocentesis. The immune globulin reduces the risk of subsequent Rh sensitization during the pregnancy, which could result in severe erythroblastosis fetalis. While chorionic villus biopsy might be an alternative to amniocentesis, it is done earlier in pregnancy, and occasionally must be followed by an amniocentesis after 14 weeks' gestation because of the possibility that maternal decidua was analyzed. Rubella immunization should be given after delivery to avoid the theoretical risk of a congenital rubella syndrome from the administration of the live vaccine. The presence of hepatitis B surface antibody suggests immunity to hepatitis B but is unrelated to amniocentesis. Intra-amniotic bleeding is a complication of amniocentesis but occurs at the time of the procedure. The amniotic fluid will appear bloody. (Cunningham et al, pp 986–987)

56. (D) The conceptus is remarkably resistant to the toxic and teratogenic effects of most drugs until about 2 postconceptual weeks (4 postmenstrual weeks). While certain drugs may be toxic to oocytes, their effect will be to prevent conception or cause an early spontaneous abortion. The developing conceptus is not exposed to maternal toxins or teratogens until after implantation and establishment of a blood supply from mother to fetus. Even after implantation, the fetus is relatively resistant to teratogens for about 1 week. Organogenesis is complete by the end of the first trimester. Congenital abnormalities are therefore unlikely in the second and third trimesters. (Cunningham et al, p 943)

57. (D) From the information in question 56, it is apparent that the fetus is relatively resistant to teratogenic effects of drugs until about 2 weeks after conception. A recommendation to abort the pregnancy cannot be made on medical probability, though the woman may choose this because she does not wish to take any chance of having an affected child. Ultrasound is incapable of detecting anomalies

until at least 12 to 14 postmenstrual weeks. The fetal warfarin syndrome does not cause chromosomal abnormalities and a genetic amniocentesis is not indicated. Vitamin K reverses the anticoagulant effects of Coumadin but does not alter the risk that the fetus will develop anomalies. (Cunningham et al, p 949)

58. (A) Nasal hypoplasia and stippled vertebral and femoral epiphyses on radiographs are the most common abnormalities associated with the fetal warfarin syndrome. Other abnormalities include hydrocephaly or microcephaly, ophthalmologic abnormalities, fetal growth restriction, and developmental delay. The period of greatest susceptibility appears to be between the sixth and ninth postmenstrual weeks. The syndrome is found in 15 to 25% of infants exposed to Coumadin at this time. (Cunningham et al, pp 949–950)

59. (C) The station of the vertex indicates that the fetal head is on the perineum. A cesarean section, either low transverse or classical, is inappropriate unless an operative vaginal delivery is unsuccessful. In women with an anthropoid pelvis, the transverse, interspinous diameter of the bony pelvis is narrow and the anteroposterior diameter of the pelvis is relatively long. In this circumstance, a forceps rotation should not be done. In women with a gynecoid pelvis, the transverse and anteroposterior diameters are more equal and rotation of the fetal head to occiput anterior would be an acceptable choice. Soft-tissue resistance to delivery is not great enough that an episiotomy will permit slight expulsive efforts by the mother to deliver the fetal head. (Cunningham et al, pp 483–484)

60. (B) Fecundability is the ability to achieve a pregnancy, and the rate per ovulation in couples with no impediment to fertility is approximately 25%. Fecundity is the ability to achieve a live birth within one ovulatory cycle. Fecundity is approximately 15% per cycle in normally fertile couples. Using the 25% fecundity rate, 25 of 100 couples will achieve a pregnancy in the first menstrual cycle of effort. In the second cycle, 25% of the remaining 75 couples will achieve a pregnancy, ap-

proximately 19 women. This is a cumulative pregnancy rate of 44%. Twenty-five percent of the remaining 56 women will conceive in the third cycle, approximately 14 women. The cumulative conception rate after three cycles is approximately 58%. However, nearly 50% of all conceptions do not progress to a live birth, ending as a very early unrecognized spontaneous abortion, a recognized first-trimester abortion, a second-trimester loss, or a third-trimester stillbirth. *(Speroff et al, pp 809–810)*

61. **(B)** Although messenger RNA for hCG is present in six- to eight-cell embryos (preimplantation), hCG cannot be detected in the maternal circulation until soon after implantation, approximately 7 days after conception or 7 days before the expected date of menses. Although hCG cannot be detected in maternal blood as early as 4 days after fertilization, maternal serum estradiol and progesterone concentrations in the luteal phase are higher in conception cycles. This is suggestive that the embryo is capable of preimplantation signaling. Clinically, pregnancy should be detected as early as possible because of the increased risk of another tubal pregnancy. If a pregnancy test is not done until 1 week following the missed menses, a transvaginal ultrasound should be done soon thereafter to ascertain if there is an intrauterine gestational sac. The serum hCG concentration must be greater than approximately 1500 mIU/mL for transvaginal ultrasonography to be reliable. Waiting 2 weeks after the expected menses to obtain a pregnancy test is too late—the risk of a ruptured tubal pregnancy and intraperitoneal hemorrhage increases with advancing gestation. *(Speroff et al, pp 241–242)*

62. **(B)** Cervical cancer is currently the only female reproductive tract cancer staged clinically according to FIGO standards. FIGO also requires that the clinical staging be based on technologies generally available worldwide, including third-world countries. For this reason, lymphangiography, angiography, CT or MR scans, laparoscopy, or hysteroscopy are not permitted to stage cervical cancer. Due to

the presence of abnormal para-aortic lymph nodes and hepatic changes consistent with metastases, she is actually a stage IVB. *(DiSaia and Creasman, pp 64–66)*

63. **(E)** Though this 46-year-old woman is staged as a IB, she should be treated as a stage IVB because of the findings on CT scan. Methods of staging that are similar allow institutions to compare results of treatment without having to account for different staging procedures and criteria. A simple TAH-BSO is appropriate therapy only for women with carcinoma in situ of the cervix (CIN III, stage 0). Women with stage I or IIA may be treated with radical hysterectomy or with radiation therapy. Beyond stage IIA, only radiation therapy is acceptable. A pelvic exenteration is indicated when there is a central recurrence after maximal dose radiation therapy. Platinum-based chemotherapy has been used for women with metastases or recurrence after radiation therapy. It is considered palliative. Recently, several have used chemotherapy as primary therapy for bulk disease. There are no randomized control trials to document that chemotherapy is superior to surgery or radiation. *(DiSaia and Creasman, pp 66–81)*

64. **(C)** Live viruses are usually contraindicated in pregnancy. Inactivated viruses are generally safe but should be given only if there is a specific indication, usually exposure to the virus. Measles, mumps, rubella, poliomyelitis, and yellow fever vaccines are all live viruses. Polio vaccine may be given if there is an increased risk of exposure. Although fetal risk from rubella vaccine has not been confirmed, the vaccine should not be used because the congenital rubella syndrome is a theoretic possibility. Tetanus toxoid in conjunction with diphtheria vaccine should be given if there has been no primary immunization or there has been no booster within 10 years. Rabies vaccine is indicated if exposure is possible or likely. Public health authorities should be consulted for indications, dosage, etc. *(ACOG Technical Bulletin, No. 160)*

65. **(C)** As many as 30% of fetuses exposed to phenytoin had minor craniofacial and digi-

tal anomalies. Cleft lip/palate, hypertelorism, broad nasal bridge, and epicanthal folds are the craniofacial anomalies observed. Hypoplasia of the distal phalanges and nails are the digital anomalies. In addition, these infants may have growth and cognitive deficiencies. Trimethadione, another anticonvulsant, causes similar anomalies. Spina bifida occurs in 1 to 2% of infants whose mothers took valproic acid during pregnancy. (*Cunningham et al, pp 951–953*)

66. **(B)** Approximately 3% of liveborn infants have a major congenital anomaly detected at birth. The incidence increases to 6 to 7% later in childhood. Chromosomal and single-gene defects account for 10 to 25% of human malformations. Fetal infections (3 to 5%), maternal disease (4%), and drugs and medications (< 1%) account for the remaining recognized causes of human malformations. Sixty-five to 75% of malformations have an unknown or multifactorial etiology. (*Cunningham et al, pp 895–896*)

67. **(B)** The main mechanism by which hemostasis is achieved following delivery is contraction of the myometrium to compress the uterine vessels that had been supplying the placenta. Lack of effective myometrial contraction (ie, uterine atony) is the major cause of postpartum hemorrhage. If the uterus is found to be firmly contracted, then other factors, such as cervical or vaginal lacerations or a coagulopathy, must be sought. (*Scott et al, pp 165–166*)

68. **(A)** Immediate management is bimanual massage and compression of the uterine fundus by placing one fist into the anterior vaginal fornix and the other hand abdominally posterior to the uterus. The uterine massage is often enough to cause myometrial contractions and slowing of the bleeding. Oxytocin or an ergot alkaloid (eg, methylergonovine) should also be administered. Insertion of a gauze pack is never indicated because it is rarely effective. It may actually worsen the bleeding by preventing contraction of the myometrium. Persistent bleeding from the uterus despite these measures may indicate

uterine rupture, retained placental fragments, or placenta accreta. If a careful curettage of the uterine lining fails to remove any placental fragments and decrease uterine bleeding, hypogastric artery ligation or a hysterectomy must be considered. (*Scott et al, pp 165–166*)

69. **(D)** Both the bloody nipple discharge and the microcalcifications are indications for an open breast biopsy. Although there are benign-appearing radiographic calcifications, clusters of calcification are associated with a 25% chance of a cancer. An open biopsy is still preferred in most centers because a fine-needle biopsy has about a 20% false-negative rate. Cytology is a screening tool. In the presence of significant risk factors for cancer, a tissue diagnosis is mandatory. Imaging studies are also screening tools with a false-negative and a false-positive rate, making such studies inappropriate for diagnosis. (*Mishell et al, pp 372–374*)

70. **(B)** The principal advantage of a fine-needle aspiration of a breast mass is that it reduces the number of open breast biopsies when it is positive for cancer. However, a negative needle biopsy is nondiagnostic (and nonreassuring), and an open biopsy is still necessary. A fine-needle biopsy does not differentiate between noninvasive and invasive cancer, nor does it delineate the extent of in situ disease. (*Mishell et al, p 372*)

71. **(E)** The factor associated with the greatest lifetime risk for developing breast cancer is a mother with a history of breast cancer—a relative risk of approximately 2.0. The relative risk is 4.0 with two first-degree relatives. Increased lifetime estrogen exposure is a minor risk factor for breast cancer. Obesity, early menarche, late menopause, and low parity are associated with an increased lifetime estrogen exposure and are minor risk factors for breast cancer. Most epidemiologic studies have concluded that menopausal estrogen replacement does not increase the risk of breast cancer. However, several such studies have observed a statistically significant increased relative risk of breast cancer with postmeno-

pausal hormone replacement, usually a relative risk of approximately 1.5. Estrogens are considered promoters of breast cancer rather than inducers of initiators. (*Mishell et al, pp 361–364*)

72. **(D)** Infiltrating ductal carcinoma accounts for approximately 80% of all breast carcinomas. Infiltrating lobular carcinoma accounts for approximately 9%, and the others 5% or less. (*Mishell et al, pp 374–375*)

73. **(A)** The best predictor of breast cancer that has spread outside the breast is the initial size of the tumor. A tumor diameter larger than 2 cm is associated with an increased probability of axillary node involvement. In turn, the presence and number of positive axillary lymph nodes is the best predictor of survival. The presence of estrogen and progesterone receptors are favorable prognostic features. A high mitotic index and a high rate of thymidine incorporation into tumor cells suggest a virulent tumor and a worse prognosis. (*Mishell et al, p 378*)

74. **(D)** Danazol, in oral doses of 100, 200, or 400 mg daily for 4 to 6 months, relieves breast pain and reduces nodularity in 90% of women. The beneficial effects often last for several months after discontinuation of the drug. Tamoxifen is a synthetic antiestrogen that competes with estrogen receptors in the breast. Relief of symptoms has been achieved in approximately 70% of women in small studies, and seems to be more effective in women with cyclic rather than continuous pain. Bromocriptine inhibits prolactin secretion, not recognized as a cause of fibrocystic breast disease and mastodynia. Oral progestins (eg, medroxyprogesterone acetate), depot medroxyprogesterone acetate (Depo-Provera), or OCs may provide symptomatic relief, but symptoms usually return after these are stopped. Hydrochlorothiazide provides unpredictable relief of symptoms. (*Mishell et al, p 359*)

75. **(D)** This is an autosomal dominant disorder. Both parents are carriers of the abnormal gene (N), which is on chromosome 17. If each

parent is a heterozygote (Nn, where n is the normal gene), 25% of their offspring will have a normal genotype, nn. Fifty percent of their offspring will be affected heterozygotes (Nn), and the remaining 25% will be homozygous affected (NN). As an autosomal disorder, there is no sex predilection; males and females are affected with equal frequency. (*Mishell et al, pp 24–25*)

76. **(A)** The normal pH of the vagina is 3.8 to 4.2. In women with a vaginal discharge, a pH less than 5.0 suggests monilial vaginitis or a physiologic discharge of normal squamous cells desquamated from the vaginal epithelium. A pH greater than 5.0 suggests some type of bacterial infection, such as bacterial vaginosis or trichomonas vaginitis. The other possibility is an atrophic vaginal epithelium. Both *Chlamydia* and gonorrhea infect the cervix and do not change the vaginal pH. (*Mishell et al, p 625*)

77. **(E)** Clue cells are shown in Figure 1–1. This indicates bacterial vaginosis. Clue cells are vaginal squamous cells with indistinct margins that are studded extensively with coccobacilli. *Trichomonas* infection is due to a unicellular protozoon. The organism on wet smear with normal saline is fusiform, slightly larger than white blood cells, and has flagella at one end. The flagella cause the motion on wet smear that is diagnostic. Monilial vaginitis is best demonstrated by placing a small amount of the discharge in 10% potassium hydroxide (KOH) and observing for branching hyphae. *Neisseria gonorrhoeae* and *Chlamydia trachomatis* cannot be seen on a wet smear. (*Mishell et al, pp 624–635*)

78. **(C)** The treatment of choice for bacterial vaginosis is metronidazole, also an effective treatment for trichomonas vaginitis. The dose is 375 to 500 mg orally twice daily for 1 week. A single daily dose of 750 mg was recently approved. Vaginal metronidazole gel or clindamycin cream are also approved forms of treatment. Concurrent therapy of the male partner is controversial. Treatment in pregnancy is recommended because there is a potential association of bacterial vaginosis and

preterm labor and delivery. *(Mishell et al, p 628; Cunningham et al, pp 804, 816)*

79. **(D)** The normal ejaculate volume is 2 to 5 mL, and the bulk of the ejaculate is from the seminal vesicles. The reduced ejaculate volume may be the result of an incomplete collection or may indicate absence of the seminal vesicles. Fructose is the reducing sugar produced by the seminal vesicles, and its absence establishes a diagnosis of congenital absence of the vasa deferentia and seminal vesicles. This explains the azoospermia (absence of sperm; aspermia is absence of an ejaculate). Men with germ cell aplasia have only Sertoli cells in their seminiferous tubules. Their ejaculate volumes are normal, and fructose is present. Likewise, men with occlusion of the vasa deferentia will be azoospermic but have a normal ejaculate volume containing fructose. Men with 17α-hydroxylase deficiency will have hypertension, be sexually infantile, and have azoospermia, because the enzyme deficiency prevents the secretion of normal amounts of cortisol, androgens, and estrogen, but an increased secretion of mineralocorticoids. Men with Klinefelter syndrome have patent vasa deferentia and seminal vesicles; their ejaculate volumes will be normal and contain fructose. *(Speroff et al, p 885)*

80. **(C)** The WHO suggests a minimal sperm concentration of 20 million/mL for normal conception rates of 15 to 20% per ovulation. However, sperm motility (percentage and velocity; > 50% with forward progression), sperm morphology (30% or more oval forms [using strict criteria]), coital frequency, and others must be considered. Stated otherwise, a sperm concentration of 10 million/mL may be associated with normal fertility if the sperm motility and morphology are better than average and coital frequency is three to four times per week. *(Speroff et al, pp 876–879)*

81. **(C)** The cycle of spermatogenesis is 73 ± 5 days. This is the time required for maturation of spermatogonia to spermatozoa. The cycle is at different stages along the seminiferous tubules, necessary to ensure the presence of

sperm in each ejaculate. Knowing this has important implications: any therapy intended to stimulate spermatogenesis must be continued for at least the duration of one spermatogenic cycle to determine whether there is a beneficial effect. *(Speroff et al, p 876)*

82. **(C)** Transit time of sperm in the epididymis and vasa deferentia is 12 to 21 days. The ability of sperm to fertilize an oocyte is greater for those sperm that have passed through the male duct system. The total time from spermatogonia to spermatozoa in the ejaculate is approximately 90 days, an important physiologic fact that must be considered when assessing the effect of an illness or treatment on spermatogenesis. *(Speroff et al, p 876)*

83. **(E)** Painful vaginal bleeding is most likely the result of placental abruption, premature separation of the placenta. Bloody show is a normal sign of impending or early labor. The bleeding is scant and intermingled with clear mucus. Bleeding from a vaginal laceration following coitus is not associated with abdominal pain. A history of coitus followed immediately by bleeding suggests this diagnosis. Bleeding from cervicitis is most often spotting and not associated with abdominal pain. Classically, bleeding with a placenta previa is painless. *(Cunningham et al, pp 745–746)*

84. **(D)** Maternal hypertension is the most common risk factor for a placental abruption. In one published report, half of the women with an abruption severe enough to kill the fetus had hypertension, and half of these had evidence of chronic vascular disease. The other choices are also risk factors for placental abruption but are not found in as many women with an abruption. *(Cunningham et al, pp 748–749)*

85. **(E)** At term, a placental abruption severe enough to cause fetal distress warrants immediate delivery. If the pregnancy is remote from term, temporizing measures may be considered, such as observation. However, delivery should be achieved if the mother becomes hemodynamically unstable. Tocolysis is ineffective in relaxing the uterus and has

the added disadvantage of causing vasodilation of an already underfilled vascular system. Amniotomy and Pitocin induction will not cause delivery rapidly enough to prevent further deterioration of the fetus. Evidence of fetal distress makes continued monitoring unacceptable. (*Cunningham et al, pp 752–755*)

86. **(A)** Cells are most sensitive to radiation during mitosis. For this reason, rapidly dividing cells are the most radiosensitive. Fractionation of radiation doses provides effective tumor treatment without increasing the rate of complications to normal tissues. (*Mishell et al, p 771*)

87. **(C)** The most common dose of radiation therapy for invasive cervical cancer is 4500 to 5000 cGy, or 45 to 50 Gy. Lower doses tend to result in treatment failures and higher doses are associated with greater complication rates. (*Mishell et al, p 853*)

88. **(A)** Each of the choices are potential complications of radiation therapy. Diarrhea and nausea may occur during the course of radiation treatment. The others are postradiation complications that usually do not occur sooner than 6 months after completing radiation. The likelihood of these complications is related to dosage, volume treated, and tissue sensitivity. Diseases that affect circulation (eg, diabetes mellitus, hypertension) and prior abdominal surgery also increase the risk of complications. (*Mishell et al, p 854*)

89. **(A)** The classic symptom of fibrocystic breast disease is cyclic bilateral breast pain. The pain and associated diffuse breast engorgement is most severe premenstrually. Cystic changes palpated premenstrually typically are smaller postmenstrually. Fibroadenomas are firm, rubbery, freely mobile, solid, and usually solitary masses. Intraductal papilloma does not cause diffuse breast symptoms. Spontaneous and intermittent nipple discharge is the classic sign of an intraductal papilloma. Intraductal carcinoma is more likely if there is a discharge from multiple ducts. Breast cancer should be suspected when a solitary firm nodule does not change throughout the menstrual cycle. A mammo-

gram is helpful, but any suspicious mass should be biopsied. Hyperprolactinemia can cause brease engorgement, but the pain is usually mild and cystic areas tend not to vary in size. (*Mishell et al, pp 357–360*)

90. **(D)** Fibrocystic disease includes a variety of histologic findings. Typical is proliferation and hyperplasia of the lobular, ductal, and acinar epithelium. Histologic variants include variable-sized cysts, adenosis, fibrosis, duct ectasia, apocrine metaplasia, and others. Ductal epithelial hyperplasia and apocrine metaplasia with atypia are the findings associated with the greatest risk of subsequent breast cancer. (*Mishell et al, pp 358–359*)

91. **(E)** Breast cancer is rare in women younger than 35 years, and the approximate incidence of breast cancer in pregnancy is 1 in 3000 deliveries. Survival rates from breast cancer in pregnancy are less than in nonpregnant women of comparable age. This may be related to delayed diagnosis because pregnant women with breast cancer and negative nodes do as well as nonpregnant women. Despite the pregnancy, the presence of a dominant mass requires histologic evaluation. Temporizing measures (choices A through C) are inappropriate in the presence of a dominant mass. Breast cytology can be difficult to interpret. (*DiSaia and Creasman, pp 470–474*)

92. **(E)** The weight of evidence is that the prognosis of early-stage breast cancer is not worsened by the massive amounts of estrogen secreted in pregnancy. With a small lesion and negative axillary nodes, a lumpectomy or segmental resection and subsequent expectant management is the management of choice. Chemotherapy and/or radiation therapy can and should be deferred until after delivery of the fetus. More advanced breast cancer carries a worse prognosis and should be treated aggressively, although there is little convincing evidence that termination of pregnancy improves the prognosis. (*DiSaia and Creasman, pp 470–474*)

93. **(A)** In late pregnancy, the large uterus commonly compresses the inferior vena cava and

impedes return of blood from the lower extremities to the heart. This may be sufficient to reduce cardiac output. In approximately 10% of women, arterial hypotension occurs, which can result in diminished uteroplacental blood flow and a decreased fetal heart rate. None of the other options occur as a result of this syndrome. Management is to have the woman roll onto her side or lean forward if she is sitting. Both these maneuvers cause the uterus to fall away from the inferior vena cava. (Cunningham et al, p 210)

94. **(C)** The strict definition of the cardinal movement of labor, called *engagement*, is given as choice C. Among other things, this means that the presenting part is fixed in the true pelvis and a prolapsed umbilical cord is unlikely to occur. Often, the fetal head is considered to be engaged when the vertex is at 0 station, the level of the ischial spines. Although engagement is conclusive evidence of an adequate pelvic inlet, its absence is not always indicative of pelvic contraction. Nevertheless, the incidence of pelvic contraction is higher in women whose presenting part is not engaged. (Cunningham et al, pp 65–66)

95. **(D)** Anti-D immune globulin should be given at the time of any vaginal bleeding, trauma, or invasive procedure (eg, amniocentesis) during pregnancy. Although maternal isoimmunization usually occurs as a result of fetomaternal transfusion at the time of delivery, a small percentage of women become isoimmunized during pregnancy. Anti-D immune globulin is routinely given to unsensitized Rh-negative women at 28 weeks' gestation to reduce this risk. Anti-D immune globulin must also be administered within 72 hours after the birth of an Rh-positive infant. Administration at 40 weeks' gestation before the onset of labor is unnecessary if the infant is Rh negative and may be ineffective if the infant is Rh positive and there is a significant fetomaternal transfusion. (Cunningham et al, pp 986–987)

96. **(B)** It is a form of passive immunization because the antibody to the Rh antigen is administered, rather than the Rh antigen itself.

The incidence of D-isoimmunization during pregnancy decreased from 1.8 to 0.07% as a result of second-trimester anti-D immune globulin administration. The combination of appropriate screening methods and the manufacturing process that inactivates the HIV virus make transmission of HIV an extremely remote possibility. It is effective if administered within 72 hours after delivery. It must be administered during and after each pregnancy because passive immunization is not permanent and each pregnancy carries a risk of Rh isoimmunization. (Cunningham et al, pp 986–987, 1305–1307)

97. **(D)** In a previously healthy woman with an uncomplicated pregnancy, the appearance of hypertension and proteinuria in the third trimester is preeclampsia. The other disorders usually are present throughout the pregnancy, may develop earlier than the third trimester, and may present with hypertension or proteinuria, but not necessarily both. (Cunningham et al, pp 694–695)

98. **(E)** The treatment of preeclampsia with a certain term pregnancy (> 37 weeks' gestation) is delivery of the infant. Induction of labor with Pitocin is the preferred method of delivery provided the preeclampsia is not severe, the HELLP syndrome (*H*emolysis, *EL*evated liver enzymes, *L*ow *P*latelets) does not develop, or fetal distress does not occur. A cesarean section should be performed if any of these develop and vaginal delivery is not imminent. (Cunningham et al, pp 714–717)

99. **(C)** The only effect of magnesium sulfate is to reduce the risk of seizures with eclampsia. While magnesium sulfate is commonly used as a tocolytic in idiopathic preterm labor, this is not its purpose in pregnant women with preeclampsia. Blood pressure is not reduced by magnesium sulfate; intravenous hydralazine is a safe antihypertensive when given in small, intermittent doses for diastolic blood pressures greater than 105 to 110 torr. Uteroplacental blood flow, decreased in preeclampsia, is unaffected by magnesium sulfate. Magnesium sulfate should be continued for 24 hours after delivery because of the

continued risk of eclamptic seizures. *(Cunningham et al, pp 714–717)*

100. **(E)** A placenta accreta must be suspected if the placenta does not separate spontaneously by 30 minutes after delivery of the infant, especially if a plane of dissection cannot be identified with attempts to manually remove the placenta. The examination immediately after birth eliminates the possibility of a cervical laceration, although the lower genital tract should be reinspected to be certain that a laceration was not overlooked. With uterine atony, the fundus is boggy and larger than expected, unlike the firm uterus found in this woman. A Couvelaire uterus occurs as a complication of placental abruption with concealed hemorrhage. Blood intravasates between myometrial fibers and diminishes the capacity of the myometrium to contract. While acute blood loss may lead to thrombocytopenia, the bleeding is the cause rather than the consequence of the low platelet count. *(Cunningham et al, pp 765–767)*

101. **(D)** Hypogastric artery ligation, angiographically directed arterial embolization, and hysterectomy are acceptable treatment options. The choice depends on the experience of the obstetrician, the rapid availability of an interventional radiology team, and the hemodynamic status of the patient. If a hypogastric artery ligation is unsuccessful, then a hysterectomy is necessary. Blood should be transfused to maintain hemodynamic stability but is never the sole treatment with placenta accreta. In one study, one fourth of the women died who had a uterine pack inserted after manual removal of the placenta. This was four times higher than in those who had an immediate hysterectomy. Administration of ergot alkaloids is a treatment option only when postpartum hemorrhage is due to uterine atony. *(Cunningham et al, pp 765–767)*

102. **(C)** Hypogastric artery ligation converts the arterial system into a venous system, thereby reducing the pulse pressure by as much as 85%. Subsequent menstrual function and fertility are normal, in part because of the rich collateral circulation to the uterus. The procedure is successful in approximately 50% of cases. The procedure is not technically easy to perform, and an intimate knowledge of the local anatomy is essential. *(Rock and Thompson, pp 862–863)*

103. **(E)** The two clues to the diagnosis of detrusor dyssynergia are the loss of urine in the recumbent position and the inability to stop the urine loss once the stream has begun. Generally, large volumes of urine are lost because of the inability to stop the flow of urine. With genuine stress incontinence (GSI), urine is lost only in the upright position when intra-abdominal and intravesical pressure exceed urethral closing pressure, such as with coughing. Women with GSI are able to voluntarily stop the flow of urine and therefore the volume of urine lost is small. With GSI, urine loss with coughing is immediate. Women with a vesicovaginal or urethrovaginal fistula will complain of a watery vaginal discharge. Women with an atonic bladder typically void small amounts and complain that the bladder still feels full (which it is). This is a disorder seen in women with neurologic dysfunction of the bladder, such as multiple sclerosis and diabetic neuropathy. *(Mishell et al, pp 590–591)*

104. **(D)** While a urine culture is a standard part of the evaluation of women with loss of urine, this woman's history is not consistent with acute cystitis. A Q-tip test is done to assess the angle the urethra makes with the horizontal in the relaxed and voiding circumstances. Though intended to differentiate GSI from other causes of incontinence, it has not proven to be sufficiently sensitive to make this distinction reliably. Urethroscopy is appropriate if a urethrovaginal fistula or urethral diverticulum is suspected. Urethrocystometry is one name for a test that measures the pressure–volume relationship in the bladder. It should be done in most women with incontinence as the most sensitive test to distinguish the various causes of incontinence. An IVP is of little value in determining the cause of incontinence. *(Mishell et al, pp 577–578)*

105. (C) Antibiotics are useful only when there is evidence of cystitis. SSRIs are antidepressants that have not been shown to improve the incontinence with detrusor dyssynergia. Surgery is of no value and may actually worsen the incontinence in women with detrusor dyssynergia. Bladder retraining, in which the patient embarks on a programmed progressive lengthening of the interval of voiding, forms the basis of therapy. While such retraining is occurring, the use of anticholinergic drugs, such as oxybutynin chloride (Ditropan), propantheline (Pro-Banthine), or flavoxate (Urispas), seems to improve the results over either alone. *(Mishell et al, p 591)*

106. (D) The cyclic pain with bulging between normal labia is the classic history for an imperforate hymen. Ninety-five percent of women with vaginal agenesis also have agenesis or hypoplasia of the uterus and do not menstruate. The cyclic pain suggests that this girl has a uterus and is menstruating back through her fallopian tubes into her abdominal cavity. The presence of a uterus and normal pubic hair excludes androgen insensitivity. Normal appearing labia exclude the possibility of labial adhesions, an uncommon disorder that almost always occurs in prepubertal girls before estrogen production begins. Transverse vaginal septa are usually found higher in the vagina; bulging and discoloration of the hymen would not be found. *(Mishell et al, pp 247–251)*

107. (D) During the embryonic period, the paired müllerian ducts fuse inferiorly and contact a plate of mesenchyme called the vaginal plate or sinovaginal bulbs. This induces elongation of the urogenital sinus from below, then eventually canalization to establish an open conduit from the uterus through the vagina. Failure of the müllerian ducts to form results in an individual with no upper vagina, cervix, uterus, or fallopian tubes. Failure of formation of the urogenital sinus causes vaginal agenesis, and agenesis or hypoplastic nonfunctioning of the uterus. Retrograde menstruation would occur only in the 5% of women with vaginal agenesis who have a functioning uterus. However, they would not have the bulging and discoloration between the labia minora. The metanephric ducts are the embryologic origin of the ureters and lower collecting system of the kidneys; abnormalities of these structures would have no direct effect on menstrual or reproductive function. *(Mishell et al, p 247)*

108. (D) A hymenotomy is done by making three or four stellate incisions in the hymen and using fine suture only to secure hemostasis. This should be done once the diagnosis of imperforate hymen is made because endometriosis is a complication of retrograde menstruation. A McIndoe vaginoplasty is done when the diagnosis is vaginal agenesis and the uterus is nonfunctioning or absent. After creating a space between the urethra and bladder anteriorly and the rectum posteriorly, a split-thickness skin graft from the buttocks is placed over a mold and inserted into this space. Within 5 to 7 days, the skin graft adheres to the walls of the created space. It is difficult to impossible to perform a McIndoe procedure and establish a permanently patent connection to a functioning uterus. For this reason, a hysterectomy is usually done in those women with vaginal agenesis who have a functioning uterus. The diagnosis in this girl is obvious enough that a laparoscopy adds nothing to the management. Girls with an imperforate hymen have a normal upper genital tract, normal ovaries, and a 46,XX karyotype. Thus, there is no indication for a gonadectomy. *(Mishell et al, pp 249–251)*

109–113. (109-A, E; 110-C, D; 111-D; 112-B; 113-C, E) The cardinal ligament is the most caudal portion of the broad ligament or parametrium. It attaches the cervix to the lateral pelvic wall and upper vagina. Blood vessels, including the uterine arteries, traverse these ligaments. The uterosacral ligaments extend from the upper, posterior portion of the cervix to the sacrum. They contain fibrous tissue and nerves but are avascular. The ovarian ligament is the avascular attachment of the ovary to the uterus. It extends from the lower pole of the ovary to the attachment of the mesosalpinx at the uterus. The round ligament originates at the top of the uterus immediately anterior and inferior to the junction of the fallopian tubes and uterus. It passes laterally to the internal inguinal ring, down the inguinal canal, to insert in the labium majus. It provides minimal support to the uterus and contains Sampson's artery. The infundibulopelvic ligament contains the ovarian artery and vein. Lymphatic channels are also present. *(Mishell et al, pp 49–51)*

114–121. (114-E, I; 115-C; 116-D; 117-B, F, K; 118-J; 119-G; 120-A, F, H; 121-F) Serous tumors recapitulate the lining of the fallopian tubes. Mucinous tumors resemble the endocervix and colonic epithelium. Endometrioid cancers are so named because they resemble the endometrium. Psammoma bodies are found in serous tumors. Germ cell tumors recapitulate embryonic and extraembryonic cells and structures. Among these, dysgerminomas are characterized by cords of lymphocytes infiltrating the stroma. Occasionally, dysgerminomas are hormonally active, usually associated with increased estrogen production. Dysgerminomas are unique in their sensitivity to radiation therapy. Endodermal sinus tumors reflect extraembryonic differentiation and resemble the yolk sac. The characteristic pathologic finding is the Schiller–Duval body, a single papillae lined by tumor cells and containing a central vessel. Immature teratomas can contain any of the three germ cell layers, but the immature elements are almost always dominated by neurectoderm. A third subtype of ovarian tumor is of sex cord/stromal derivation. Granulosa cell tumors often produce and secrete estrogen and are noted for their propensity for late recurrence (10 to 15 years). The distinctive architectural pattern are rosettes of a single layer of granulosa cells surrounding proteinaceous material, Call–Exner bodies. Sertoli–Leydig cell tumors usually secrete androgens, seemingly in proportion to the number of Leydig cells with the tumor. *(Mishell et al, pp 901–935)*

REFERENCES

ACOG Technical Bulletin. *Immunization During Pregnancy.* Number 160. October 1991.

Creasy RK, Resnik R. *Maternal–Fetal Medicine: Principles and Practice,* 3rd ed. Philadelphia: WB Saunders; 1994.

Cunningham FG, MacDonald PC, Gant NF, et al. *Williams Obstetrics,* 20th ed. East Stamford, CT: Appleton & Lange; 1997.

DiSaia PJ, Creasman WT. *Clinical Gynecologic Oncology.* St. Louis: Mosby, 1997.

Mishell DR Jr., Stenchever MA, Droegemueller W, Herbst AL. *Comprehensive Gynecology,* 3rd ed. St. Louis: Mosby; 1997.

MMWR Morbidity and Mortality Weekly Report. Recommendations and Reports. *1998 Guidelines for Treatment of Sexually Transmitted Diseases.* Volume 47, No. RR-01. January 23, 1998. U.S. Department of Health and Human Services.

Rock JA, Thompson JD. *TeLinde's Operative Gynecology,* 8th ed. Philadelphia: Lippincott-Raven; 1997.

Scott JR, DiSaia PJ, Hammond CB, Spellacy WN, eds. *Danforth's Obstetrics and Gynecology,* 7th ed. Philadelphia: JB Lippincott; 1994.

Speroff L, Glass RH, Kase NG. *Clinical Gynecologic Endocrinology and Infertility,* 5th ed. Baltimore: Williams & Wilkins; 1994.

Sweet RL, Gibbs RS. *Infectious Diseases of the Female Genital Tract,* 3rd ed. Baltimore: Williams & Wilkins; 1995.

Yen SSC, Jaffe RB. *Reproductive Endocrinology: Physiology, Pathophysiology and Clinical Management,* 3rd ed. Philadelphia: WB Saunders; 1991.

Subspecialty List:
Obstetrics and Gynecology

74. Gynecology: breasts
75. Approach to the patient
76. Gynecology
77. Gynecology
78. Gynecology
79. Reproductive endocrinology
80. Reproductive endocrinology
81. Reproductive endocrinology
82. Reproductive endocrinology
83. Obstetrics: abnormal
84. Obstetrics: abnormal
85. Obstetrics: procedures
86. Approach to the patient
87. Neoplasia
88. Neoplasia
89. Neoplasia
90. Gynecology: breasts
91. Gynecology: breasts
92. Gynecology: breasts
93. Gynecology: breasts
94. Obstetrics: abnormal
95. Approach to the patient
96. Obstetrics: procedures
97. Obstetrics: procedures
98. Obstetrics: abnormal

99. Obstetrics: procedures
100. Obstetrics: abnormal
101. Obstetrics: abnormal
102. Obstetrics: procedures
103. Obstetrics: procedures
104. Gynecology
105. Gynecology: procedures
106. Gynecology
107. Approach to the patient
108. Approach to the patient
109. Gynecology: procedures
110. Approach to the patient
111. Approach to the patient
112. Approach to the patient
113. Approach to the patient
114. Approach to the patient
115. Neoplasia
116. Neoplasia
117. Neoplasia
118. Neoplasia
119. Neoplasia
120. Neoplasia
121. Neoplasia
122. Neoplasia

Pediatrics
Questions

Patricia Lye, MD

DIRECTIONS (Questions 122 through 229): Each of the numbered items or incomplete statements in this section is followed by answers or completions of the statement. Select the ONE lettered answer or completion that is BEST in each case.

122. The type of exercise most likely to cause exercise-induced bronchospasm is

    (A) 5-kilometer run (25 minutes)
    (B) 100-yard sprint
    (C) playing football
    (D) moderate-intensity walk (30 minutes)
    (E) swimming butterfly style (25 yards)

123. Atopy primarily is mediated via which type of immunologic reaction as classified by Gell and Coombs?

    (A) type I (anaphylactic reactions)
    (B) type II (cytotoxic reactions)
    (C) type III (Arthus or immune complex reactions)
    (D) type IV (cell-mediated reactions)
    (E) all of the above

124. In an adolescent presenting with pityriasis rosea, which of the following would be an appropriate blood test to order?

    (A) Veneral Disease Research Laboratory (VDRL)
    (B) complete blood count
    (C) hepatitis A immunoglobulin M (IgM)
    (D) fluorescent antinuclear antibody (FANA)
    (E) glucose

125. Which of the following statements regarding the transmission of varicella-zoster virus is true?

    (A) Children with chickenpox are infectious only during the period of time when skin lesions are present.
    (B) Children with chickenpox are infectious for a few days after crusting of skin lesions has occurred.
    (C) Susceptible individuals cannot contract chickenpox from patients with zoster (shingles).
    (D) Transmission of the virus from an acutely infected patient to a susceptible host elsewhere in the hospital via an immune intermediary has been reported.
    (E) Varicella-zoster immune globulin (VZIG) should be administered to susceptible immunocompromised individuals who are exposed to a patient with chickenpox.

126. Which of the following statements regarding the gross motor development of an infant is true?

    (A) By 6 months, most infants are able to assume a sitting position without help.
    (B) By 7 months, most infants are able to creep or crawl.
    (C) By 15 months, most infants are able to walk alone.
    (D) By 16 months, most infants are able to walk down stairs with one hand held.
    (E) By 16 months, most infants are able to walk up stairs with one hand held.

127. Which of the following statements regarding hepatitis A infection in children is true?

   (A) Most children with hepatitis A will develop clinically apparent jaundice.
   (B) The most rapid test for diagnosis is viral culture of nasopharyngeal secretions.
   (C) All household and sexual contacts should receive immune globulin.
   (D) The incubation period is 10 to 21 days.
   (E) Immunity to hepatitis A virus is short lived.

128. In which of the following children would the use of live oral poliovirus vaccine (OPV) be contraindicated?

   (A) one who developed a fever of 39°C following the previous administration of OPV
   (B) one with diarrhea
   (C) one with an upper respiratory infection and low-grade fever
   (D) one whose sibling has acquired immune deficiency syndrome (AIDS)
   (E) one with Hirschsprung's disease

129. The fragile X syndrome is characterized by

   (A) multiple fractures of long bones
   (B) easy bruising and poor wound healing
   (C) mental retardation
   (D) small testes
   (E) recurrent bacterial infection

130. A 2-month-old infant is brought to the emergency department with irritability and lethargy. The parents state that he was well until he rolled off the couch onto the floor yesterday. On examination, he is inconsolable and afebrile. The fontanels are full and tense. He has a generalized tonic–clonic seizure. The most important initial diagnostic study to do is

   (A) serum calcium, phosphorus, and magnesium levels
   (B) analysis of cerebrospinal fluid (CSF)
   (C) cranial computed tomography (CT) scan
   (D) serum ammonia level
   (E) serum acetaminophen level

131. Which of the following statements regarding child sexual abuse is correct?

   (A) Most instances occur outside the child's home.
   (B) Diagnostic physical findings most often are present.
   (C) The perpetrators most often are females.
   (D) The perpetrators most often are known by the victim prior to the incident.
   (E) The victims most often are males.

132. Which of the following statements concerning sensorineural hearing loss in children with bacterial meningitis is true?

   (A) It occurs rarely (< 5% of cases).
   (B) It occurs more commonly when *Hemophilus influenzae* type B rather than *Streptococcus pneumoniae* is the causative organism of the meningitis.
   (C) Its onset often is late in the clinical course, after discontinuation of antimicrobial therapy.
   (D) Prompt institution of antimicrobial therapy appears not to influence the incidence.
   (E) Evoked-response audiometry is indicated only if there is clinically evident hearing loss.

133. An increased incidence of inguinal hernia is associated with

   (A) female gender
   (B) congenital heart disease
   (C) post-term delivery
   (D) cryptorchidism
   (E) celiac disease

134. Which of the following statements about congenital toxoplasmosis is true?

   (A) Microcephaly and hydrocephalus may occur.
   (B) Subsequent infants are frequently affected.
   (C) The full impact of the disease can be predicted at birth.

(D) Abdominal wall defects may occur.

(E) Infected mothers are usually ill, with fever, headache, and malaise.

135. Which of the following, when given in excess, would most likely cause pseudotumor cerebri?

(A) vitamin A

(B) vitamin B

(C) vitamin C

(D) vitamin D

(E) zinc

136. Aniridia and hemihypertrophy are associated with

(A) Wilms' tumor

(B) neuroblastoma

(C) acute lymphoblastic leukemia

(D) Hodgkin's disease

(E) retinoblastoma

137. Which of the following malignant neoplastic processes has the highest rate of spontaneous regression?

(A) neuroblastoma

(B) Ewing's sarcoma

(C) Wilms' tumor

(D) acute myelogenous leukemia

(E) Hodgkin's disease

138. Which of the following conditions is the leading cause of death in the United States in infants (birth to 12 months)?

(A) bacterial meningitis

(B) unintentional injuries

(C) congenital malformation syndromes

(D) prematurity and its complications

(E) sudden infant death syndrome (SIDS)

139. A 3-month-old infant is brought to your office in the winter with a history of one day of vomiting, followed by 3 days of diarrhea. She has had six to eight stools per day, which are loose and foul-smelling. On exam, she looks well. Which of the following viruses is the most likely cause of her illness?

(A) adenovirus

(B) enterovirus

(C) human herpesvirus, type 6

(D) respiratory syncytial virus

(E) rotavirus

140. On rounds, a patient is presented who has chronic granulomatous disease. As you listen to the history, you remember that the immune deficiency in this disease is a

(A) B-cell defect

(B) bactericidal defect of neutrophils

(C) complement deficiency

(D) T-cell dysfunction

(E) T- and B-cell deficiency

Questions 141 and 142

141. A 10-year-old boy comes to your office in the winter with a sore throat for 2 days. He has had fever, headache, and abdominal pain at home. He does not have any allergies to medications. On exam, he has a temperature of 38.6°C, an erythematous pharynx, and tender cervical adenopathy. Which of the following would be the most appropriate antimicrobial agent to use?

(A) erythromycin

(B) penicillin

(C) trimethoprim–sulfamethoxazole

(D) azithromycin

(E) cefaclor

142. The same child returns to your office the next day. He has taken the medication you prescribed. He is feeling a little better. His fever has resolved, but he has developed a rash. His exam is unchanged except that he is afebrile and he has a fine, papular rash over his body, which is accentuated in his axilla and groin. Which of the following is the most likely cause of his rash?

    (A) allergic reaction to the antibiotic
    (B) rash from the antibiotic seen in patients with mononucleosis
    (C) scarlet fever
    (D) serum sickness
    (E) viral exanthem typical of enterovirus

Questions 143 and 144

An 8-year-old girl presents for a checkup. She is new to your practice. The mother states that she has always been small for her age; otherwise, she has been well. On physical exam, she is short and has a height age of 4 years, 4 months. You note some abnormalities in her general appearance (Figure 2–1).

143. Which of the following is the most likely diagnosis?

    (A) Marfan syndrome
    (B) Noonan syndrome
    (C) trisomy 21
    (D) Turner syndrome
    (E) Williams syndrome

144. As you continue your physical exam, you remember that congenital heart disease is common in this particular syndrome. Which of the following is the most likely congenital heart defect in patients with this syndrome?

    (A) supravalvular aortic stenosis
    (B) atrioventricular (AV) canal defects
    (C) coarctation of the aorta
    (D) pulmonary valvular stenosis
    (E) mitral valve prolapse

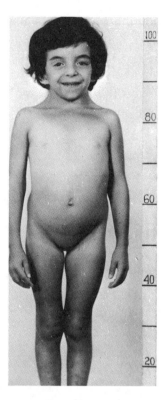

Figure 2–1. Phenotypic 8-year-old female. *(From Grumbach, Barr.* Recent Prog Horm Res *14:255, 1958.)*

Questions 145 and 146

A 12-year-old boy comes to the clinic for a sports physical. He is new to your practice. He comes with his foster mother, who states that he was recently placed in her care because of his mother's problems with drug abuse. Although a complete medical history is not available, she knows that he has not received regular care. He does not have any chronic medical problems. She also knows that his father died of heart disease when he was 35. On physical exam, the boy's height is greater than the 95th percentile. His arm span exceeds his height.

145. Which of the following is the most likely cause of his tall stature?

    (A) Ehlers–Danlos syndrome
    (B) Kleinfelter syndrome
    (C) Marfan syndrome
    (D) Noonan syndrome
    (E) Williams syndrome

146. As you continue your physical exam, you remember that congenital heart disease is common in this particular syndrome. Which of the following is the most likely congenital heart defect in patients with this syndrome?

    (A) supravalvular aortic stenosis
    (B) AV canal defects
    (C) coarctation of the aorta
    (D) pulmonary valvular stenosis
    (E) mitral valve prolapse

147. A 17-year-old girl comes to the clinic with several weeks of joint pain and rash. The joint pain is most prominent in the hands. She states that the pain is most severe in the morning and tends to improve over the day. She has noted some swelling of her fingers. She has also had a rash on her face that becomes more prominent when she is outside. She states that the sunlight tends to bother her eyes. On further questioning, she states that she has not felt well for several months. She has had intermittent fever, has been more tired than usual, and has lost weight even though she has not been dieting. On physical exam, she looks tired. She has lost 5 pounds since her last visit one year ago. She has an erythematous rash on her cheeks. She has several shallow ulcers in her mouth. She has fusiform swelling of her fingers and pain with movement of her fingers. Which of the following in the most likely diagnosis?

    (A) systemic lupus erythematosus (SLE)
    (B) dermatomyositis
    (C) juvenile rheumatoid arthritis
    (D) rheumatic fever
    (E) Lyme disease

Questions 148 and 149

You are called by one of your colleagues about a patient who is moving to your city. She states that he is a 3-year-old boy with Arnold–Chiari malformation. As you listen to her description of the patient and his recent issues, you remember that Arnold–Chiari malformation is a congenital anomaly often associated with hydrocephalus.

148. Which of the following is the mechanism that causes hydrocephalus?

    (A) excessive CSF secretion
    (B) aqueductal stenosis
    (C) inflammation of the ependymal lining
    (D) displacement of the brain stem and cerebellum caudally
    (E) blockage of the foramen of Monro

149. As you continue to listen, you remember that Arnold–Chiari malformation is often associated with other congenital anomalies. Which of the following anomalies is often associated with this syndrome?

    (A) agenesis of the corpus callosum
    (B) cleft palate
    (C) meningomyelocele
    (D) renal agenesis
    (E) ventricular septal defect

150. A cephalosporin is the drug of first choice in treating infections due to

    (A) *Neisseria gonorrhoeae*
    (B) methicillin-resistant *Staphylococcus aureus*
    (C) *Chlamydia trachomatis*
    (D) *Mycoplasma pneumoniae*
    (E) *Streptococcus pyogenes* group A

151. Which of the following is associated with café au lait spots?

    (A) Chédiak–Higashi syndrome
    (B) Hippel–Lindau syndrome
    (C) Marfan syndrome
    (D) neurofibromatosis
    (E) Sturge–Weber syndrome

152. Of the following diseases or conditions, which is transmitted via a tick bite?

    (A) Kawasaki disease
    (B) brucellosis
    (C) ehrlichiosis
    (D) leptospirosis
    (E) psittacosis

153. Which of the following is characteristic of pneumonia caused by *Mycoplasma pneumoniae?*

(A) occurrence among preschool-aged children

(B) elevated peripheral white blood cell (WBC) count

(C) presence of cold agglutinins in the serum

(D) lifelong immunity after an infection

(E) sudden onset of fever, sore throat, and a dry, hacking cough

154. Which of the following statements concerning Kawasaki disease is correct?

(A) It occurs almost exclusively in teenagers and young adults.

(B) Fever is an invariable feature of the disease.

(C) Thrombocytopenia frequently occurs late in the course of illness.

(D) The most common serious complication is central nervous system (CNS) hemorrhage.

(E) Oral or intravenous corticosteroid therapy is indicated.

155. A 5-year-old febrile child presents with swelling of the right eyelid. Proptosis and limitation of ocular movements is noted. The most likely diagnosis is

(A) retinoblastoma

(B) orbital cellulitis

(C) periorbital cellulitis

(D) neuroblastoma

(E) hyphema

156. Which of the following diseases or conditions results in a conjugated ("direct") hyperbilirubinemia?

(A) Gilbert's disease

(B) Crigler–Najjar syndrome

(C) breast milk jaundice

(D) physiologic jaundice

(E) congenital biliary atresia

157. Which of the following statements regarding *Pneumocystis carinii* infection in infants and children is correct?

(A) It is a common cause of pneumonia in children in daycare centers.

(B) The most common manifestation is reactive airway disease.

(C) Extrapulmonary infection is common.

(D) It is an important pathogen in children with AIDS.

(E) The organism can be cultured from sputum.

158. Otitis media occurring during the first 8 weeks of life deserves special consideration because the bacteria responsible for infections during this time may be different from those that affect older infants and children. Which of the following organisms is the most likely to cause otitis media in these infants?

(A) *Chlamydia trachomatis*

(B) *Escherichia coli*

(C) *Neisseria gonorrhoeae*

(D) *Treponema pallidum*

(E) *Toxoplasma gondii*

159. Among the conditions that cause edema of the eyelids is orbital cellulitis. This is a serious infection that must be recognized early and treated aggressively if complications are to be avoided. Which of the following features is useful in differentiating orbital cellulitis from periorbital (preseptal) cellulitis?

(A) proptosis

(B) elevated WBC count

(C) fever

(D) lid swelling

(E) conjunctival inflammation

160. A 6-month-old infant is diagnosed with her first episode of otitis media. She does not have any allergies to medications. Which of the following medications would be the recommended initial therapy for this infant?

(A) amoxicillin

(B) amoxicillin–clavulanic acid

(C) cephalexin

(D) ceftriaxone

(E) erythromycin

161. In pediatric patients, the risk of developing post-traumatic epilepsy is significantly increased by

(A) a brief loss of consciousness

(B) an acute intracranial hemorrhage

(C) retrograde amnesia

(D) post-traumatic vomiting

(E) a linear skull fracture

162. A 4-year-old previously healthy but unimmunized boy presents with sudden onset of high fever, inspiratory stridor, and refusal to drink. Of the following causes of inspiratory stridor, which best fits this clinical scenario?

(A) epiglottitis

(B) vascular ring

(C) croup

(D) foreign body aspiration

(E) laryngeal tumor

163. A dominant inheritance pattern has been described for

(A) astrocytoma

(B) acute lymphoblastic leukemia

(C) neuroblastoma

(D) rhabdosarcoma

(E) Wilms' tumor

164. The leading cause of death among adolescents aged 15 to 19 years is

(A) cancer

(B) AIDS

(C) suicide

(D) homicide

(E) unintentional injuries

165. The most common cause of amenorrhea or abnormal uterine bleeding in an adolescent is

(A) infection

(B) depression

(C) anorexia

(D) hypothyroidism

(E) pregnancy

166. Air leak syndrome (pneumothorax and pneumomediastinum) in newborns may correctly be described as

(A) rarely affecting term newborn infants

(B) having a high incidence in infants with meconium aspiration syndrome

(C) invariably symptomatic

(D) due to congenital anomaly of the lungs

(E) limited to newborn infants receiving positive-pressure ventilation

167. Vitamin D toxicity may produce

(A) bone pain

(B) diarrhea

(C) hypercalcemia

(D) hypophosphatemia

(E) increased intracranial pressure

168. A child appears to be suffering from minimal change nephrotic syndrome. Which of the following findings would support this diagnosis?

(A) blood urea nitrogen (BUN) of 50 mg/mL

(B) blood pressure of 140/95

(C) clinical response to steroid therapy

(D) macroscopic hematuria

(E) normal serum level of C3

169. Cyanosis in newborns may be caused by

(A) atrial septal defect

(B) hypoplastic left heart

(C) patent ductus arteriosus

(D) pulmonary stenosis

(E) total anomalous pulmonary venous return

170. Which of the following statements regarding intraventricular hemorrhage in newborn infants is correct?

  (A) It is most common in term infants.
  (B) Vascular events, especially changes in blood pressure, are a major etiologic factor.
  (C) Most patients have some bleeding diathesis.
  (D) CT is necessary for diagnosis in most cases.
  (E) Lumbar puncture should be avoided if the diagnosis is suspected.

171. Acetaminophen poisoning is correctly described by which of the following statements?

  (A) CNS symptoms are an early clue to prognosis.
  (B) Administration of specific antidote must be guided by a timed blood level.
  (C) Activated charcoal should not be used.
  (D) Death most commonly results from renal insufficiency.
  (E) Small children are more likely than adolescents to suffer serious adverse effects.

172. A 5-week-old bottle-fed boy presents with persistent and worsening projectile vomiting, poor weight gain, and hypochloremic metabolic alkalosis. Of the following diagnostic modalities, which would most likely reveal the diagnosis?

  (A) ultrasound of abdomen
  (B) barium enema
  (C) evaluation of stool for ova and parasites
  (D) testing well water for presence of nitrites
  (E) serum thyroxine

173. Your next patient is a 4-month-old infant who is returning to have her ear checked. You diagnosed her with otitis media 2 weeks ago and she has taken 10 days of amoxicillin. She is feeling well, and her mother's only concern is that she has developed a diaper rash over the last 3 days. The mother has been using emollient creams on it, which

have not helped. On physical exam, there are no abnormal findings except for the rash (Figure 2–2). Which of the following is the most likely diagnosis?

  (A) allergic dermatitis
  (B) bullous impetigo
  (C) *Candida* dermatitis
  (D) irritant dermatitis
  (E) seborrheic dermatitis

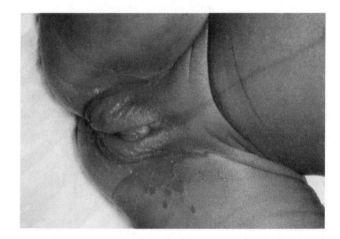

Figure 2–2. Diaper dermatitis. *(Photograph courtesy of Neil S. Prose.)*

174. A 7-year-old boy presents with a rash. His mother states that he was well until 3 days ago when he developed fever and malaise. The next day, the rash started as papules on the trunk, which rapidly changed to vesicles. The lesions have spread all over the body. On physical exam, he has no fever and appears well. You note numerous vesicles all over the body, some of which have crusted over. Which of the following is the most likely diagnosis?

  (A) chickenpox
  (B) Kawasaki disease
  (C) measles
  (D) rubella
  (E) staphylococcal scalded skin syndrome

175. A 10-year-old boy presents with a 1-day history of fever, cough, and chest pain. He has not been eating and has been listless. He does not have any previous history of health problems. On physical exam, his temperature is 40°C and he is tachypneic. He looks ill. He has rales on his left posterior lower lung fields. You order a chest x-ray (Figure 2–3). Which of the following organisms is most likely responsible for his pneumonia?

(A) *Hemophilus influenzae*
(B) *Mycoplasma pneumoniae*
(C) *Pneumocystis carinii*
(D) *Staphylococcus aureus*
(E) *Streptococcus pneumoniae*

176. An 18-month-old girl is brought to the hospital with a history of 6 days of bloody diarrhea. She has been drinking well but has not been wetting her diaper. She has been irritable. On physical exam, she has periorbital edema. She appears pale and is tachycardic. Her complete blood count (CBC) shows a hemoglobin of 6 g/dL, and a platelet count of 100,000/mm³. Her BUN is 50 mg/dL

and creatinine is 5.5 mg/dL. Her urinalysis shows gross hematuria. Which of the following is the most likely causative organism for her clinical problem?

(A) *Escherichia coli* 0157:H7
(B) group A streptococci
(C) group B streptococci
(D) *Staphylococcus aureus*
(E) the cause of this illness is not known

177. Which of the following childhood immunizations is given to reduce the possible exposure of pregnant women to children with a disease that causes birth defects?

(A) hepatitis B
(B) *Hemophilus influenzae*, type B
(C) MMR (measles, mumps, rubella)
(D) polio
(E) tetanus

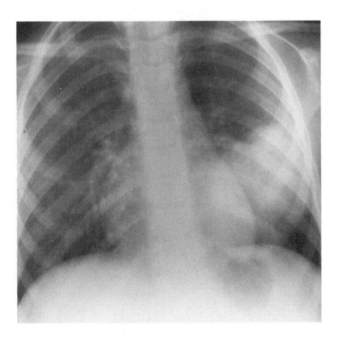

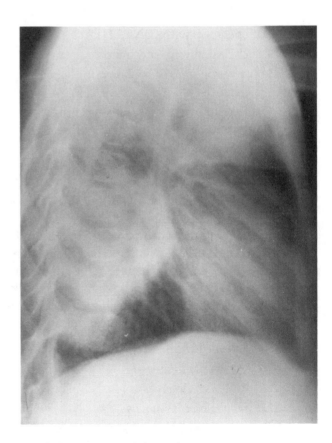

Figure 2–3. Chest x-ray of a 10-year-old boy with high fever, cough, and chest pain.

178. A 9-year-old boy presents with a several-day history of progressive arm and leg weakness. He has been well except for an upper respiratory infection 2 weeks ago. The patient is alert and oriented. On repeated examination, the heart rate varies between 60 and 140 beats/min and the blood pressure varies between 90/60 and 140/90 mm Hg. Respirations are shallow, with a rate of 50/min. There is symmetric weakness of the face and all four extremities. Deep tendon reflexes are absent. Sensation is intact. The most likely diagnosis is

(A) polymyositis
(B) myasthenia gravis
(C) transverse myelitis
(D) Guillain–Barré syndrome
(E) viral encephalitis

179. An 18-month-old boy is brought to the clinic for a checkup. As part of his routine care, a serum lead level is obtained. It is 25 μg/mL. The most appropriate next step in his management is

(A) chelation with $CaNa_2EDTA$
(B) chelation with succimer
(C) investigation of his home for lead hazards
(D) reassurance that this level is not a problem
(E) repeating the level in 6 months

180. A 6-year-old girl presents with a 2-week history of a tender, swollen inguinal lymph node. She has no other symptoms. On physical exam, an ulcerated papule is noted on the child's ipsilateral lower leg. The parents deny cat exposure but remember removing a tick from the child's leg approximately 2 weeks prior. Which of the following organisms is most likely to cause this clinical picture?

(A) *Bartonella henselae*
(B) *Francisella tularensis*
(C) *Rickettsia rickettsii*
(D) *Staphylococcus aureus*
(E) *Streptococcus pyogenes*

181. A 7-year-old child is scheduled for an elective tonsillectomy. The most important instruction to the parents should be to make sure that the child

(A) avoids contact with other children
(B) discontinues antibiotics 72 hours before surgery
(C) avoids aspirin and antihistamines for 2 weeks before surgery
(D) does not drink from siblings' cups
(E) eats iron-laden foods for 3 weeks before surgery

182. Routine examination of an otherwise healthy kindergarten child with a history of asthma reveals a blood pressure (BP) of 140/90 mm Hg. The most likely cause of the hypertension is

(A) theophylline toxicity
(B) chronic lung disease
(C) renal disease
(D) coarctation of the aorta
(E) obesity

183. A 13-year-old girl presents with lethargy, fever, severe headache, and a stiff neck. On examination, a unilateral fixed, dilated pupil and papilledema are noted. Which of the following is the most appropriate initial step in managing this patient?

(A) administration of intravenous (IV) cefotaxime
(B) administration of IV mannitol
(C) CT of the head
(D) intubation and hyperventilation
(E) performance of a lumbar puncture

184. A newborn infant requires repeated resuscitations in the delivery room because of failure to breathe and cyanosis. During spells of crying, which appear to alleviate the cyanosis, his breath and heart sounds are normal, as is direct laryngoscopy. Vigorous respira-

tory movements appear ineffectual. Immediate management of this infant consists of

(A) obtaining a chest x-ray

(B) obtaining an electrocardiogram (ECG)

(C) arterial blood gas determinations

(D) inserting an oropharyngeal airway

(E) administration of naloxone

185. A 7-year-old boy is brought to a physician's office after falling from his bicycle and striking his head on the sidewalk. No adult was present, and his friends are unable to give a reliable history. Neurologic examination reveals no abnormalities; there is a 3- to 4-cm abrasion on the left forehead. Reasonable management would include

(A) obtaining a CT scan

(B) admitting him overnight for observation

(C) obtaining a skull x-ray and discharging the patient if normal

(D) instructing the mother to observe the patient's neurologic status during the next 24 to 48 hours at home

(E) obtaining a CT scan and admitting him for observation

186. An adolescent is treated in the emergency department because she ingested a fistful of her brother's theophylline tablets after a family argument. A reasonable treatment approach for this patient would be to

(A) empty the stomach and check the theophylline level; if it is < 40 mg/mL, the patient may be discharged

(B) empty the stomach, administer activated charcoal, and check the theophylline level; if it is < 40 mg/mL, the patient may be discharged

(C) admit the patient and monitor her theophylline level for the next 48 hours

(D) empty the stomach and begin charcoal hemoperfusion

(E) empty the stomach; administer activated charcoal; send a urine specimen for a toxic screen; obtain a theophylline level and repeat the theophylline level in 4 hours

187. Children with sickle cell anemia are at increased risk of developing overwhelming infection with certain microorganisms. Which of the following is the most reasonable step to prevent such infection?

(A) periodic injections of gamma globulin

(B) injection of VZIG after exposure to varicella

(C) withholding live virus vaccines

(D) prophylactic administration of oral penicillin daily

(E) early use of amoxicillin at home for episodes of fever

188. In most of the United States, which of the following individuals would usually be considered capable of giving valid informed consent for his or her own medical treatment?

(A) a 10-year-old who needs a transfusion

(B) a 12-year-old with a sore throat

(C) a 15-year-old who might be pregnant

(D) a 17-year-old with asthma away at boarding school

(E) a 17-year-old with cancer needing chemotherapy

189. A 14-year-old child with diabetes mellitus is seen for routine follow-up. The child is being maintained with two injections of neutral protamine Hagedorn (NPH) and regular insulin a day. The patient's daily records show that blood glucose levels are consistently between 120 and 150 before breakfast, before dinner, and before bedtime. You should

(A) decrease the dose of NPH insulin

(B) increase the dose of NPH insulin

(C) decrease the dose of regular insulin and order a glycosylated hemoglobin (Hb) test

(D) increase the dose of regular insulin and order a glycosylated Hb test

(E) maintain the same dose of insulin and order a glycosylated Hb test

190. A previously well 2½-year-old child is seen because of a brief generalized seizure, which apparently lasted 1 minute or less. One hour before the seizure, the mother had noted the child to feel hot but had not taken his temperature. There is no family history of seizures. The child is noted to be alert and active, and physical and neurologic examinations are within normal limits except for a temperature of 40°C (104°F) and bilateral otitis media. Management at this time should include

    (A) immediate reduction of body temperature by administration of aspirin and the use of ice and alcohol sponging
    (B) institution of phenobarbital therapy to be maintained for a minimum of 1 year
    (C) institution of phenytoin therapy to be maintained for a minimum of 1 year
    (D) reassurance and instructions regarding taking the child's temperature and administration of acetaminophen
    (E) an electroencephalogram (EEG) in 3 to 5 days

191. A 7-month-old presents with a history of constipation for one month. He has one hard stool every week. He has been well otherwise. His physical exam is normal. Which of the following is the most likely cause of his problem?

    (A) hypothyroidism
    (B) lead poisoning
    (C) functional constipation
    (D) Hirschsprung's disease
    (E) hypocalcemia

192. An 11-month-old boy presents with pallor. On examination, he is noted to be a tachycardic but happy baby whose height is at the 25th percentile and weight is at the 95th percentile. His diet mainly consists of whole milk and pureed fruits. Which of the following diagnostic test results is most likely?

    (A) decreased free erythrocyte protoporphyrin
    (B) decreased iron-binding capacity

    (C) elevated mean corpuscular volume
    (D) low serum ferritin levels
    (E) normal hemoglobin

193. A specific pattern of abnormalities has been identified among infants born to mothers who consume moderate to large amounts of alcohol during their pregnancies. Which of the following abnormalities is characteristic of these infants

    (A) cataracts
    (B) developmental dysplasia of the hip
    (C) gonadal dysgenesis
    (D) neural tube defects
    (E) mental retardation

194. A 4-year-old girl presents to the emergency department with fever and a petechial rash. A sepsis workup is performed and IV antibiotics are administered. Gram-negative diplococci are identified in the CSF. Which of the following is true of this condition?

    (A) Antibiotic prophylaxis of fellow daycare attendees is not necessary.
    (B) The most common neurologic residual is seizures.
    (C) The presence of meningitis decreases the survival rate.
    (D) Shock is the usual cause of death.
    (E) Vancomycin administered intravenously is the treatment of choice.

195. A 3-year-old boy suddenly begins choking and coughing while eating peanuts. On physical examination, he is coughing frequently. He has inspiratory stridor and mild intercostal and suprasternal retractions. Initial management would include

    (A) back blows
    (B) abdominal thrusts
    (C) blind finger-sweeps of the hypopharynx
    (D) permitting him to clear the foreign body by coughing
    (E) emergency tracheostomy

196. During a well-child visit, the grandmother of an 18-month-old patient is concerned because the child's feet turn inward. She first noticed this when her grandson began to walk. It does not seem to bother the child. On examining his gait, his knees point forward and his feet turn inward. Which of the following is the most likely cause of this condition?

(A) adducted great toe
(B) femoral anteversion
(C) Legg–Calvé–Perthes disease
(D) medial tibial torsion
(E) metatarsus adductus

197. A 13-year-old girl presents with parental concerns of poor posture. She has not had any back pain. On examination, she has unequal shoulder height, asymmetric flank creases, and a forward-bending test that shows rib asymmetry. The physical exam is otherwise normal. Which of the following is the most likely cause of her condition?

(A) congenital scoliosis
(B) leg length inequality
(C) idiopathic scoliosis
(D) postural roundback
(E) Scheuermann kyphosis

198. After 10 days of nasal congestion and rhinorrhea, a 3-month-old infant develops a severe hacking cough during which he repeatedly turns dusky and appears to choke on or to vomit profuse thick, clear nasopharyngeal mucus. For 7 days, the coughing continues unabated. On physical exam, he is afebrile and his lungs are clear. His chest x-ray is normal. His WBC count is 24,000/mm^3, with 15% polymorphonuclear cells, 82% lymphocytes, and 3% monocytes. Which of the following antibiotics should be used to treat this patient?

(A) amoxicillin
(B) amoxicillin–clavulanic acid
(C) erythromycin
(D) tetracycline
(E) no antibiotics are necessary

199. Which of the following orally administered antibiotics is appropriate for initial therapy of acute sinusitis in children?

(A) ciprofloxacin
(B) amoxicillin–clavulanic acid
(C) cephalexin
(D) penicillin V
(E) dicloxacillin

200. A 16-year-old girl presents with a history of primary amenorrhea. On examination, short stature and a short neck with a low posterior hairline are noted. Chromosomal analysis most likely would reveal

(A) fragile X
(B) trisomy 18
(C) trisomy 21
(D) 45,XO
(E) XXY

201. A beekeeper's previously healthy 6-month-old son develops gradual onset of lethargy, poor feeding, constipation, and generalized weakness. On taking a history, you determine that the child has recently been placed on a homemade formula consisting of evaporated milk, water, and honey. The most likely explanation for this symptom complex is

(A) sodium intoxication
(B) Hirschsprung's disease
(C) hypothyroidism
(D) spinal cord tumor
(E) botulism

202. Which of the following conditions potentially is preventable by the current universally recommended vaccines of childhood?

(A) meningitis due to *Neisseria meningitidis*
(B) meningitis due to *Streptococcus pneumoniae*
(C) meningitis due to *Hemophilus influenzae* type B
(D) otitis media due to nontypeable *H influenzae*
(E) pneumonia due to respiratory syncytial virus

203. A 4-year-old child manifests symptoms of fever, sore throat, and swollen lymph nodes. The spleen tip is palpable. Throat culture and rapid slide (Monospot) test results are negative. The next logical diagnostic procedure would involve

(A) rapid streptococcal antigen test
(B) heterophil titer
(C) Epstein–Barr virus (EBV) titer
(D) chest x-ray
(E) bone marrow examination

204. A 2-year-old is brought to the emergency department with sudden onset of unresponsiveness, miosis, bradycardia, and muscle fasciculations. These findings are most suggestive of poisoning with

(A) acetaminophen
(B) organophosphates
(C) salicylates
(D) tricyclic antidepressants
(E) vitamin A

205. A 2-year-old boy presents with refusal to use his right arm for one day. He is otherwise well. His mother states she pulled upward on his arm the evening prior in order to keep him from tripping down the stairs. The most likely diagnosis is

(A) Colles' fracture
(B) fractured clavicle
(C) greenstick fracture of the humerus
(D) rotator cuff injury
(E) subluxation of the radial head

206. A 4-year-old child presents with an enlarged submandibular node that is 4 cm in diameter, nontender, and not fluctuant. The node has been enlarged for about 4 weeks, and there is no history of fever or contact with any person who was ill. A CBC is normal, and a Mantoux test with 5 tuberculin units of purified protein derivative shows 6 mm of induration. The most likely diagnosis is

(A) cat scratch fever
(B) acute pyogenic lymphadenitis

(C) acute lymphoblastic leukemia
(D) tuberculous lymphadenitis
(E) atypical mycobacteria lymphadenitis

207. A 4-year-old child with grade III vesicoureteral reflux who has recurrent urinary tract infections despite adequate antibiotic prophylaxis should have

(A) IV antibiotic treatment for 2 weeks
(B) repeat renal scan
(C) renal arteriogram
(D) antireflux surgery
(E) addition of vitamin C (ascorbic acid) to the treatment regimen

208. A 7-year-old is prescribed a phenothiazine for nausea and vomiting. He develops torticollis and facial muscle spasms. The most appropriate management would be to administer

(A) diazepam
(B) diphenhydramine
(C) epinephrine
(D) naloxone
(E) steroids

209. The most appropriate evaluative procedure for an otherwise normal 7-day-old boy with perineal hypospadias is

(A) renal ultrasonography
(B) serum creatinine determination
(C) cystography
(D) circumcision
(E) intravenous pyelography (IVP)

210. A 2-week-old presents with hepatosplenomegaly and a thick, purulent, bloody nasal discharge. Coppery, oval, maculopapular skin lesions are present in an acral distribution. The neurologic examination is normal, including head circumference. Which of the following is the most likely cause of this congenital infection?

(A) cytomegalovirus (CMV)
(B) herpes simplex virus (HSV)

(C) group B streptococci (GBS)

(D) *Toxoplasma gondii*

(E) *Treponema pallidum*

211. A 7-month-old presents with a history of 3 days of fever to 104°F, which resolved the same day that an exanthem erupted. The exanthem is prominent on the neck and truck. It is macular, with discrete lesions 3 to 5 mm in diameter. The most likely diagnosis is

(A) erythema infectiosum

(B) measles

(C) roseola infantum

(D) rubella

(E) scarlet fever

212. A 2-week-old is brought to the clinic for a checkup. She has been breast feeding well, and her parents have no concerns. Her physical exam is normal except for mild icterus. Her serum bilirubin is 5 mg/dL (all unconjugated). Which of the following is the most likely cause of her condition?

(A) breast milk jaundice

(B) congenital biliary atresia

(C) Crigler–Najjar syndrome

(D) Gilbert's disease

(E) physiologic jaundice

213. A few hours after eating Christmas dinner, a previously well 7-year-old boy and his parents develop vomiting, abdominal cramps, and diarrhea. Differential diagnosis of the cause of these gastrointestinal symptoms should include

(A) *Clostridium difficile*

(B) *Campylobacter*

(C) *Enterobius vermicularis* (pinworms)

(D) *Staphylococcus aureus* exotoxin

(E) *Clostridium botulinum*

214. Separation anxiety most often develops at

(A) 4 to 6 months of age

(B) 6 to 8 months of age

(C) 8 to 10 months of age

(D) 10 to 12 months of age

(E) 12 to 14 months of age

215. A 1-day-old infant who received silver nitrate eye drops in the delivery room is suffering from bilateral purulent conjunctival discharge. The most likely cause of this child's condition would be

(A) *Neisseria gonorrhoeae* infection

(B) herpes simplex infection

(C) nasolacrimal duct obstruction

(D) chemical irritation

(E) *Pseudomonas* infection

216. Otitis media in children beyond the neonatal period is commonly caused by

(A) *Streptococcus pneumoniae*

(B) *Staphylococcus aureus*

(C) *Mycoplasma pneumoniae*

(D) *Escherichia coli*

(E) group A streptococcus

217. A kindergarten student complains of nausea and vague abdominal pain after breakfast. On two occasions you have seen this child, and complete physical examinations have disclosed no abnormalities. You suspect the child may have a school-related emotional disorder. Physical illness that could mimic this pattern includes

(A) seizure disorder

(B) peptic ulcer

(C) pinworm infestation

(D) lactose intolerance

(E) Crohn's disease

218. A few weeks after a presumed viral respiratory infection, a 4-year-old girl presents with bruising and petechiae. Bone marrow examination reveals increased numbers of megakaryocytes, but is otherwise normal. Hb is 13.5 g/100 mL. Platelet count is 30,000/mm^3. Which of the following would be appropriate for this child at this time?

(A) daily prednisone

(B) a transfusion of packed red blood cells (RBCs) and platelets

(C) intravenous gamma globulin

(D) splenectomy

(E) no specific therapy

219. A 4-month-old presents with a 2-day history of vomiting and intermittent irritability. On exam, "currant jelly" stool is noted in the diaper, and a sausage-shaped mass is palpated in the right upper quadrant of the abdomen. The condition most likely to cause this is

(A) appendicitis

(B) diaphragmatic hernia

(C) giardiasis

(D) intussusception

(E) rotavirus gastroenteritis

220. A 7-year-old girl presents with a history of sexual abuse 2 weeks prior. At that time, a vaginal fluid culture yielded *Neisseria gonorrhoeae*. Subsequently, she received ceftriaxone intramuscularly. She now has a watery, mucoid vaginal discharge. After additional studies are obtained, the most appropriate antibiotic to administer is

(A) acyclovir

(B) ciprofloxacin

(C) erythromycin

(D) penicillin

(E) tetracycline

221. An 18-month-old boy has received 5 days of amoxicillin for otitis media. He continues to have fever and on physical exam the right tympanic membrane is bulging with purulent fluid behind it. Which of the following is the best antibiotic to use?

(A) amoxicillin–clavulanic acid

(B) dicloxacillin

(C) cephalexin

(D) erythromycin

(E) penicillin

Questions 222 and 223

A 13-year-old boy presents for evaluation of short stature. His growth chart from ages 2 through 12 years is shown in Figure 2–4. His growth in the first 2 years of life was typically at the 25th percentile. He has been healthy, has a good appetite, and is doing well in school. He lives with his parents and is an only child. His parents' heights are both at the 50th percentile. His father states that he grew several inches after he completed high school. A complete physical exam is normal. His Tanner stage is 1.

222. Which of the following is the most likely cause of this patient's short stature?

(A) constitutional delay

(B) deprivational dwarfism

(C) familial short stature

(D) growth hormone deficiency

(E) hypothyroidism

223. Which of the following tests is the most appropriate next step in the care of this patient?

(A) bone age

(B) cranial imaging

(C) growth hormone stimulation

(D) thyroid function tests

(E) no tests are necessary

BOYS: 2 TO 18 YEARS
PHYSICAL GROWTH
NCHS PERCENTILE

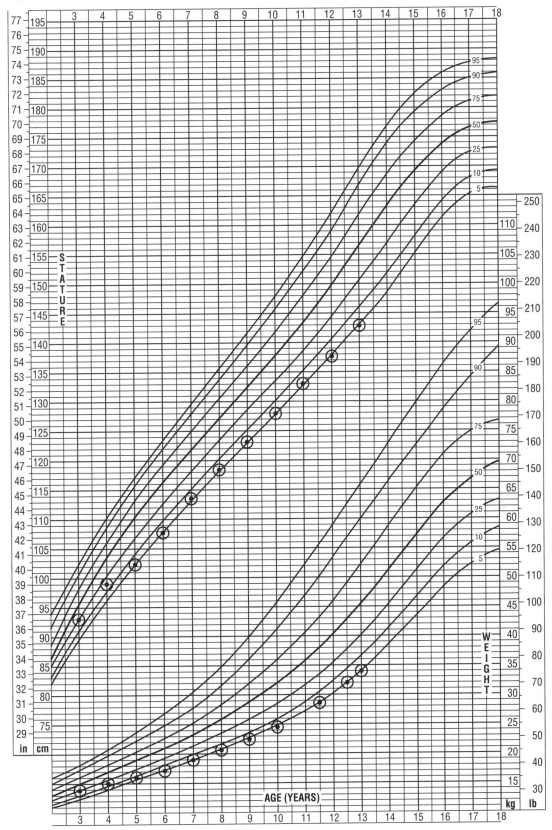

Figure 2–4. Boys: 2 to 18 years—Physical Growth NCHS Percentiles.

Questions 224 and 225

A 12-year-old girl presents with chest pain when she plays basketball. The pain is substernal, is associated with dyspnea, and occurs after she has been playing vigorously. The pain does not radiate. The pain and dyspnea resolve with rest. She does not have palpitations or any lightheadedness associated with the pain. She does not have pain or dyspnea at other times. There is no history of early cardiac deaths or unexplained deaths of young people in her family. Her physical exam is normal except for a grade 2/6 systolic vibratory murmur heard at the left lower sternal border.

224. Which of the following is the most likely cause of her symptoms?

   (A) angina
   (B) asthma
   (C) costochondritis
   (D) esophagitis
   (E) mitral valve prolapse

225. Which of the following tests should be ordered for this patient?

   (A) chest x-ray
   (B) echocardiogram
   (C) pulmonary function tests
   (D) 24-hour Holter monitoring
   (E) no tests are necessary

Questions 226 and 227

A 4-month-old girl presents for well-child care. She has had a low-grade fever at home and some rhinorrhea. On physical exam, she has a temperature of 38.0°C and clear rhinorrhea, and the rest of her exam is normal. Her immunization history is:

Patient Age	Immunizations Received
Birth	Hepatitis B (Hep B)
1 month	Hep B
2 months	Diphtheria, tetanus, acellular pertussis (DTaP), *Hemophilus influenzae* type B (HIB), inactivated polio vaccine (IPV)

226. Which are the most appropriate immunizations to give to this patient?

   (A) DTaP, HIB, IPV
   (B) DTaP, HIB
   (C) DTaP
   (D) Hep B
   (E) no immunizations should be given

227. Which of the following would be a reason to not give pertussis immunization to this patient?

   (A) She has had 5 days of diarrhea.
   (B) She was born to a mother who is positive for human immunodeficiency virus (HIV).
   (C) She was born 8 weeks prematurely.
   (D) She has a family history of seizures.
   (E) She has a progressive neurologic disorder.

Question 228

An 18-month-old boy presents with a history of fever to 39.0°C for 5 days. He has also been irritable and has not been drinking well. Associated symptoms include red eyes, a rash, and some trouble walking. On physical exam, he has a temperature of 39.5°C. He has bilateral bulbar conjunctivitis, a strawberry tongue, an inflamed oral pharynx, edema of the hands and feet, a morbilliform rash, and cervical lymphadenopathy. He is very irritable. His CBC shows a WBC of 15,000/mm^3 with 60% neutrophils, 35% lymphocytes, and 5% monocytes. His hemoglobin is 12.0 g/dL and platelet count is 500,000/mm^3.

228. Which of the following is the most likely diagnosis?

   (A) erythema infectiosum (Fifth disease)
   (B) Kawasaki disease
   (C) rubella
   (D) rubeola (measles)
   (E) rheumatic fever

Question 229

An athletic 12-year-old boy complains of left knee pain when he runs and plays sports. The pain resolves when he rests. He has otherwise been well. His physical exam is normal except for swelling and increased prominence over the left tibial tubercle. A radiograph of the left knee is normal.

229. Which of the following is the most likely diagnosis?

    (A) Legg–Calvé–Perthes disease

    (B) Osgood–Schlatter disease

    (C) patellar subluxation

    (D) popliteal cyst

    (E) slipped capital femoral epiphysis

DIRECTIONS (Questions 230 through 234): For each item, select the ONE best lettered option that is most closely associated with it. Each lettered heading may be selected once, more than once, or not at all.

For each of the following patients with possible congenital heart disease, select the most likely diagnosis.

    (A) aortic stenosis

    (B) atrial septal defect

    (C) atrioventricular canal defect

    (D) carotid bruit

    (E) coarctation of the aorta

    (F) mitral stenosis

    (G) mitral valve prolapse

    (H) peripheral pulmonic stenosis

    (I) pulmonic stenosis

    (J) Still's murmur

    (K) transposition of the great arteries

    (L) tetralogy of Fallot

    (M) truncus arteriosus

    (N) venous hum

    (O) ventricular septal defect

230. A newborn full-term infant develops cyanosis shortly after birth. On exam, the infant is in no distress, is well perfused, has a normal cardiac exam including no obvious murmurs, and has no organomegaly. The pulse oximeter is 77%. The ECG is normal, and chest x-ray reveals a normal heart size with a narrow mediastinum and normal pulmonary vascularity.

231. A 4-year-old boy with normal growth, development, and physical activity is noted to have a murmur at a checkup. On exam, he has no abnormal findings except for a 2/6 musical systolic ejection murmur at the lower sternal border, which is softer when he sits up.

232. A 5-year-old boy with normal growth, development, and physical activity is in the clinic for a checkup. His physical exam is totally normal except for a widely split second heart sound and a 2/6 systolic ejection murmur at the upper left sternal border that does not radiate.

233. A 2-month-old who is growing and developing normally is noted to have a murmur at a checkup. The physical exam is entirely normal except for a 2/6 systolic ejection murmur heard over the entire chest, especially in the axilla and back.

234. A 18-month-old who is growing and developing normally has a murmur noted at a checkup. The physical exam is entirely normal except for a 2/6 holosystolic murmur at the left sternal border.

Answers and Explanations

122. **(A)** Exercise-induced bronchospasm (EIB) can be demonstrated in 10 to 15% of the general population, and in greater than 85% of children with typical asthma. The type of exercise most likely to induce EIB is high in intensity, continuous, and prolonged in duration (usually > 5 or 6 minutes). Simultaneous environmental factors, such as cold, dry air or pollutants and allergens may contribute to the likelihood of EIB. *(Bar-Or, pp 88–108)*

123. **(A)** Atopy consists of a syndrome of dermatitis, allergic rhinitis, and asthma. A specific patient may have one, two, or all three clinical manifestations as his or her symptom complex. However, each of these entities has an immunoglobulin E (IgE)-dependent mechanism. Hence, atopy is a Gell and Coombs type I reaction. *(Oski et al, pp 209–211)*

124. **(A)** Pityriasis rosea is a papulosquamous eruption consisting of multiple oval-shaped scaling lesions, which are truncal in distribution. This eruption resembles the papulosquamous eruption of secondary syphilis, although the rash of secondary syphilis often involves the palms and soles. The etiology of pityriasis rosea is unknown but is felt to be viral. It is a self-limiting illness lasting several weeks to a few months, and there is no adequate treatment other than symptomatic treatment of pruritus, when necessary. *(Oski et al, pp 904–905)*

125. **(E)** Children with chickenpox may be infectious for 1 or 2 days before the appearance of the rash. Once skin lesions have crusted, the patient is no longer infectious. Suscep-

tible individuals can contract chickenpox from patients with zoster. In the cases of both chickenpox and zoster, transmission is thought to occur by the respiratory route rather than by direct contact. The virus can travel long distances in the air and remain viable. Transmission from one hospital patient to other susceptible hospitalized patients has been reported to occur through air vents. VZIG should be given within 3 or 4 days of exposure to varicella-susceptible individuals who are immunocompromised. *(Oski et al, pp 1220–1223; American Academy of Pediatrics, pp 578–579)*

126. **(C)** Although there are variations in gross motor development, most infants will be able to walk by 15 months of age. The ability to walk up steps (18 months) usually precedes the ability to walk down steps (20 months). Most infants can assume the sitting position without help by 8 to 9 months and crawl by 9 to 10 months. *(Behrman, pp 40–45)*

127. **(C)** Children, especially those in daycare, commonly are infected with the hepatitis A virus. Unlike adults, children most often are asymptomatic. Frequently, outbreaks of hepatitis A in a daycare center are not recognized until a daycare worker or parent of an attendee becomes ill. An elevated hepatitis A IgM is the most rapid and reliable confirmation of diagnosis. The incubation period is 15 to 50 days, with an average of 25 to 30 days. Household and sexual contacts who are exposed should receive immunoglobulin. *(American Academy of Pediatrics, pp 237–246)*

128. **(D)** Oral poliovirus vaccine contains live attenuated polioviruses that are shed in the vaccinee's stool for weeks. Susceptible or immunocompromised caretakers and household contacts are at risk of contracting paralytic disease due to the vaccine strains. Hence, prior to administering OPV, health care providers must determine the status of caretakers and household contacts. Inactivated poliovirus vaccine (IPV), may be administered in such cases. A mild infection such as diarrhea or an upper respiratory infection is not a contraindication to receiving an immunization. A fever following previous vaccinations is not a contraindication. *(American Academy of Pediatrics, p 432)*

129. **(C)** The fragile X syndrome is an X-linked chromosomal abnormality characterized by mental retardation, macro-orchidism, and certain inconsistent facial characteristics. The enlarged testes usually are not evident until puberty. The disorder must be considered in the differential diagnosis whenever there is mental retardation in more than one male member of a family. The term fragile X refers to the fact that the chromosomal abnormality is discernible only by special laboratory techniques, for example, growing the patient's cells in a medium with low concentrations of folic acid. *(DeArce and Kearns, pp 84–91)*

130. **(C)** Though infection must be considered as an etiology, acute trauma is more likely in this scenario. This case represents the classic picture of the shaken baby syndrome, which produces intracranial trauma without obvious external findings. This infant is critically ill and lacks preceding illness or constitutional symptoms. The tense fontanels reflect increased intracranial pressure. A cranial CT scan may show diffuse edema or a localized lesion, such as a subdural hemorrhage. Metabolic causes of seizures do not cause increased intracranial pressure. Acetaminophen toxicity does not cause CNS symptoms. *(Kliegman, pp 518–521; Rudolph et al, pp 145–147)*

131. **(D)** For several reasons, physical findings are lacking in most cases of sexual abuse. Many instances of sexual abuse do not involve vaginal or rectal penetration, most cases are reported weeks to months after the event(s), and the tissues involved can heal remarkably well. Victims, usually females, most often are acquainted with the perpetrator, usually male, prior to the sexual assault. In most cases, the abuse occurs in the home of the child. Health care providers must maintain a high degree of suspicion for this widespread psychosocial problem, and should be well versed in the evaluation of children alleged to be sexually abused. Complex or difficult cases should be referred to a multidisciplinary team for evaluation. *(Behrman, pp 117–119)*

132. **(D)** Sensorineural hearing loss is detected by evoked-response audiometry in between 5 and 10% of children with bacterial meningitis. Up to 30% of children with meningitis caused by *S pneumoniae* will have hearing deficits. Hearing loss generally is noted early in the course of bacterial meningitis and occurs despite prompt initiation of appropriate antimicrobial therapy. All children with bacterial meningitis should have hearing assessment by evoked-response audiometry before or soon after hospital discharge. *(Oski et al, p 1127)*

133. **(D)** Several conditions are associated with an increased incidence of inguinal hernias. Prematurity and male gender are the most common associations. Certain connective tissue disorders (Marfan syndrome and Ehlers–Danlos syndrome) as well as other congenital anomalies (abdominal wall defects, hypospadias, cryptorchidism, etc) also are seen in the presence of an inguinal hernia. *(Rowe et al, pp 446–449)*

134. **(A)** Congenital toxoplasmosis occurs only in infants whose mothers are primarily or initially infected with *Toxoplasma gondii*. The mothers are almost always asymptomatic, and subsequent offspring are not affected. The severely affected fetus may be stillborn, born prematurely, or born alive at full term. Clinical manifestations include hydrocephalus, microcephaly, maculopapular rash, hepatosplenomegaly, micro-ophthalmia, and chorioretinitis. The full impact of the disease on the infant's development may not become apparent for months. *(Rudolph et al, pp 768–772)*

135. **(A)** Pseudotumor cerebri, or benign intracranial hypertension, is characterized by increased intracranial pressure, normal or small ventricles, and normal cerebrospinal fluid. Symptoms include headache, irritability, nausea, disturbances of visual acuity, dizziness, and tinnitus. Often, it is a manifestation of hypervitaminosis A. Although it is thought of as benign, progressive visual field and acuity loss may occur. *(Oski et al, pp 594, 897)*

136. **(A)** Wilms' tumor is a malignant embryonal neoplasm of the kidney. It is the second most common solid tumor of childhood. Girls are affected more frequently than boys (2:1). The incidence of Wilms' tumor peaks at 1 to 3 years of age. The classic presentation is a painless abdominal mass that is usually hard, smooth, and unilateral. Hematuria occurs in 12 to 25% of children with Wilms' tumor, and hypertension has been reported in up to 60% of patients. Aniridia or hemihypertrophy may be observed in patients with Wilms' tumor. *(Oski et al, pp 1723–1726)*

137. **(A)** Neuroblastoma is a malignant neoplasm arising from sympathetic nervous tissue and may occur anywhere such tissue is found. It is a uniquely pediatric process, occurring almost exclusively in the first 6 years of life. The diagnosis is most often made during evaluation of an abdominal mass. Advanced stages of the disease are accompanied by systemic symptoms such as fever, anemia, and weight loss. The diagnosis is almost always suggested by increased urinary excretion of vanillylmandelic acid or homovanillic acid, or both. Treatments include surgery, radiation, and chemotherapy. Prognosis depends on the patient's age and the extent to which the disease has spread. Younger patients fare especially well. Of great interest is the fact that neuroblastoma has the highest rate of spontaneous regression of any of the malignancies that afflict humankind. *(Rudolph et al, pp 1286–1289)*

138. **(C)** The four leading causes of infant death in 1996 were (in order) congenital malformations, disorders related to short gestation, SIDS, and respiratory distress syndrome. These four accounted for more than half of all the infant deaths. SIDS rates have fallen by 38% since 1992, when recommendations were made to place infants on their backs or sides to sleep. *(Guyer et al, pp 905–918)*

139. **(E)** Because many childhood viral illnesses have seasonal presentations, the etiologic agent may be suspected on the basis of clinical and seasonal presentation. Yearly winter outbreaks of bronchiolitis and pneumonia are associated with respiratory syncytial virus. Summer outbreaks of gastroenteritis are associated with enterovirus, while winter outbreaks are associated with rotavirus. Although adenovirus can cause diarrhea, it more commonly causes respiratory symptoms. Human herpesvirus type 6 is the etiologic agent in roseola infantum. *(Oski et al, pp 1300–1302, 1309–1311, 1330–1331, 1346–1347, 1583–1586)*

140. **(B)** Chronic granulomatous disease has as its underlying defect the inability of neutrophil leukocytes and monocytes to kill some phagocytized bacteria. Affected infants may suffer recurrent infections with bacteria and fungi that rarely cause disease in normal children. These organisms include *Pseudomonas, Serratia marcescens, Klebsiella,* and *Aspergillus fumigatus. Staphylococcus aureus* is also a frequent pathogen. *(Rudolph et al, pp 1230–1231)*

141. **(B)** Penicillin remains the drug of choice for treatment of streptococcal pharyngitis. Amoxicillin, macrolides, and cephalosporins are acceptable alternatives. *(Oski et al, pp 1201–1202, 1234, 1355–1357)*

142. **(C)** Scarlet fever is caused by toxins made by group A streptococci. It is usually seen in patients with strep throat. The rash is papular and described as sandpaper-like. Sometimes it is easier to feel it than to see it. An allergic rash would be urticarial. More than 80% of patients with EBV infection develop a maculopapular rash if given amoxicillin. This patient's clinical course is not typical for EBV,

which presents more gradually, and patients often have posterior cervical adenopathy and splenomegaly. Patients with serum sickness often have urticarial rashes, sometimes progressing to angioedema. They may also have arthritis, myalgias, and lymphadenopathy. The rash in enteroviral infections is typically macular. (Rudolph et al, pp 477, 640, 930)

143. **(D)** Patients with Turner syndrome have a 45,X karyotype. The classic physical features are illustrated in this case. Patients have short stature, a webbed neck, ptosis, triangular faces, prominent brow, hypertelorism, low-set ears, and pectus excavatum. (Rudolph et al, p 1785)

144. **(C)** Turner syndrome is associated with coarctation of the aorta and aortic stenosis. Williams syndrome is associated specifically with supravalvular aortic stenosis. In Noonan syndrome, the cardiac defect most often is pulmonary valvular stenosis or an atrial septal defect. Marfan syndrome is associated with mitral valve prolapse and aortic root dilatation. Septal defects, primarily endocardial cushion defects, are the most common heart defects among children with Down syndrome. (Rudolph et al, pp 1782–1783)

145. **(C)** Marfan syndrome is a genetic disorder of connective tissue. It is transmitted in an autosomal dominant manner. Patients have tall stature and skeletal disproportion, where the arm span exceeds the height. Other important clinical features include subluxation of the ocular lens, which occurs in 50 to 80% of patients. Progressive dilatation of the aortic root and ascending aorta can lead to dissection or rupture. (Rudolph et al, pp 392–393)

146. **(E)** Marfan syndrome is associated with mitral valve prolapse and aortic root dilatation. (Rudolph et al, pp 392–393)

147. **(A)** SLE is an autoimmune disorder that affects multiple organs. The diagnosis is based on the presence of four or more major criteria. These include malar rash, oral ulcers, arthritis, and photosensitivity. This patient has all of these symptoms, as well as the systemic symptoms often seen at presentation. The disorder is predominately a disease of women, and in the pediatric population is a disease of adolescence. Chronic renal disease is an important and common cause of morbidity and mortality among patients with SLE. (Rudolph et al, pp 486–488)

148. **(D)** Noncommunicating hydrocephalus refers to blockage of cerebrospinal fluid flow within the ventricular system. Aqueductal stenosis is a common cause of congenital noncommunicating hydrocephalus. In communicating hydrocephalus, there is blockage to CSF flow outside the ventricular system or its exit foramina. Bacterial meningitis or congenital infection may produce inflammatory scarring of the arachnoid villi, disrupting the normal CSF absorptive process and thereby producing communicating hydrocephalus. Hydrocephalus secondary to excessive secretion of CSF is unusual and, when it occurs, generally is associated with a functioning choroid plexus papilloma. Arnold–Chiari malformation is a hindbrain anomaly characterized by caudal displacement of the cerebellum and brain stem. (Rudolph et al, pp 1870–1874)

149. **(C)** Anomalies associated with Arnold–Chiari malformation include meningomyelocele and other malformations in the central nervous system, but not absence of the corpus callosum. (Rudolph et al, pp 1870–1874)

150. **(A)** Ceftriaxone, a third-generation cephalosporin, is the drug of choice for therapy in gonorrhea. It is administered intramuscularly. It is not effective against *Chlamydia trachomatis* or *Mycoplasma pneumoniae*. Penicillin remains the drug of choice for the treatment of group A streptococcal disease. Cephalosporins are not effective against methicillin-resistant strains of *Staphylococcus aureus*. (Feigin and Cherry, pp 549–550, 2183–2186)

151. **(D)** Café au lait spots are discrete macular skin lesions with light brown pigmentation that usually present within the first year of life. Common "birthmarks," they often occur as an isolated finding. The presence of five or more café au lait spots should prompt

consideration of neurofibromatosis, one of the four or five neurocutaneous syndromes. Sturge–Weber and Hippel–Lindau have vascular lesions. Patients with Chediak–Higashi syndrome have oculocutaneous albinism. Marfan syndrome has no typical dermatologic manifestations. *(Rudolph et al, pp 392–393, 2044)*

152. **(C)** Kawasaki disease is an acute vasculitis of unknown etiology. Humans contract brucellosis by direct contact with infected animals or by drinking unpasteurized milk. Ehrlichosis is transmitted by ticks. Leptospiriosis is obtained from exposure to the urine of infected animals. Psittacosis is obtained from exposure to bird feces. *(American Academy of Pediatrics, pp 693–696)*

153. **(C)** *Mycoplasma pneumoniae* is the most common cause of pneumonia in school-aged children and adults in the outpatient setting. It is an uncommon cause of pneumonia among infants and young children. Common clinical findings include fever, malaise, sore throat, and cough, which develop gradually over several days. The chest roentgenogram often reveals perihilar and lower lobe infiltration. The peripheral WBC count usually is normal. Cold agglutinins are found in the serum in about 50% of cases by the end of the second week of the illness. *(American Academy of Pediatrics, pp 370–371)*

154. **(B)** Centers for Disease Control and Prevention (CDC) criteria require fever of at least 5 days' duration for a clinical diagnosis of Kawasaki disease. According to these criteria, patients also must have at least four of five other findings, including bilateral conjunctival infection, one or more changes of the oral mucous membranes (eg, pharyngeal erythema; dry, fissured, and erythematous lips; and "strawberry" tongue), one or more changes of the extremities (eg, erythema, edema, and desquamation), rash, and cervical lymphadenopathy. Kawasaki disease occurs most commonly during the first 2 years of life. Thrombocytosis, rather than thrombocytopenia, is an almost invariable feature late in the course of illness. The most common se-

rious complication of Kawasaki disease is coronary artery aneurysm formation, which can result in thrombosis, aneurysmal rupture, or other cardiac effects. *(Oski et al, pp 1422–1426)*

155. **(B)** Orbital (also referred to as postseptal) cellulitis is a medical emergency. It is a bacterial infection of the orbit. It must be distinguished from periorbital (also referred to as preseptal) cellulitis by the presence of proptosis or limitations of extraocular movements. When orbital cellulitis is suspected, cultures of blood and CSF should be obtained, appropriate antibiotics should be administered intravenously, an ophthalmologist should be consulted, and CT films should be obtained to delineate the extent of the infectious process. Both retinoblastoma and battered child syndrome may present with lid edema. Typically, these children are afebrile and nontoxic in appearance. Hyphema is hemorrhage into the anterior chamber of the eye and is caused by trauma. Twenty percent of patients with neuroblastoma present with eye symptoms from metastasis. Proptosis is one of the possible presentations and can be of relatively acute onset. In general, other systemic symptoms are present and have developed more gradually. *(Oski et al, pp 654–655, 887, 1734)*

156. **(E)** Virtually all neonates manifest a benign, self-limited elevation of unconjugated bilirubin during the first week of life. This is termed physiologic jaundice and is thought to be due to low levels of glucuronyl transferase activity. Breast milk jaundice is also unconjugated and seen in the first few weeks of life in breast-fed babies. Gilbert's disease and Crigler–Najjar syndrome are hereditary (autosomal dominant) defects in bilirubin conjugation. Both result in an indirect hyperbilirubinemia. Crigler–Najjar syndrome is associated with a complete lack of glucuronyl transferase and is often fatal. In Gilbert's disease, a partial defect in glucuronyl transferase results in mild elevations of serum indirect bilirubin levels and requires no therapy. Congenital biliary atresia typically presents in infants 3 to 6 weeks of age with per-

sistent direct hyperbilirubinemia. Persistent direct hyperbilirubinemia in a neonate constitutes a medical emergency and requires immediate evaluation. (*Oski et al, pp 427–429, 455–456*)

157. **(D)** *Pneumocystis carinii* infection in children is almost completely restricted to those with immunologic abnormalities. Such abnormalities may include congenital or acquired immunodeficiency states, such as cancer, immunosuppressive drugs, or malnutrition. Infection with HIV, as in AIDS, is one of the major settings in children in which *P carinii* infection is encountered. The manifestation of such infection often is that of a diffuse, interstitial pneumonia; reactive airway disease has not been reported. *P carinii* pneumonitis has not been shown to occur in normal children, whether or not in a daycare setting. Extrapulmonary manifestations occur uncommonly with this organism. Definitive diagnosis of *P carinii* pneumonia requires microscopic examination of lung biopsy or bronchoalveolar lavage specimens. (*Rudolph et al, pp 775–776*)

158. **(B)** *Chlamydia trachomatis* is considered an unusual cause of otitis media at any age. *Neisseria gonorrhoeae* causes conjunctivitis in the newborn. Syphilis and toxoplasmosis cause congenital infections. *E coli* is one of the neonatal pathogens that also causes otitis media in neonates. The symptoms of otitis media in newborns are often similar to those of sepsis; they are subtle and nonspecific and may include poor feeding, lethargy, vomiting, or diarrhea. Once the diagnosis is established, the initial therapy should be similar to that for neonatal sepsis, such as parenteral ampicillin and cefotaxime. Under ideal circumstances, the results of cultures obtained by tympanocentesis may then allow further treatment with a more specific antibiotic of low toxicity. Older infants may respond well to oral therapy but require frequent observation. (*Feigin and Cherry, pp 908–909*)

159. **(A)** Proptosis and limitation of extraocular motility distinguish orbital cellulitis from periorbital cellulitis. Fever, lid swelling, redness of the eye, and leukocytosis generally are present in either condition. Orbital cellulitis (infection within the orbit) may follow directly from a wound near the orbit or may result from bacteremia, but the most common source involves extension from the paranasal sinuses. The organisms most frequently implicated as pathogens are *Hemophilus influenzae*, *Staphylococcus aureus*, group A beta-hemolytic streptococci, and *Streptococcus pneumoniae*. The risk of complication is great, with extension resulting in cavernous sinus thrombosis, meningitis, or brain abscess. Prompt hospitalization and parenteral antibiotic therapy are indicated. (*Oski et al, p 857*)

160. **(A)** *H influenzae*, *S pneumoniae*, and *Moraxella catarrhalis* are the most common bacterial pathogens in otitis media of children. Amoxicillin is still the initial drug to use in uncomplicated otitis media because of its good coverage, except for beta-lactamase–positive organisms, and its excellent safety profile. The other drugs (except for erythromycin) are acceptable second-line medications. (*Oski et al, pp 974–976*)

161. **(B)** Late post-traumatic epilepsy is diagnosed when a seizure occurs for the first time more than 1 week after a head injury. Factors that correlate with an increased risk of developing post-traumatic epilepsy include presence of a depressed skull fracture, acute intracranial hemorrhage, cerebral contusion, or unconsciousness lasting more than 24 hours. Because the risk of a subsequent seizure is approximately 75%, acute and chronic treatment with anticonvulsants is indicated. Loss of consciousness, retrograde amnesia, and vomiting are relatively common immediate consequences of head trauma. They are usually transient and are not highly correlated with a risk of subsequent post-traumatic seizures. (*Rudolph et al, p 1950*)

162. **(A)** Croup and epiglottitis have similar presentations but need to be distinguished immediately. Croup usually results from a viral infection of the larynx, and epiglottitis from a bacterial (*H influenzae* type B) infection of the epiglottis. Children with epiglottitis tend to

be toxic in appearance. Croup involves the airway and epiglottitis involves the airway and the digestive tract. Children with croup usually will swallow and drink. Children with epiglottitis most often will refuse to drink and may even drool as a result of their refusal to swallow saliva. Patients with foreign bodies in their upper airways do not typically have fever. Patients with vascular rings and laryngeal tumors have more gradual onset of symptoms. *(Oski et al, pp 822–823, 981–984)*

163. **(E)** Wilms' tumor, a renal neoplasm, is second only to lymphoma as the most common intra-abdominal neoplasm in the pediatric age group. Approximately 40% of these tumors, including all bilateral tumors, are hereditary. The overall survival rate is 70 to 80%. Other neoplasms that may have a dominant inheritance pattern are pheochromocytoma, medullary carcinoma of the thyroid, and retinoblastoma. *(Rudolph et al, pp 1284–1285, 1748, 1771, 2105)*

164. **(E)** Unintentional injuries is the leading cause of death among adolescents ages 15 to 19 years, accounting for 46.3% of all deaths. The second and third most common causes of death in this population are homicide (19.6%) and suicide (16.7%). Cancer is the fourth, accounting for 4.6%. *(Guyer et al, pp 905–918)*

165. **(E)** Pregnancy is the most common cause of amenorrhea or abnormal uterine bleeding in an adolescent. Among adolescent girls aged 15 to 19 years, the annual risk of pregnancy is 10%. Through adolescence, the cumulative risk of pregnancy is nearly 40%. *(McAnarney et al, pp 659–671)*

166. **(B)** About 1 to 2% of all newborn infants delivered at term develop pneumothorax. Very high transpulmonary pressures generated during the initial breaths, in combination with obstruction of the airways by fluid, may cause the air leak syndrome. It can also be produced by excessive positive pressures applied during resuscitation in the delivery room. Some pneumothoraces can be asymp-

tomatic. When a newborn develops sudden increase in respiratory distress with retractions, poor air entry in the chest, cyanosis, irritability, hypotension, and either tachycardia or bradycardia, an air leak syndrome should always be suspected. Auscultating the chest, obtaining a chest x-ray, or transilluminating the chest with a fiberoptic light can be useful in detecting air in the chest. When pneumomediastinum is suspected, a lateral chest x-ray should always be taken; the collection of air can be seen anterior to the heart. Spontaneous pneumothorax can be asymptomatic and resolves spontaneously. If it causes severe respiratory distress, chest tube drainage may be necessary. *(Rudolph et al, pp 1611–1612)*

167. **(C)** The only recognized toxic effect of any vitamin D preparation is hypercalcemia, which may or may not be symptomatic. Symptoms may include abdominal pain, vomiting, polyuria, headaches, hypertension, and seizures. Serum phosphate remains normal. *(Norman, pp 947–971)*

168. **(C)** Minimal change nephrotic syndrome is the most common form of nephrotic syndrome. Features that favor this diagnosis include the absence of azotemia, hypertension, and hematuria. Complement levels are usually normal. Approximately 90% of patients with this diagnosis respond to steroid therapy compared to a much smaller percentage for children with nephrotic syndrome secondary to focal segmental glomerulosclerosis or membranoproliferative glomerulonephritis. *(Rudolph, pp 1366–1369)*

169. **(E)** Cyanosis in newborn infants is associated with major right-to-left shunts. Total anomalous pulmonary venous return results in a right-to-left shunting through an interatrial communication, usually a patent foramen ovale. Patent ductus arteriosus and atrial septal defect, when unaccompanied by other cardiovascular abnormalities, cause left-to-right shunt that do not produce cyanosis. Coarctation of the aorta does not typically cause symptoms in the newborn. Hypoplastic left heart presents with signs of failure in

the newborn period. *(Rudolph et al, pp 1462–1485)*

170. **(B)** Intraventricular and periventricular hemorrhages occur almost exclusively in premature infants. Current evidence suggests that vascular events, especially hypotension followed by hypertension, are a major factor in producing the hemorrhage. Many of these infants were asphyxiated at birth, and this is thought to be one predisposing factor. Although bleeding disorders certainly can predispose to intraventricular hemorrhage, the great majority of afflicted infants do not have any discernible abnormalities of hemostasis. Ultrasonography is a safe and effective way of diagnosing intraventricular hemorrhage in neonates. Lumbar puncture is avoided only if clinical signs suggest imminent brain or brain stem herniation. *(Rudolph et al, p 224)*

171. **(B)** Acetaminophen causes liver injury by forming a metabolite that exhausts the supply of glutathione by conjugating to it, thereby exposing the liver to oxidative damage from the metabolite itself and from other free radicals. Guided by a blood level timed from the estimated time of ingestion, the compound acetylcysteine (Mucomyst) must be given to restore glutathione levels. There is no clinical evidence that activated charcoal inhibits the efficacy of acetylcysteine. CNS symptoms are not characteristic of the early course of acetaminophen poisoning; should they occur, ingestion of a combination of drugs must be suspected. The early phases of acetaminophen ingestion may be deceptively asymptomatic, with the occurrence of fatal liver failure on the third to fifth day after ingestion. Of those individuals who ingest enough acetaminophen to produce blood levels in the toxic range, adults and adolescents are more likely than children to suffer hepatotoxicity. *(Ellenhorn, pp 181–187)*

172. **(A)** The case presented is classic of pyloric stenosis. This results from hypertrophy and hyperplasia of smooth muscle in the stomach causing a narrowed, even, obstructed outlet. Persistent projectile vomiting causes ongoing losses of calories and electrolytes, resulting in growth failure and hypochloremic metabolic alkalosis. Hyponatremia and hypokalemia may also be associated. Often, the diagnosis can be made by physical examination alone. However, if an olive-shaped mass is not palpated, an abdominal ultrasound may confirm the diagnosis. *(Behrman et al, pp 1060–1062)*

173. **(C)** Diaper dermatitis is a very common problem in infants. The infant's rash is due to *Candida*. *Candida* dermatitis is red, without bullae, and has satellite lesions at the margins. It is common in infants, especially when they have been on antibiotics. In bullous impetigo, the skin is initially erythematous and then bullae develop. Allergic dermatitis and irritant dermatitis are the most prominent on the convex areas and are intensely red. In seborrheic dermatitis, children tend to have the rash on the scalp, neck, and face also. It is scaly and more prominent in the intertriginous areas. *(Hurwitz, pp 27–29)*

174. **(A)** This is a typical presentation of chickenpox. A prodrome of fever and malaise is followed by the rapid eruption of papules that turn to vesicles and crust over. The rash in measles, rubella, and Kawasaki disease are macular or maculopapular. In staphylococcal scalded skin syndrome, a diffuse, tender erythroderma develops. *(Jensen et al, pp 664–665)*

175. **(E)** This is a "round pneumonia," most commonly caused by *S pneumoniae*. Onset of this disease is relatively acute. *H influenzae* type B is an uncommon cause of systemic infections because of routine immunization. *Mycoplasma* is the most common cause of community-acquired pneumonia in this age group. Patients typically have a more gradual onset of symptoms. *Pneumocystis* does not cause pneumonia in otherwise healthy children. *S aureus* can cause pneumonia in healthy children but it is not as common as *S pneumoniae* or *Mycoplasma*. *(Jensen, pp 988–992)*

176. **(A)** The child most likely has hemolytic–uremic syndrome. This illness is most common in children less than 2 years old. They present with a prodromal illness, bloody diarrhea, and then a sudden onset of lethargy

and pallor when the hemolytic anemia occurs. Coincident with this is the development of acute renal failure, often with low urine output. *E coli* 0157:H7 is the most common organism in this country. Group A streptococci are associated with poststreptococcal acute glomerulonephritis. Thrombocytopenia and anemia are not seen in this disease. (*Rudolph et al, pp 1356–1362*)

177. **(C)** Most childhood immunizations are given to prevent illnesses in childhood. The only exceptions to this are hepatitis B and rubella. Hepatitis does not cause a congenital infection. (*American Academy of Pediatrics, pp 18–49*)

178. **(D)** Progressive, symmetric motor weakness, areflexia, and autonomic instability, with mild or absent sensory signs, are typical features of Guillain-Barré syndrome. Frequently, there is a history of infection (often respiratory) in the several weeks preceding clinical onset of the syndrome. Supportive evidence for the diagnosis includes elevation of CSF protein concentration with a mild (10 or fewer cells/mL) mononuclear pleocytosis, and slowing of nerve conduction velocities. In polymyositis, deep tendon reflexes would be intact. Myasthenia gravis is characterized by weakness aggravated by repetitive movement. In transverse myelitis, sensation would also be lost. Viral encephalitis is characterized by mental status abnormalities. (*Oski et al, pp 2071–2073*)

179. **(C)** The Centers for Disease Control and Prevention (CDC) has identified lead poisoning as one of the most common and preventable childhood health problems in the United States. Recent data indicate that undesirable behavioral and cognitive deficits can occur at levels previously thought to be "safe." Screening all children ages 6 to 72 months, by questionnaire or blood lead level, is suggested. Children at greatest risk for lead poisoning include young inner-city children who live in housing constructed prior to 1960; children living near lead processing smelters, battery recycling plants, or other industry which releases lead; or children with siblings or playmates diagnosed with lead

poisoning. Eliminating the lead source is the cornerstone of treatment. Chelation therapy generally is reserved for those children with blood lead levels greater than 45 µg/dL. (*CDC, pp 51–65; Committee on Drugs, pp 155–160*)

180. **(B)** Lymphadenitis is a common finding in pediatrics. When evaluating a tender or enlarged lymph node, obtain a pointed history, then search upstream. Often, a previously unrecognized skin lesion will be helpful in making the correct diagnosis. *Streptococcus pyogenes* and *Staphylococcus aureus* singularly or simultaneously are the most common causes of skin infection and lymphadenitis in children. However, they present more acutely. The presence of an ulcerated papule and the history of tick exposure indicate this child may have the ulceroglandular form of tularemia. Tularemia, caused by *F tularensis*, is a systemic infection most often transmitted by tick or rabbit exposure. Of the six clinical syndromes caused by *F tularensis*, the ulceroglandular form is the most common and accounts for 75% of cases. The incubation period for tularemia is 3 to 21 days, which also supports this diagnosis. Though lack of parental knowledge of cat exposure makes the diagnosis of cat scratch disease (caused by *Bartonella henselae*) less likely, it by no means eliminates the diagnosis. Infection with *R rickettsii* results in a systemic illness, Rocky Mountain spotted fever, in which fever, headache, rash, and myalgias are common findings. (*Feigin and Cherry, pp 220–230, 1085–1086, 1316–1320, 1848–1853; Koehler, pp 1–27*)

181. **(C)** Aspirin and antihistamines have been shown to adversely affect platelet aggregation, leading to increased bleeding time. Moreover, this effect may persist for 7 to 10 days after discontinuing these medications. When possible, children undergoing surgery should not be receiving aspirin or antihistamines. The use of antibiotics would not be a contraindication to elective surgery. Children undergoing elective surgery should be free of respiratory infection. It is prudent to counsel the parents in ways to minimize infection, but avoiding social contacts and shared eating utensils would likely have little effect in

the case described in the question. A child should be free of anemia before elective surgery, but eating iron-rich foods would not significantly elevate Hb in a short period of time. *(Rudolph et al, pp 1244–1245; Champion et al, pp 653–656)*

182. **(C)** The most common causes of hypertension in young children are renal in origin. Polycystic kidney disease, congenital vascular anomalies, tumors, and infections all are causes. Urologic evaluation is imperative for the child described in the question. Theophylline toxicity that is severe enough to significantly elevate BP would be unlikely in the absence of jitteriness, nausea, or tachycardia. Chronic lung disease would not elevate the systemic BP in an otherwise healthy child. Coarctation of the aorta is a less common cause of hypertension in this age group. BPs taken on all extremities would be helpful in the diagnosis. *(Rudolph et al, pp 1543–1547)*

183. **(D)** This case most likely represents an adolescent with meningitis who has developed increased intracranial pressure. Intubation and hyperventilation is indicated immediately. Hyperventilation is the most appropriate immediate, nonsurgical treatment of intracranial hypertension. By hyperventilating this patient, you will decrease the P_{CO_2}, resulting in vasoconstriction in the central nervous system. Decreasing the P_{CO_2} 5 to 10 mm Hg will decrease intracranial pressure 25 to 30%. Administering antibiotics, preferably after blood cultures are obtained, is appropriate. Obtaining a CT scan of the head may reveal intracranial lesions, which require additional therapy. Mannitol given intravenously also is a highly effective means for lowering intracranial pressure. Mannitol does not cross the blood–brain barrier. It remains in the capillaries and creates an osmotic gradient, causing fluid to shift from intracellular spaces to the vasculature, thereby decreasing intracranial pressure. Although a lumbar puncture may be necessary eventually, it is contraindicated as initial management because of the possibility of brain stem herniation. *(Oski et al, pp 1125–1132, 2042–2043)*

184. **(D)** The presence of a congenital membranous or bony septum between the nose and pharynx is called choanal atresia. Most newborns are obligatory nose breathers and breathe effectively only through their noses. Therefore, if choanal obstruction is unilateral, breathing difficulty may not occur until the first respiratory infection. On the other hand, those newborns with bilateral atresia who are also obligatory nose breathers will make vigorous attempts to inspire with sucking in of their lips, or may promptly become apneic and cyanotic, requiring resuscitation. Those who are able to mouth breathe may have difficulty when feeding or manifest persistent mouth breathing and cyanosis that is relieved by crying. Treatment consists of surgical correction. *(Rudolph et al, pp 214, 1580–1581)*

185. **(D)** In most instances of mild head trauma, skull films are not useful or indicated. Mild head trauma has a low likelihood of producing a skull fracture. If such a fracture is found, no specific treatment is indicated unless the fracture is basilar in location or is depressed, in which case additional special views are needed. The trauma that requires actual treatment is injury to blood vessels or to brain tissue itself. This is usually diagnosed on the basis of a history of abnormal neurologic status (unconsciousness or seizures) or abnormalities found on neurologic examination. Should any of these be present, a CT scan, rather than skull x-rays, is more likely to show an abnormality and is therefore the preferred study. In an individual who has no abnormality by history or on physical examination, an intracranial bleed or severe brain injury is not likely; if present, it would be expected to produce symptoms within several hours of the injury. Thus, it makes sense to instruct parents to check for specific neurologic findings such as vomiting, seizures, somnolence, severe headaches, or anisocoria. *(Tecklenburg and Wright, pp 40–47)*

186. **(E)** Although serious toxic symptoms from theophylline are rare at levels of less than 40 mg/mL, they can occur. Adolescents sometimes ingest long-acting preparations, which may produce continued absorption and ris-

ing levels for as long as 16 to 24 hours. Repeated blood levels should be checked until a decrease is demonstrated. Adolescents making suicidal gestures frequently ingest whatever they find in the medicine cabinet. Thus, checking for the presence of other toxic compounds in the blood is always wise. Finally, treatment should include aggressive emptying of the gastrointestinal tract. Activated charcoal has been shown to enhance body clearance of theophylline and should be used in anyone who has taken a significant overdose. Indications for hemoperfusion include intractable seizures, persistent hypoperfusion unresponsive to fluids and vasopressors, uncontrollable dysrhythmias, and levels exceeding 100 μg/mL. (Ellenhorn et al, pp 828–834)

187. **(D)** Children with sickle cell disease develop functional asplenia, presumably from repeated splenic infarction. This results in vulnerability to bacteremia and overwhelming infection, especially with encapsulated bacteria. The organism most commonly involved is *Streptococcus pneumoniae*. Daily prophylactic oral penicillin is indicated for young children. Because of the risk of bacteremia, these patients need careful medical evaluation when they develop fever. There are no data to support the use of gamma globulin in these children. They are not at higher risk for complications from live virus vaccines or from varicella. (Rudolph et al, pp 1203–1207)

188. **(C)** In most states, a person attains the age of maturity at 18 years of age and then has the right to give consent to medical treatment. State laws give adolescents the power to consent to some medical treatment, including diagnosis and treatment of sexually transmitted diseases, pregnancy, psychiatric care, and substance abuse treatment. Absence from home during camp or boarding school does not confer an emancipated status, and parents retain both control over and responsibility for the medical care of such youngsters if they are younger than 18 years. (Traugott and Alpers, pp 922–927)

189. **(E)** Although a patient's records reflect almost perfect control of blood sugar, this may

not be the case. If the child is snacking during the day, there may be periods of hyperglycemia between the times of testing. Additionally, adolescent patients are notorious for problems of compliance. A perfect daily log always should make the physician suspicious of fabrication and noncompliance. Measurement of glycosylated Hb (Hb A$_1$C) in the blood provides a measure of the mean blood glucose concentration through the life span of the circulating RBCs, which is approximately 2 months. This test is based on the fact that glucose attaches to the Hb molecule in a nonreversible manner. Therefore, the percentage of glycosylated Hb is proportionate to the mean blood glucose concentration over a period of time. This test is extremely helpful in evaluating long-term control and probably is indicated routinely in the management of patients with insulin-dependent diabetes. It certainly would be indicated in the patient described in the question. (Nathan et al, 341–346; Oski et al, pp 1981–1986)

190. **(D)** The child described in the question appears to have had a simple febrile seizure. Febrile seizures almost always are benign and carry an excellent prognosis. This is especially true of those that are classified as simple—lasting less than 20 minutes and without focal features. Although the risk of a second seizure during this febrile illness is small, attempts to reduce body temperature are appropriate. Acetaminophen and ibuprofen are preferable to aspirin for many reasons, not the least of which is the possible association of aspirin with Reye syndrome. Additionally, sponging is generally not effective and, if undertaken, it should be done with lukewarm water rather than ice water, and alcohol should not be used. Inhalation of alcohol vapor has led to neurologic depression and coma. Continuous prophylaxis with phenobarbital or phenytoin is not indicated for simple febrile seizures. An EEG is not necessary. Reassurance about a good outcome is appropriate, as are instructions regarding the proper way to take the child's temperature and the proper dosage of acetaminophen or ibuprofen for fever. (Lorin, pp 153–180)

191. **(C)** Hypocalcemia is not a cause of constipation. On the contrary, it increases irritability of nerve cells and may result in diarrhea. Hypothyroidism, lead poisoning, and Hirschsprung's disease all may be associated with constipation. Congenital hypothyroidism and Hirschsprung's disease (a congenital disorder characterized by regional absence of ganglion cells from the myenteric plexus of the colon) present at birth. Lead poisoning is more common after the child becomes mobile. Functional constipation is the most common cause of constipation at this age. It is usually due to dietary factors. *(Oski et al, p 1845)*

192. **(D)** Iron deficiency anemia is the most common hematologic disorder in infancy. Heralded by a microcytic hypochromic anemia, it usually is precipitated by inadequate iron intake. Excessive intake of iron-poor foods such as whole milk, along with inadequate intake of iron-fortified foods such as cereal, can result in the clinical picture described. This is reflected in a decrease in the serum iron. The body attempts to compensate by producing more transferrin, the protein that binds serum iron. The level of serum ferritin, the iron-binding protein of tissues, provides a relatively accurate estimate of the body's iron stores. Free erythrocyte protoporphyrins are precursors of hemoglobin and are increased because hemoglobin synthesis is rate-limited by a deficiency of iron. Decreased amounts of hemoglobin per RBC result in small cells (microcytes). Other common causes of hypochromic microcytic anemia in childhood include lead poisoning and thalassemia. *(Rudolph et al, pp 1176–1180)*

193. **(E)** The characteristics of fetal alcohol syndrome include (1) persistent deficient growth affecting weight, height, and head circumference and beginning in utero; (2) facial abnormalities such as micrognathia, short palpebral fissures, and a thin upper lip; (3) cardiac abnormalities, commonly septal defects; (4) minor limb abnormalities with some restriction of mobility and some alteration in palmar crease patterns; and (5) mental deficiency ranging from mild to severe. There is a decided relationship between the extent of abnormalities and the degree of mental retardation. Affected infants may present with hypoglycemia and alcohol withdrawal symptoms, which may last for 48 to 72 hours. Immediate management of these infants consists of correction of the hypoglycemia. Ongoing monitoring of the child's development is essential. Prevention by restriction of alcohol consumption during pregnancy is advised. *(Rudolph et al, pp 419–420)*

194. **(D)** Meningococcemia is a fulminant systemic rapidly progressing infection that results in shock and is followed by death in 20% of afflicted children. The presence of meningitis has been shown to increase the survival rate to approximately 95%. Sensorineural deafness is the most common residual following bacterial meningitis. Penicillin, ampicillin, or a third-generation cephalosporin would be an appropriate antibiotic to choose for treatment. Vancomycin's spectrum of activity is limited to gram-positive organisms. *(Oski et al, pp 1199–1203; American Academy of Pediatrics, p 360)*

195. **(D)** In the management of foreign body aspiration, it is generally felt that if the victim can speak, breathe, or cough, all interventions are unnecessary and potentially dangerous. When intervention is required, the first maneuver is a series of abdominal thrusts (for children > 1 year of age) or back blows (for children 1 year of age or younger). When obstruction persists, foreign bodies sometimes can be removed from the oral cavity or pharynx if they can be seen, but blind fingersweeps of the hypopharynx are not recommended. Emergency tracheostomy, preferably performed by an experienced clinician, is employed only in cases of critical airway obstruction unrelieved by other maneuvers. *(Oski et al, p 643)*

196. **(D)** Adducted great toe, metatarsus adductus, medial tibial torsion, and femoral anteversion can result in intoeing. In most cases, this is a benign condition that requires only observation. In this child, because the child's knees are straight, the rotational deformity is below this joint. In metatarsus adductus, the forefoot is adducted compared to the hindfoot. Idiopathic avascular juvenile necrosis of the femoral head, or Legg–Calvé–Perthes disease, most commonly is seen in 4- to 8-year-old boys. Loss of hip medial rotation is an early sign. *(Berkowitz, pp 300–305)*

197. (C) Idiopathic scoliosis is the most common back deformity in children. The incidence peaks in early adolescence and is much more common in girls. Screening for scoliosis should be part of every well check and sports physical in children at Tanner (II–V) stages. Congenital scoliosis is caused by failure of formation or fusion of the ossific nuclei of the vertebrae. It can present at any age, depending on the degree of curvature, and is much less common than idiopathic scoliosis. Patients with leg length inequality present with limp. Patients with Scheuermann kyphosis usually present with back pain and have a sharp kyphotic angulation with forward bending. Postural roundback is an exaggerated kyphotic appearance often seen in adolescents. *(Rudolph et al, pp 2149–2156)*

198. (C) Whooping cough, or pertussis, tends to have a prolonged course, with a 2-week prodrome of undifferentiated upper respiratory infection followed by approximately 2 weeks of a paroxysmal, machine gun–like cough and nasopharyngeal mucus that is strangling, thick, and clear. The typical whoop, a stridorous inspiratory gasp at the end of each paroxysm, is often absent in infants younger than 6 months. Post-tussive vomiting more likely will be found in this age group. The diagnosis should be suspected in children with a paroxysmal, harsh cough and absolute lymphocytosis. Specific inquiry into the history of a severe or long-lasting cough in adult caretakers should be sought. The diagnosis is made by culture of the organism (*Bordetella pertussis*) or by an immunofluorescent study of throat swab material. Erythromycin is the drug of choice. It has little effect on the illness course after paroxysms are established and is used primarily to limit spread of infection to others. *(American Academy of Pediatrics, pp 394–396)*

199. (B) Amoxicillin–clavulanic acid is active against the major pathogens of acute sinusitis in children: *Streptococcus pneumoniae, Moraxella catarrhalis,* and nontypeable *Hemophilus influenzae.* Both *M catarrhalis* and *H influenzae* may produce beta-lactamase. The fixed combination of amoxicillin and potassium clavulanate (a beta-lactamase inhibitor) is active against most beta-lactamase–producing isolates of *M catarrhalis* and *H influenzae.* Ciprofloxacin, a quinolone antibiotic, is not recommended for routine use in children. The quinolones have been found to damage growing cartilage in some immature animals. Cephalexin (a first-generation cephalosporin), penicillin V, and dicloxacillin (an antistaphylococcal penicillin) lack useful activity against *M catarrhalis* and *H influenzae.* *(Oski et al, pp 951–957)*

200. (D) Turner syndrome (usually 45,XO karyotype) occurs in 1 of 3000 live births. The hallmark of this genetic disease is gonadal dysgenesis. Though sexual maturation usually does not occur, a girl with Turner syndrome occasionally will have menstrual periods but rarely will be fertile. Treatment may include estrogen replacement or growth hormone utilization. Psychosocial support is extremely important. *(Oski et al, pp 779–782, 2198–2199)*

201. (E) The child described in the question appears to be afflicted with infant botulism. *Clostridium botulinum* spores are commonly found in honey, and the toxin responsible for the symptoms described is produced in the infant gastrointestinal tract. Children younger than 1 year should therefore not be fed honey. Hypernatremic dehydration may show some similarities to infant botulism, but the skin and mucous membranes are characteristically dry. Serum sodium level is often greater than 160. Hirschsprung's disease would explain constipation but not the other findings listed. Congenital hypothyroidism shows a more insidious onset, with prolonged constipation and weakness. In addition, developmental retardation would likely be present. *(Rudolph et al, pp 555–558)*

202. **(C)** Though vaccines against meningococcal and pneumococcal disease are available, they currently are recommended only for certain high-risk groups. A vaccine against respiratory syncytial viral disease currently is not licensed. The *H influenzae* conjugate vaccines are recommended for universal use in infancy and childhood. They are effective in inducing protective antibody responses for the type B strains, which cause meningitis, sepsis, and other infectious syndromes. However, the vaccine is not effective in preventing otitis media which is most often due to unencapsulated nontypeable *H influenzae*. (*American Academy of Pediatrics, pp 15–71*)

203. **(C)** Infectious mononucleosis may affect children of all ages. The rapid slide (Monospot) test response is positive in approximately 90% of infected persons; however, younger children with mononucleosis may have a negative result. Moreover, many younger children have poor antibody response to the heterophil titer test. The specific serodiagnostic test for EBV, the agent responsible for most cases of infectious mononucleosis, confirms the diagnosis. A repeat throat culture, even if positive for beta-hemolytic streptococcus, may be of only partial value since both infectious mononucleosis and streptococcal pharyngitis may be present simultaneously. Bone marrow examinations potentially are painful and contribute little to the correct diagnosis. (*Oski et al, pp 1204–1207*)

204. **(B)** Organophosphate poisoning is a leading cause of fatal ingestions of nonpharmaceutical compounds. Common components of insecticides, organophosphates are readily absorbed across skin and mucous membranes. They bind irreversibly to cholinesterase, which results in prolongation of the effects of acetylcholine, centrally and peripherally. Symptoms include muscle fasciculations, paralysis (nicotinic effect) and miosis, salivation, diarrhea, bradycardia, lacrimation (muscarinic effect) and obtundation, seizures, or apnea (central effect). Acetaminophen ingestion can present with vomiting and then later signs of liver failure if it is severe enough. Patients with salicylate overdose

present with hypoglycemia, respiratory alkalosis followed by metabolic acidosis, hypokalemia, and mental status changes. Tricyclic antidepressants poisoning causes arrhythmias, mental status changes, and anticholinergic symptoms. Patients with acute vitamin A toxicity have mental status changes, nausea, and vomiting. (*Ellenhorn, pp 184, 210–219, 622, 1021, 1615*)

205. **(E)** Nursemaid's elbow, or subluxation of the radial head, occurs in children following longitudinal traction on a pronated extended elbow. When attempting to restrain a child, an uninformed caretaker may jerk on a child's upper extremity. The result is a painful subluxed elbow which is easily reduced by simultaneous flexion and supination of the forearm. (*Oski et al, p 1037*)

206. **(E)** Nontuberculous lymphadenitis (atypical mycobacteria) is characterized by nontender lymphadenitis. Affected persons are usually afebrile, and the CBC is usually normal. Unlike tuberculous lymphadenitis, a history of contact with a tuberculous individual is lacking, and the reaction to 5 tuberculin units of purified protein derivative is almost always less than 10 mm of induration. Cat scratch fever is characterized by tender, fluctuating nodes and low-grade fever. Acute lymphadenitis is characterized by tender nodes that may fluctuate. The WBC count is often elevated, and there is frequently a shift to the left on the differential. In addition, the sufferer is often febrile. Acute lymphoblastic leukemia may present as lymphadenitis, but the CBC is usually abnormal, with blasts present on the peripheral smear. (*Feigin and Cherry, pp 220–230, 1085–1086, 1354–1356*)

207. **(D)** Vesicoureteral reflux is the most common anatomic abnormality associated with recurrent urinary tract infection in children. Many cases of reflux are the result of an inadequate length of submucosal ureter immediately proximal to its opening into the bladder lumen, a condition that sometimes requires surgical correction. However, in other children, reflux often appears to result from the direct effects of infection on ureteral tone and peristalsis. Thus, many children may outgrow mild degrees of reflux if they are maintained on prophylactic antibiotics. Moderate to severe degrees of reflux frequently require surgery. Failure of adequate antibiotic treatment to prevent infection is also a prime indication for surgery. Repeating an IVP or performing a renal arteriogram on an already diagnosed case would not be useful, although a radionuclide scan may be very helpful to determine the present degree of reflux with a minimum of radiation exposure. Vitamin C, although reportedly useful in acidifying the urine to help prevent infection, does not enhance adequate antibiotic prophylaxis. IV antibiotics would be necessary only if oral antibiotics were not successful in eradicating infection. (*Rudolph et al, pp 1398–1399*)

208. **(B)** Infants and children are especially sensitive to phenothiazines. Extrapyramidal signs (spasmodic torticollis, hyperirritability, tremors, dysphagia, opisthotonus, etc) may occur after relatively small doses. Higher doses may result in hypotension, seizures, coma, and death. Diphenhydramine reverses only the extrapyramidal signs. Diazepam would be indicated only if the patient develops seizures. Naloxone is used to reverse the effects of opiates. Epinephrine is used for anaphylactic reactions. (*Ellenhorn, pp 89–92*)

209. **(A)** Children with more severe cases of hypospadias have an increased incidence of concomitant urinary tract anomalies and require careful evaluation. Ultrasonography is a safe and noninvasive procedure that is sensitive in the diagnosis of neonatal urinary tract pathology. It is a better choice than either IVP or cystography, which use contrast media and radiation. Serum creatinine determinations are a measure of renal function and are unnecessary in an otherwise healthy child. Circumcision is not indicated in children with hypospadias. In fact, it may be contraindicated in cases of second- or third-degree hypospadias, in which the prepuce can be used to construct an absent distal segment of urethra. (*Rudolph et al, pp 1403*)

210. **(E)** Transplacental passage of *T pallidum* causes widespread disease in the fetus. Organs most severely affected include brain, bone, liver, and lung. Hepatosplenomegaly, rare in neonates with GBS or HSV infections, occurs in 90% of neonates with congenital syphilis. Mucocutaneous lesions produce a persistent, purulent, often bloody nasal discharge which is termed *snuffles*. This nasal discharge is highly infectious. Skin rash is uncommon in CMV and GBS infections. The acral distribution described is characteristic of congenital syphilis. Congenital toxoplasmosis characteristically presents with neurologic abnormalities. The classic triad includes hydrocephalus, chorioretinitis, and diffuse intracranial calcifications. (*Oski et al, pp 540–551, 1240–1243*)

211. **(C)** Roseola infantum, or sixth disease, is a common acute illness of young children. Human herpesvirus-6 is the most common etiologic agent. The rash of erythema infectiosum presents initially on the face. It is intensely red with a "slapped-cheek" appearance. Rubella and measles are not commonly seen because of routine vaccination. The rash of scarlet fever is on the trunk and is described as sandpaper-like. (*Feigin and Cherry, pp 1789–1791*)

212. **(A)** Virtually all neonates manifest a benign, self-limited elevation of bilirubin during the first week of life. This is termed physiologic jaundice, and is thought to be due to low levels of glucuronyl transferase activity. Gilbert's disease and Crigler–Najjar syndrome are hereditary (autosomal dominant) defects in bilirubin conjugation. Both result in an indirect hyperbilirubinemia. In Crigler–Najjar syndrome, bilirubin levels are usually above 10 mg/dL. Gilbert's disease usually manifests itself at an older age. Congenital biliary atresia typically presents in infants 3 to 6 weeks of age with persistent direct hyperbilirubinemia. Breast milk jaundice occurs in 10 to 30% of breast-fed infants. It presents as prolonged, unconjugated hyperbilirubinemia in the first few weeks/months of life. (*Rudolph et al, pp 1134–1135; Gartner, pp 422–432*)

213. (D) The simultaneous occurrence of similar symptoms in several family members suggests a point source of illness. Diarrhea produced by the exotoxin of *S aureus* often occurs within a few hours after ingestion of contaminated ham, poultry, or eggs. It is characterized by vomiting, abdominal cramps, and diarrhea. Although diarrhea caused by *C difficile* exotoxin is not rare, it generally is associated with the use of antibiotics and is not considered a cause of diarrhea de novo. *Campylobacter* and *Clostridium botulinum* both can produce vomiting and diarrhea, but the incubation is considerably longer than the several hours described in the case scenario. Pinworms do not cause diarrhea. *(Rakel, pp 60–62)*

214. (B) By the end of the sixth month of life, normal infants will develop clear preferences for social contact with the persons giving them the most care. By the ages of 6 to 8 months, most normal infants will display anxiety when persons outside their circle of caretakers approach them. *(Behrman, pp 20–21)*

215. (D) Silver nitrate, the traditional prophylactic treatment for the neonate's eyes, is very effective against gonorrheal ophthalmitis. These drops are not effective against the most common cause of neonatal conjunctivitis, *Chlamydia trachomatis*, which requires erythromycin or tetracycline for eradication. Silver nitrate is commonly associated with the sterile purulent discharge of chemical conjunctivitis. Herpes simplex virus can cause neonatal conjunctivitis, but its occurrence on the first day of life would be unusual. *Pseudomonas* conjunctivitis generally is hospital acquired, occurring in ill infants receiving mechanical ventilation. Nasolacrimal duct obstruction is a transient structural anomaly that may be accompanied by persistent tearing and occasional purulent discharge. The condition is usually unilateral and clears within 6 to 9 months after birth. Rarely, duct probing or surgery is necessary because of persistent stenosis beyond 1 year of age or for repeated infections. *(Oski et al, p 812)*

216. (A) Nontypeable *H influenzae, S pneumoniae,* and *Moraxella catarrhalis* are the most common bacterial pathogens in otitis media of children. *S aureus, E coli,* and group A streptococci each account for 2% or less of all cases of otitis media in children beyond the neonatal period. *Mycoplasma* is thought to be an uncommon cause of otitis media. *(Oski et al, pp 974–976)*

217. (D) A seizure equivalent such as abdominal epilepsy presenting solely with abdominal pain is most unusual. Recurrent headache and abdominal pain with no relationship to meals or time of day are the norm. An EEG is not always helpful in making this diagnosis, because 14 and 16/sec positive spikes may occur in apparently normal children. Pinworms are an unusual cause of abdominal pain, especially in the morning after meals. There seems to be no relationship between the presence of abdominal pain in children and whether or not they have pinworm infestation. Peptic ulcer disease in children may present in subtle ways, and vague abdominal pain, often relieved by meals, is common. Other signs such as weight loss, vomiting, pallor and other signs of anemia, and gastrointestinal (GI) hemorrhage are clues to the diagnosis. Stool examination for occult blood and endoscopy are useful diagnostic tools, particularly because upper GI x-ray studies may show no abnormalities in 25% of children with duodenal ulcers. Crohn's disease may produce lower abdominal pain, sometimes in association with recurrent fevers, impaired linear growth, weight loss, or diarrhea. Lactose intolerance, causing vague recurrent abdominal pain and gas, is a common problem. Children with a relative deficiency of the enzyme lactase are especially likely to have symptoms after consuming quantities of yogurt and milk. The lactose hydrogen breath test confirms the diagnosis. Lactose-free diets almost totally alleviate symptoms. *(Rudolph et al, pp 1031–1034)*

218. (E) Most cases of idiopathic thrombocytopenic purpura (ITP) in children are preceded by viral infections and, in contrast to adults, the great majority of children recover spontaneously. Although not all patients require therapy, most authorities suggest treating when the platelet count is less than 20,000. Standard treatment has been oral prednisone. Recently, IV gamma globulin has been shown to be effective. However, this agent is expensive and less convenient than oral prednisone. The child described in the question might reasonably be treated with either agent. Because the child's Hb is 13.3 g/100 mL, there is no indication for transfusion of RBCs. Although the platelet count is very low, platelet transfusions are short lived and generally are indicated only in the presence of serious bleeding, as, for example, from the GI tract. Thus, platelet transfusions are not indicated in this patient. Splenectomy is reserved for the very rare child who does not respond to conservative therapy or who develops chronic ITP. *(Rudolph et al, pp 1241–1242, Kliegman, pp 841–848)*

219. **(D)** Intussusception, or telescoping of the bowel into a more distal section of bowel, is the most common cause of intestinal obstruction in infants aged 3 to 12 months. The case presented represents the classic presentation. Giardiasis presents less acutely and would not be associated with a mass. In gastroenteritis, frequent loose stools without blood would be the major symptom. Diaphragmatic hernia occurs in newborns and the major symptom is respiratory distress. Although appendicitis can occur in infants, it is very unusual. *(Oski et al, pp 1856–1858)*

220. **(C)** Sexually transmitted diseases occur in 5 to 20% of sexually abused children. Like adults, children with one sexually transmitted disease frequently have a second. *Chlamydia trachomatis*, the most commonly isolated sexually transmitted agent, likely is the cause of this child's symptoms. Though both erythromycin and tetracycline are effective therapeutic antimicrobials, erythromycin is the drug of choice because of the age of this patient. Tetracyclines are deposited in growing bones and teeth. This may result in depression of linear bone growth and dental staining. This effect is dose related and extends up to 8 years of age. *(Oski et al, pp 788, 864)*

221. **(A)** Patients with persistent otitis media after 5 days of amoxicillin likely have resistant *Streptococcus pneumonia*, or a beta-lactamase positive *Moraxella catarrhalis* or *Haemophilus influenzae*. Cephalexin, erythromycin, dicloxacillin, and penicillin would not cover the beta-lactamase positive organisms. Some would recommend that the patient would benefit from a higher dose of the amoxicillin component in the combination antibiotic to provide better coverage for resistant *Streptococcus pneumoniae*. *(Behrman, p 1816)*

222. **(A)** Constitutional delay is a normal pattern of growth, characterized by a relatively late pubertal growth spurt. It is recognized most commonly in boys. Patients typically show a moderate degree of short stature in early to middle childhood. The growth pattern is often similar to one or both parents. Final adult height is within the expected genetic potential. The children are otherwise well. Familial short stature is also a normal growth pattern in a short but otherwise normal family. One or both parents are typically 1 to 2 standard deviations below mean height for adults. The growth pattern parallels the normal growth curve at a percentile consistent with genetic potential. Deprivational dwarfism is due to psychosocial factors. It typically presents at a younger age, and weight is affected more than the height so that these children are not proportionately small. Hypothyroidism can affect growth but would cause a decrease in growth velocity when it occurred. The patient's height curve would flatten out, instead of paralleling the normal curves. Short stature from growth hormone deficiency typically presents by 3 years. *(Kliegman, pp 1023–1034)*

223. **(E)** Given that this is a classic case of constitutional growth delay, no diagnostic studies are indicated. Close monitoring of growth would be indicated. A bone age, if performed, would be less than chronologic age, demonstrating the growth potential for the patient. Cranial imaging would be indicated if the patient had evidence for onset of secondary hypopituitarism. *(Kliegman, pp 1023–1034)*

224. (B) Chest pain in adolescents is a common problem. It is rarely associated with serious illness. In this patient, with onset with exercise, resolution with rest, and a family history of asthma, exercise-induced asthma is the most likely cause. Angina is a rare cause of chest pain in adolescents, and with a normal cardiac exam and no family history of cardiac disease, this is unlikely. Costochondritis is a common cause of chest pain but typically has an insidious onset and does not resolve with rest. Esophagitis is a common cause of chest pain but is typically impacted by eating, not exercise. Mitral valve prolapse can cause chest pain, although most pediatric patients with mitral valve prolapse are asymptomatic. On exam, they often have a systolic click. *(Kliegman, pp 183–193)*

225. (E) In a patient with symptoms and signs consistent with exercise-induced asthma, a therapeutic trial of inhaled albuterol is the first line of therapy and diagnosis. If there is evidence of cardiac disease on history or physical exam, then one should proceed with the indicated tests. Pulmonary function tests could be used to confirm the diagnosis and are used in cases in which the diagnosis is uncertain or if patients fail the therapeutic trial. *(Kliegman, pp 183–193)*

226. (A) According to the 1997 immunization schedule, this patient should receive the second dose of DTaP, HIB, and IPV. A low-grade fever and rhinorrhea is not a contraindication to any of these immunizations. *(American Academy of Pediatrics, pp 18–19, 404–407, 583)*

227. (E) The contraindications to this vaccination are an immediate anaphylactic reaction to the vaccine and onset of encephalopathy unexplained by another cause within 7 days of administration. Children with a progressive neurologic disorder characterized by developmental delay or neurologic findings, including those known to have or suspected of having a condition that predisposes to seizures, such as tuberous sclerosis, should not receive any pertussis immunizations. Premature infants should receive their vaccines according to the usual schedule. Infants with HIV should not receive OPV or varicella vaccine. *(American Academy of Pediatrics, pp 18–19, 404–407, 583)*

228. (B) Kawasaki disease is an acute febrile illness of unknown etiology that typically affects young children, usually those less than 5 years of age. There are six clinical criteria used for diagnosing this disease. The presence of 5 days or more of fever, in addition to four of the five additional criteria, establishes the diagnosis. The five additional criteria are bilateral bulbar nonexudative conjunctivitis, rash, hand and foot changes (edema followed by desquamation), oral changes such as strawberry tongue and erythema, and cervical lymphadenopathy. Erythema infectiosum presents with a prodrome of malaise and myalgia and then with local erythema of the cheeks (slapped cheeks). Rubella and rubeola are unusual because of the MMR vaccination. Rubeola presents with the 3 "Cs"—cough, coryza, and conjunctivitis—followed by the oral inflammation and the pathognomonic Koplik spots, rash, and fever. Rubella is typically a mild disease characterized by low-grade fever and a maculopapular rash. Rheumatic fever is also unusual. It tends to present in children over 3 years of age after an infection with group A streptococci, with transient migratory arthritis, carditis, chorea, rash, and nodules. Diagnosis is made according to the Jones criteria. *(Kliegman et al, pp 749, 936–944)*

229. (B) Osgood–Schlatter results from microfractures and inflammation of the tibial tubercle where the patellar tendon inserts. It is most commonly seen in young adolescents who are involved in athletics. Legg–Calvé–Perthes disease is idiopathic avascular necrosis of the capital femoral epiphysis and presents between the ages of 2 and 12 with a painless limp. Patellar subluxation is usually due to a congenital deficiency within the patellofemoral joint. On exam, these patients have tenderness over the inferior surface of the patella and terminal subluxation of the patella when the knee is fully extended. Popliteal cysts are usually asymptomatic and present with a fluid-filled mass in the popliteal fossa. The symptoms of slipped capital femoral epiphysis are variable but typically involve hip pain and limp. On exam, patients have limitation of motion in the hip. It is most common in obese adolescents. *(Behrman et al, pp 1936–1942)*

230–234. (230-K, 231-J, 232-B, 233-H, 234-O) Transposition of the great arteries is the most common cause of cyanotic heart disease in the neonate. Cyanosis usually appears in the first day of life. Cardiac findings are often otherwise normal, although patients may have a single S_2. The classic chest x-ray shows a normal heart size with a narrow mediastinum (egg on a string). Other causes of cyanotic congenital heart disease are tetralogy of Fallot and truncus arteriosus. The chest x-ray in truncus arteriosus shows increased pulmonary flow and in tetralogy of Fallot decreased pulmonary flow. Murmurs are commonly heard in children with normal hearts. This is particularly true in young children with relatively thin chest walls where the normal flow murmurs arising from the pulmonary and aortic roots are easily heard on the anterior chest. To label a murmur as normal, patients should be free of any cardiac symptoms. The rest of the cardiovascular exam should also be normal. One of the typical flow murmurs in young children is the Still's murmur. The murmur is musical or vibratory. It is a systolic ejection murmur and is usually heard best at the left lower sternal border. Atrial septal defect is one of the common congenital heart lesions with a left-to-right shunt. Patients are usually asymptomatic, and the problem is usually diagnosed when the murmur is detected. Murmurs are due to increased flow across normal valves. The systolic murmur is due to increased flow across the right ventricular outflow tract. The widely split second heart sound is due to the increased right ventricular diastolic volume and a prolonged ejection time across the pulmonary valve. Peripheral pulmonic stenosis is an ejection murmur heard best at the upper sternal border with transmission to the axilla and the back. It is caused by the sharp angle between the main pulmonary artery and its branches. It is heard in infants only and should disappear by 6 months of age. Ventricular septal defects are the most common congenital heart lesions. The most important characteristic about the murmur is that it begins early in systole, often obscuring S_1. Depending on the size of the defect, the murmur will be longer or shorter. Atrioventricular canal detected after the newborn period can present with a similar sounding murmur. It is much less common than a ventricular septal defect but would be a strong possibility if the patient had Down syndrome. *(Kliegman et al, pp 204–209, 221–227)*

REFERENCES

American Academy of Pediatrics. *Report of the Committee on Infectious Diseases,* 24th ed. Evanston: American Academy of Pediatrics; 1997.

Bar-Or O. *Pediatric Sports Medicine for the Practitioner,* 1st ed. New York: Springer-Verlag; 1983.

Behrman RE, Miegman RM, Arvin AM. *Nelson Textbook of Pediatrics,* 15th ed. Philadelphia: WB Saunders; 1996.

Berkowitz CD. *Pediatrics: A Primary Care Approach.* Philadelphia: WB Saunders; 1996.

Centers for Disease Control. *Preventing Lead Poisoning in Young Children.* October 1991.

Champion LAA, Schwartz AD, Luddy RE, Schindler S. The effects of four commonly used drugs on platelet function. *J Pediatr* 1976;89: 653–656.

Committee on Drugs. Treatment guidelines for lead exposure in children. *Pediatrics* 1995;96: 155–160.

DeArce MA, Kearns A. The fragile X syndrome: the patients and their chromosomes. *J Med Genet* 1984;21:84–91.

Ellenhorn MJ. *Ellenhorn's Medical Toxicology: Diagnosis and Treatment of Human Poisoning,* 2nd ed. Baltimore: Williams & Wilkins; 1997.

Feigin RD, Cherry JD. *Textbook of Pediatric Infectious Diseases,* 3rd ed. Philadelphia: WB Saunders; 1992.

Gartner LM. Neonatal jaundice. *Pediatr Rev* 1994; 15:422–432.

Guyer B, Martin J, MacDorman M, Anderson R,

Strobino D. Annual Summary of Vital Statistics—1996. *Pediatrics* 1997;100:905–918.

Hurwitz S. *Clinical Pediatric Dermatology: A Textbook of Skin Disorders of Childhood and Adolescence.* Philadelphia: WB Saunders; 1981.

Jenson HB, Baltimore RS. *Pediatric Infectious Diseases: Principles and Practice,* 1st ed. Stamford, CT: Appleton & Lange; 1995.

Kliegman RM. *Practical Strategies in Pediatric Diagnosis and Therapy.* Philadelphia: WB Saunders; 1996.

Koehler JE. Bartonella infections. *Adv Pediatr Infect Dis* 1996;11:1–27.

McAnarney ER, Kreipe RE, Orr DP, et al. *Textbook of Adolescent Medicine.* Philadelphia: WB Saunders; 1992.

The Medical Letter on Drugs and Therapeutics: Drugs for Treatment of Acute Otitis Media in Children. New Rochelle; Medical Letter, Inc; 1994;36:19–21.

Norman ME. Vitamin D in bone disease. *Pediatr Clin North Am* 1982;29:947–971.

Oski FA, DeAngelis CD, Feigin RD, et al. *Principles and Practice of Pediatrics,* 2nd ed. Philadelphia: JB Lippincott; 1994.

Rowe MI, O'Neill JA, Grosfeld JL, et al. *Essentials of Pediatric Surgery.* St. Louis: Mosby; 1995.

Rudolph AM, Hoffman JIE, Rudolph CD. *Pediatrics,* 20th ed. Stamford, CT: Appleton & Lange; 1996.

Tecklenburg FW, Wright MS. Minor head trauma in the pediatric patient. *Pediatr Emerg Care* 1991; 7:40–47.

Traugott L, Alpers A. In their own hands. *Arch Pediatr Adolesc Med* 1997;151:922–927.

Subspecialty List: Pediatrics

190. Neurological
191. Gastroenterology
192. Growth and development; Hematology
193. Toxic; Congenital
194. Infection; Epidemiology
195. Respiratory
196. Growth and development, Orthopedics
197. Adolescent medicine; Growth and development; Orthopedics
198. Infection; History taking; Management
199. Infection; Iatrogenic; Management
200. Adolescent medicine; Genetics
201. Infection; Endocrine/Metabolic; Nutritional
202. Prevention; Infection
203. Infection
204. Poisoning
205. Orthopedics
206. Infection
207. Structural; Infection
208. Poisoning; Management
209. Structural; Iatrogenic
210. Neonatology; Infection
211. Infection
212. Neonatology; Gastroenterology
213. Infection; Gastroenterology
214. Growth and development
215. Infection; Toxic
216. Infection
217. Infection; Psychosocial; Metabolic; Idiopathic
218. Management
219. Gastroenterology
220. Gynecology; Epidemiology
221. Infection; Management
222. Growth and development
223. Growth and development
224. Respiratory; Cardiology; Orthopedics
225. Diagnostic testing
226. Prevention; Infection
227. Prevention; Infection
228. Infection; Epidemiology
229. Orthopedics
230. Cardiology
231. Cardiology
232. Cardiology
233. Cardiology
234. Cardiology

CHAPTER 3

Internal Medicine
Questions

Rebekah Wang Cheng, MD

DIRECTIONS (Questions 235 through 297): Each of the numbered items or incomplete statements in this section is followed by answers or completions of the statement. Select the ONE lettered answer or completion that is BEST in each case.

Questions 235 Through 237

235. You evaluate a 70-year-old man who complains of muscle weakness. His appearance is remarkable for periorbital heliotrope rash with edema and erythema on his upper chest, neck, and face (Figure 3–1) What will you most likely find on exam?

(A) proximal muscle weakness
(B) distal muscle weakness
(C) ataxic gait
(D) hyperactive deep tendon reflexes
(E) inflamed small joints

236. What is the most likely diagnosis?

(A) polymyositis
(B) dermatomyositis
(C) spinocerebellar degeneration
(D) vasculitis
(E) rheumatoid arthritis

237. Which of the following blood parameters is likely to be elevated?

(A) serum creatinine
(B) serum potassium
(C) serum sodium
(D) rheumatoid factor
(E) creatinine phosphokinase

238. Early treatment of travelers' diarrhea is now preferred over prophylaxis. Which of the following antibiotics is the drug of choice?

(A) ciprofloxacin
(B) erythromycin
(C) tetracycline
(D) cephalexin
(E) metronidazole

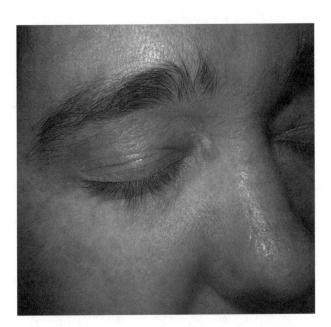

Figure 3–1. Heliotrope erythema on face and eyelid. *(Reprinted with permission from Hurwitz RM.* Pathology of the Skin. *Stamford, CT: Appleton & Lange, 1998.)*

239. What is the likely diagnosis for the ulcerated lesion on the person's cheek shown in Figure 3–2?

(A) squamous cell carcinoma
(B) malignant melanoma
(C) benign ulcerated nevus
(D) basal cell carcinoma
(E) hemangioma

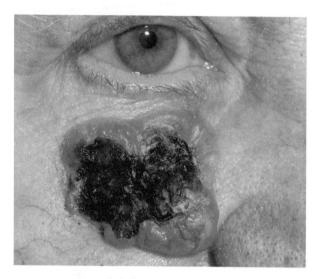

Figure 3–2. *(Reprinted with permission from Fitzpatrick TB.* Color Atlas and Synopsis of Clinical Dermatology, *2nd ed. New York: McGraw-Hill, 1994.)*

Questions 240 Through 243

A dentist asks you to evaluate a 42-year-old woman prior to tooth extraction.

240. Which of the following would prompt you to prescribe prophylactic antibiotics?

(A) midsystolic click at the left sternal border
(B) insulin-dependent diabetes
(C) a holosystolic murmur at the apex
(D) a history of congestive heart failure
(E) S_4 gallop

241. What would be the prophylactic antibiotic of choice for dental procedures?

(A) amoxicillin
(B) vancomycin

(C) cephalexin
(D) penicillin
(E) clindamycin

242. In patients who are not intravenous (IV) drug users and who do not have prosthetic valves, what organism is the most common cause of bacterial endocarditis?

(A) *Enterococcus*
(B) *Streptococcus*
(C) *Staphylococcus*
(D) *Candida*
(E) *Pseudomonas*

243. Which of the following is true regarding prophylaxis against bacterial endocarditis?

(A) Bacterial endocarditis has a low mortality of less than 5%.
(B) Endocarditis is extremely rare in the absence of underlying heart disease.
(C) An atrial septal defect carries a greater risk than a ventricular septal defect.
(D) Patients with previous endocarditis are not at high risk for a second episode.
(E) Penicillin-allergic patients should receive vancomycin and erythromycin.

Questions 244 Through 246

You make the diagnosis of Marfan syndrome in a very tall 22-year-old man with long, thin extremities.

244. What other finding is associated with this disease?

(A) family history in 100% of the patients
(B) upward subluxation of the lenses
(C) mental retardation
(D) malar rash
(E) increased length of trunk compared with the limbs

245. The major cause of morbidity and mortality in Marfan patients is cardiac. Which of the following is a common complication?

(A) pulmonary stenosis
(B) ventricular septal defect (VSD)

(C) pulmonary hypertension

(D) aortic root dilatation

(E) coronary artery disease (CAD)

246. What is the best way to monitor these patients for cardiovascular changes?

(A) electrocardiogram (ECG)

(B) chest x-ray

(C) angiography

(D) pulmonary function tests

(E) echocardiography

247. A 73-year-old woman undergoes colonic resection and ileostomy for carcinoma of the colon. What is a potential complication after the ileostomy becomes established?

(A) cholelithiasis

(B) hepatitis

(C) calcium depletion

(D) pancreatitis

(E) hyperkalemia

248. A 72-year-old woman complains of infrequent, hard stools and a feeling of incomplete evacuation. Which of the following may be a likely contributing cause?

(A) frequent use of antacids

(B) oral iron therapy

(C) thyrotoxicosis

(D) diverticulosis

(E) too much dietary fiber

249. A 59-year-old woman complains of shortness of breath and aching left-sided chest pain that radiates to the left shoulder. Physical examination shows no abnormalities; her chest x-rays are shown in Figure 3–3. Which of the following statements is true concerning this disease?

(A) This tumor frequently metastasizes to distant sites.

(B) Direct exposure to asbestos is required.

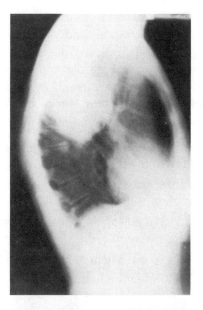

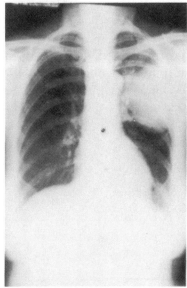

Figure 3–3. Chest x-rays of 59-year-old woman.

(C) Most cases are associated with recent, massive exposure to asbestos.

(D) Diffuse forms may be cured by chemotherapy alone.

(E) Localized forms may be cured by surgery alone.

250. A 23-year-old woman presents with "skipped heartbeats" and on cardiac examination is found to have a midsystolic click followed by a late systolic murmur. Echocardiogram shows prolapse of the mitral valve. Which of the following is true about this condition?

(A) Mitral valve prolapse is present in up to 10% of the population.
(B) Mitral valve prolapse is more common in men.
(C) Prophylaxis against bacterial endocarditis is not required.
(D) Risk of pulmonary embolism is high.
(E) Ventricular arrhythmias do not occur.

251. A 57-year-old man complains of worsening headache, nausea, and vomiting for 2 months. On examination, he is lethargic, confused, and has right-sided weakness. While waiting for a computed tomography (CT) scan, he develops status epilepticus, suffers cardiorespiratory arrest, and dies. His brain at autopsy is shown in Figure 3–4. What is the most likely diagnosis?

(A) glioma
(B) meningioma
(C) craniopharyngioma

(D) pituitary adenoma
(E) acoustic neuroma

252. A 19-year-old high school senior complains of feeling "fat and ugly" despite being extremely thin. She takes small amounts of food at meals and occasionally gags herself to induce vomiting after meals. Which of the following is commonly associated with this disorder?

(A) menorrhagia
(B) metrorrhagia
(C) loss of body hair
(D) bradycardia
(E) thrombocytopenia

Questions 253 and 254

A 59-year-old woman had a left modified radical mastectomy for intraductal carcinoma 2 years previously. She presents with confusion, lethargy, and thigh pain. X-rays reveal a lytic lesion in the shaft of the femur.

253. Which of the following blood abnormalities is likely?

(A) high glucose
(B) low calcium
(C) high potassium

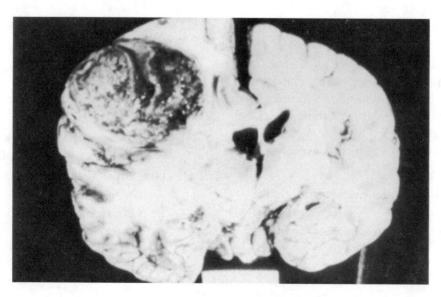

Figure 3–4. CT scan of a 57-year-old man.

(D) high calcium

(E) low magnesium

254. Which of the following is the appropriate initial therapy?

(A) radiotherapy to the femur

(B) vigorous saline infusion

(C) tamoxifen

(D) chemotherapy

(E) glucocorticoids

255. A 55-year-old retired policeman has had hypertension for about 15 years for which he takes hydralazine. He has a 35-pack year tobacco history and continues to smoke one pack a day. On his visit, he complains about the appearance of his nose (Figure 3–5) and asks if something can be done to decrease the redness. Which of the following statements is correct?

(A) Hydralazine does not play a role in his nasal erythema.

(B) Smoking probably aggravates the dilatation of the blood vessels on his nose.

(C) He should avoid alcohol and spicy foods.

(D) There is no effective topical therapy.

(E) Laser therapy will worsen the erythema.

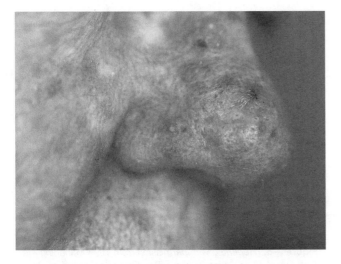

Figure 3–5. Rosacea. *(Reprinted with permission from Hurwitz.* Pathology of the Skin. *Stamford, CT: Appleton & Lange, 1998.)*

256. A 46-year-old attorney is noted to have normal cholesterol levels but a very high fasting triglyceride level of 1600. He is otherwise healthy and has no risk factors for CAD. Which of the following statements is correct?

(A) Hypertriglyceridemia is a strong independent risk factor for premature CAD.

(B) Dietary modification is usually sufficient.

(C) High triglyceride levels are associated with elevated high-density lipoprotein (HDL) levels.

(D) Hypertriglyceridemia is usually associated with skin lesions.

(E) Control of triglyceride levels can prevent attacks of acute pancreatitis in patients with extreme hypertriglyceridemia.

257. A 60-year-old patient with long-standing diabetes has a creatinine of 3.6, which has been stable for several years. Which of the following antibiotics requires the most dosage modification in chronic renal failure?

(A) tetracycline

(B) gentamicin

(C) erythromycin

(D) nafcillin

(E) chloramphenicol

258. A 57-year-old man is on maintenance hemodialysis for chronic renal failure. Which of the following metabolic derangements can be anticipated?

(A) hypercalcemia

(B) hypophosphatemia

(C) osteomalacia

(D) vitamin D excess

(E) hypoparathyroidism

259. A 72-year-old woman is receiving transdermal estrogen therapy. By not using oral estrogen, which of the following complications may be avoided?

    (A) endometrial cancer
    (B) hypertension
    (C) breast cancer
    (D) stroke
    (E) hypertriglyceridemia

260. A 25-year-old man was admitted to the intensive care unit with a severe head injury, with fracture of the base of the skull. Approximately 18 hours after the injury, he developed polyuria. Urine osmolality was 150 mOsm/L and serum osmolality was 350 mOsm/L. Intravenous fluids were stopped, and 3 hours later urine output and urine osmolality remained unchanged. Five units of vasopressin were intravenously administered. Urine osmolality increased to 300 mOsm/L. What is the most likely diagnosis?

    (A) central diabetes insipidus
    (B) nephrogenic diabetes insipidus
    (C) water intoxication
    (D) solute overload
    (E) syndrome of inappropriate antidiuretic hormone secretion (SIADH)

261. A 43-year-old executive is concerned about his risk for heart disease, because he is under a lot of stress from his position. Which of the following is a proven risk factor for premature CAD?

    (A) type A behavior pattern
    (B) low-density lipoprotein (LDL) cholesterol > 110 mg/100 mL
    (C) HDL cholesterol < 35 mg/100 mL
    (D) a family history of coronary disease before the age of 60 in a first-degree relative
    (E) type O blood group

262. A 52-year-old business woman has a strong family history of CAD. Because of this, you recommend that she begin estrogen/progestin therapy. She is reluctant because of

fears of cancer. You outline the risks and benefits of hormone replacement therapy (HRT) in postmenopausal women for her. Which of the following do you tell her about combination HRT?

    (A) increases bone density
    (B) does not affect hot flushes
    (C) increases endometrial carcinoma risk
    (D) decreases vaginitis
    (E) decreases breast cancer risk

263. A 20-year-old female presents to the office complaining that her right eye has been itchy and watery. The patient reports that the onset was abrupt. The patient is noted to be afebrile with normal vital signs. Examination discloses a red eye with watery discharge. Minimal preauricular adenopathy is also found on examination. Tonometry is normal. Profuse tearing is noted (Figure 3–6). The most likely diagnosis is

    (A) viral conjunctivitis
    (B) bacterial conjunctivitis
    (C) foreign-body reaction
    (D) allergic conjunctivitis
    (E) acute open-angle glaucoma

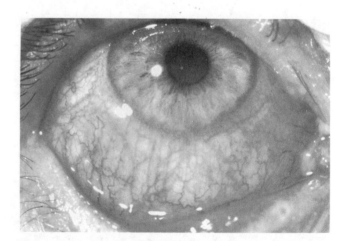

Figure 3–6. *(Reprinted with permission from 1994 Managing the Red Eye: A Slide Script Program, San Francisco, American Academy of Ophthalmology, from Jenson HB, Baltimore RS.* Pediatric Infectious Diseases. *Stamford, CT: Appleton & Lange, 1995.)*

264. A 22-year-old man complains of low back pain and stiffness that is worse on arising and improves with exercise. On examination, he is found to have limited mobility of the sacroiliac joints and lumbar spine. A serum test for histocompatibility antigen HLA-B27 is positive. What is the most common extraskeletal manifestation of this disease?

(A) premature cataracts

(B) splenomegaly

(C) acute iritis

(D) aortic insufficiency

(E) pulmonary fibrosis

Questions 265 and 266

A 54-year-old man presents to the emergency department complaining of epigastric discomfort, which began while he was walking his dog after dinner about one-half hour earlier. He has not received medical care for several years. On exam, he is moderately obese and in obvious discomfort and seems restless. His blood pressure (BP) is 160/98, and his exam is otherwise unremarkable. His ECG is seen in Figure 3–7.

265. What is your clinical diagnosis?

(A) gastroesophageal reflux

(B) costochondritis

(C) gastroenteritis

(D) inferior wall myocardial infarction

(E) anterolateral myocardial infarction

266. What is your next step in management?

(A) trial of antacid immediately

(B) reassurance and arrange outpatient follow-up

(C) arrange for cardiac intensive care bed

(D) begin thrombolytic therapy in the emergency department

(E) arrange for cardiac catheterization

267. A 70-year-old woman who lives independently and has been doing well is hospitalized for pneumonia. She is begun on ceftriaxone and erythromycin but continues to deteriorate and have high fevers 4 days after admission. Which of the following factors is a poor prognostic sign in community-acquired pneumonia?

(A) age > 50

(B) systolic BP > 160

(C) leukocytosis > 15,000

(D) altered mental status

(E) infection with *mycoplasma pneumonia*

268. A 32-year-old woman is referred to you by her dermatologist for further evaluation. She developed these changes gradually in the last year. Her hands are seen in Figure 3–8. What other associated disease is likely?

(A) acquired immune deficiency syndrome (AIDS)

(B) Addison's disease

(C) lymphoma

(D) primary biliary cirrhosis

(E) Hashimoto's thyroiditis

269. A 75-year-old man who developed diabetes within the last 6 months was found to be jaundiced. He has remained asymptomatic, except for weight loss of about 10 pounds in 6 months. On physical examination, he is found to have a nontender, globular, right-upper-quadrant mass that moves with respiration. A CT scan shows enlargement of the head of the pancreas, with no filling defects in the liver. What is the most likely cause of his painless jaundice?

(A) malignant biliary structure

(B) carcinoma of the head of the pancreas

(C) choledocholithiasis

(D) cirrhosis of the liver

(E) pancreatitis

270. Which of the following is a useful clue to the diagnosis of *Legionella* pneumonia?

(A) diarrhea

(B) rash

(C) pedal edema

(D) elevated serum glucose

(E) photophobia

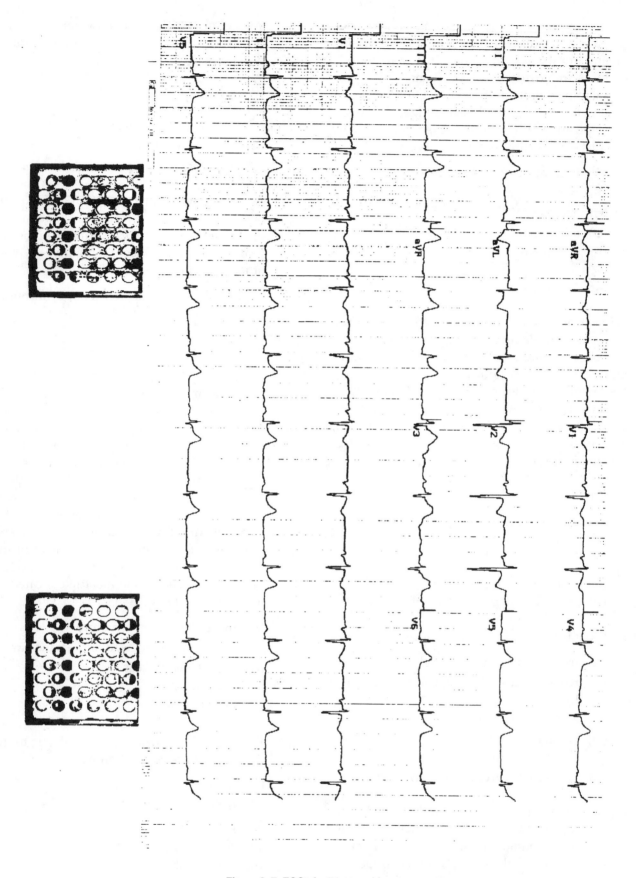

Figure 3–7. ECG of a 54-year-old man.

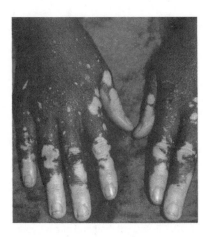

Figure 3–8. *(Reprinted with permission from Bondi.* Dermatology Diagnosis & Therapy. *Stamford, CT: Appleton & Lange, 1991.)*

271. A 60-year-old previously healthy man presents with massive rectal bleeding. What is the most likely diagnosis?

    (A) diverticulosis of the colon
    (B) ulcerative colitis
    (C) external hemorrhoid
    (D) ischemic colitis
    (E) carcinoma of the colon

272. A 24-year-old man runs a marathon on an unusually hot and muggy day. Several hours later he becomes ill, with fever, weakness, and painful swollen legs and passes dark brown urine. Which of the following is a common finding with this disorder?

    (A) urine ortho-toluidine (Hematest) reaction will be negative
    (B) serum will be pink
    (C) serum creatine phosphokinase levels will be elevated
    (D) elevated serum haptoglobin levels
    (E) low serum potassium levels

273. While examining a 46-year-old woman, you hear a diastolic murmur that is increased when the patient is in the left lateral decubi-

tus position. You ask her to run in place for 3 minutes, and the murmur is found to be accentuated as well by exercise. What is the most likely valvular defect?

    (A) aortic regurgitation
    (B) mitral stenosis
    (C) tricuspid stenosis
    (D) pulmonic regurgitation
    (E) VSD

Questions 274 and 275

A 44-year-old secretary complains of abdominal pain in the epigastric area that awakens her in the early morning and is also present when she is hungry. Eating food or taking antacids relieves the pain. Being reprimanded by her boss and stress at work make the pain worse. She takes no regular medications other than occasional ibuprofen for headaches. Her exam is unremarkable and her stool is heme positive in two of three samples. Upper endoscopy reveals a duodenal ulcer.

274. What is the most likely etiology of her ulcer?

    (A) nonsteroidal use
    (B) stress at work
    (C) gastrin-secreting tumor
    (D) *Helicobacter pylori* infection
    (E) *Clostridium difficile* infection

275. Which of the following is most effective for treatment and healing of the ulcer?

    (A) liquid antacid
    (B) amoxicillin
    (C) ranitidine
    (D) omeprazole
    (E) combination clarithromycin and omeprazole

276. A 73-year-old man has been experiencing increasing drowsiness and incoherence. He has a history of arrhythmias and has fallen twice in the past 2 weeks. There are no focal deficits on neurologic examination. A contrast CT scan of the head is shown in Figure 3–9. What is the treatment of choice?

(A) parenteral antibiotics

(B) antifungal therapy

(C) neurosurgical evacuation of the clot

(D) observation and a repeat CT scan in 1 month

(E) fibrinolytic therapy

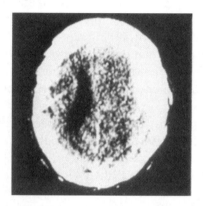

Figure 3–9. CT scan of the head of a 73-year-old man.

277. A 63-year-old man complains of sudden onset of right-sided headache while at work. He rapidly becomes confused and lethargic. On examination, he is hemiparetic and has bilateral Babinski's signs. A CT scan of the head is shown in Figure 3–10. What is the patient most likely to have?

(A) an arteriovenous malformation

(B) a carotid occlusion

(C) hypertension

(D) an underlying malignancy

(E) abnormal clotting studies

278. A 54-year-old woman is noted to have BP in the range of 135/85 on several occasions. This is considered the "high-normal" stage for hypertension. All patients in this range would be encouraged in lifestyle modification. For her, drug therapy is indicated as well. Which of the following would be an indication for drug therapy?

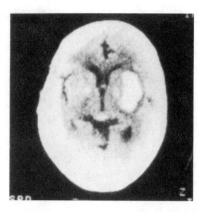

Figure 3–10. CT scan of the head of a 63-year-old man.

(A) obesity

(B) diabetes

(C) high cholesterol

(D) family history of heart disease

(E) smoking

279. A 44-year-old man undergoes evaluation for worsening headaches. His posteroanterior and lateral arteriograms are shown in Figure 3–11. What is the patient most likely to develop?

(A) hypopituitarism

(B) subarachnoid hemorrhage

(C) hypercalcemia

(D) tentorial herniation

(E) chronic meningitis

Questions 280 Through 282

A 35-year-old pharmacist complains of "hurting all over." Her pain is particularly bad in her upper back and shoulders, and she notes morning stiffness. On exam, her joints are not inflamed, but she has symmetric "tender points" in the posterior neck, anterior chest, lateral buttocks, medial knees, and lateral elbows. Your preliminary diagnosis is fibromyalgia.

280. What is another characteristic symptom associated with this syndrome?

(A) sleep disturbance

(B) fever

(C) rash on the extremities

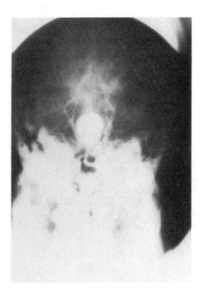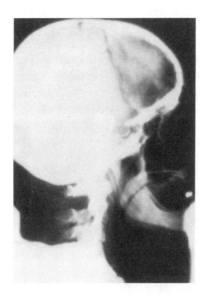

Figure 3–11. Posteroanterior and lateral arteriograms of a 44-year-old man.

(D) muscle weakness

(E) migratory joint inflammation

281. What diagnostic testing will you order?

(A) Lyme titers

(B) electromyelography

(C) sedimentation rate

(D) spine radiographs

(E) screening test for depression

282. What therapeutic recommendation will you make?

(A) avoid most physical activity

(B) trial of amoxicillin

(C) benzodiazepine in low doses for sleep

(D) low-dose steroid

(E) low-dose antidepressant

283. A 62-year-old man is undergoing neurologic evaluation. His arteriogram demonstrates the lesion shown in Figure 3–12. Which of the following deficits would be compatible with this lesion?

(A) diplopia

(B) transient monocular blindness

(C) ataxia

(D) vertigo

(E) dysarthria

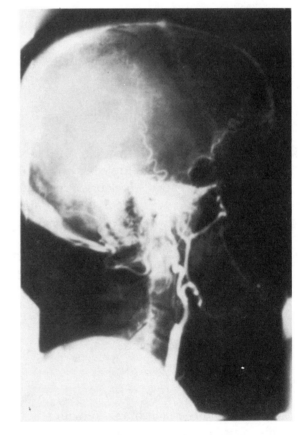

Figure 3–12. Arteriogram of a 62-year-old man.

Questions 284 and 285

A 30-year-old woman who had been human immunodeficiency virus (HIV) positive for 4 years was recently diagnosed with AIDS.

284. Which of the following meets the criteria for the case definition?

(A) oral thrush
(B) herpes zoster
(C) persistent lymphadenopathy
(D) peripheral neuropathy
(E) pulmonary tuberculosis

285. Which of the following immunologic abnormalities would be expected?

(A) increased numbers of CD4+ (helper) T cells
(B) increased number of CD8+ (suppressor) T cells
(C) cutaneous anergy to usual skin test antigens
(D) normal B-cell function
(E) increased natural killer cell function

286. When you examine the back of an elderly gentleman, you note multiple brown papules and nodules having a "stuck on" appearance. These are shown in Figure 3–13. The patient tells you they have been there for years. What is the most likely diagnosis?

(A) melanocytic nevi
(B) actinic keratoses
(C) seborrheic keratoses
(D) seborrheic dermatitis
(E) malignant melanoma

Questions 287 and 288

A 58-year-old man is establishing care with you because his insurance changed. His old records have not yet arrived, but he is complaining of palpitations and lightheadedness, so you order the ECG shown in Figure 3–14.

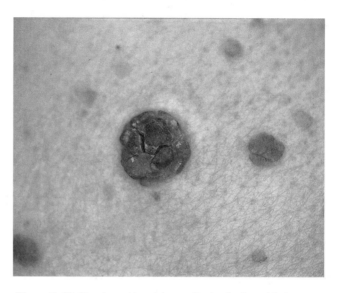

Figure 3–13. Papules and nodules on the back of an elderly gentleman. *(Reprinted with permission from Hurwitz. Pathology of the Skin. Stamford, CT: Appleton & Lange, 1998.)*

287. What is the underlying abnormality?

(A) right bundle branch block (RBBB)
(B) left bundle branch block (LBBB)
(C) accelerated junctional rhythm
(D) left anterior fascicular block
(E) intraventricular conduction delay

288. What is the most likely problem associated with this pattern?

(A) congenital heart disease
(B) severe aortic valve disease
(C) hypokalemia
(D) atrial septal defect
(E) ventricular septal defect

289. A 48-year-old man complains of joint pain and stiffness for the past 3 months. Both hands and feet are warm and the joints are swollen. Which of the following suggests the diagnosis of rheumatoid arthritis (RA)?

(A) early morning stiffness lasting 1 hour
(B) numbness and blanching of fingers on exposure to cold
(C) symmetric involvement of the distal interphalangeal joints
(D) facial rash in the malar region
(E) synovial fluid with high viscosity and 30,000 lymphocytes/mm^3

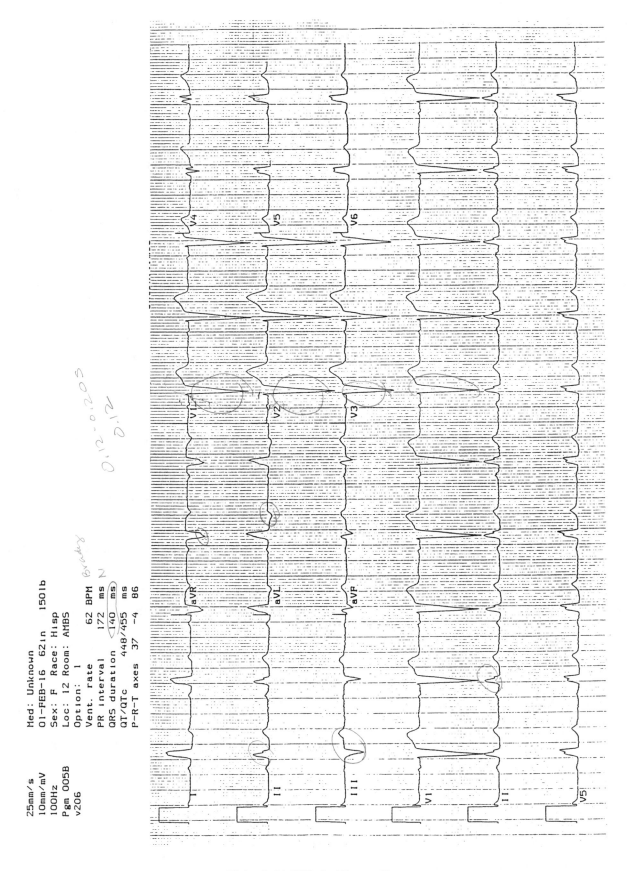

Figure 3–14. ECG of a 58-year-old man.

290. During a routine checkup, a 45-year-old executive is found to have hypercalcemia. Subsequent workup reveals elevated parathormone, decreased phosphorus, elevated chloride, and normal blood urea nitrogen (BUN) and creatinine in serum. Urinary calcium is above normal levels. What is the most likely etiology?

(A) multiple myeloma
(B) primary hyperparathyroidism
(C) hypervitaminosis D
(D) sarcoidosis
(E) milk alkali syndrome

291. A 26-year-old woman comes to your office in the winter complaining of a stuffy nose. She has no pets. On exam, her nasal mucosa is somewhat pale and boggy. What is the most likely cause of her nonseasonal allergic rhinitis?

(A) ragweed
(B) dust mites
(C) aerosol spray
(D) cigarette smoke
(E) houseplants

Questions 292 and 293

A 72-year-old man has the sudden onset of suprapubic pain and oliguria. His temperature is 38.0°C (100.4°F), pulse is 100/min, respirations are 12/min, and BP is 110/72 mm Hg. Abdominal examination is remarkable only for a tender, distended urinary bladder.

292. What should the immediate management of this patient be?

(A) plain x-ray of the abdomen
(B) abdominal ultrasonography
(C) urethral catheter
(D) intravenous furosemide
(E) intravenous pyelogram (IVP)

293. Which of the following is a likely cause of this condition?

(A) urinary tract infection
(B) prostatic hypertrophy

(C) posterior urethral valves
(D) renal carcinoma
(E) renal arterial occlusion

294. A 42-year-old woman is noted to have a multinodular goiter on exam. She has no symptoms and is clinically euthyroid. Which of the following statements about Hashimoto's thyroiditis is true?

(A) The condition is associated with prior radioactive exposure.
(B) Patients diagnosed with this disorder have an increased incidence of thyroid cancer.
(C) Corticosteroids are helpful in controlling the progression of the disease.
(D) Antinuclear antibodies are pathognomonic for this disease.
(E) Hashimoto's thyroiditis is an autoimmune disease.

Questions 295 and 296

A 24-year-old college student complains of fatigue, arthralgias, mucosal ulcerations, and a "butterfly" facial rash. Biopsy of the rash reveals linear deposition of immunoglobulin G (IgG) and complement at the dermal–epidermal junction.

295. Which of the following is true concerning this disease?

(A) Women and men are equally affected.
(B) Skin biopsy findings are usually pathognomonic.
(C) Biopsy specimen of noninvolved skin will be normal.
(D) Serum complement levels decrease with disease flares.
(E) The erythrocyte sedimentation rate (ESR) is a reliable guide to disease activity.

296. What is the most specific test for this disease?

(A) antinuclear antibodies (ANA)
(B) anti-Sm

(C) anti-RNP

(D) anti-Ro

(E) antihistone

297. A 60-year-old man with easy fatigability was found to have hypercalcemia, decreased parathormone level, normal BUN and creatinine, and increased urinary excretion of calcium. A chest x-ray showed an irregular density in the right upper lobe of the lung. What is the most likely etiology of his hypercalcemia?

(A) multiple myeloma

(B) excessive thiazide ingestion

(C) paraneoplastic syndrome

(D) prolonged immobilization

(E) secondary hyperparathyroidism

DIRECTIONS (Questions 298 through 311): Each set of matching questions in this section consists of a list of 5 lettered options followed by several numbered items. For each item, select the ONE best lettered option that is most closely associated with it. Each lettered heading may be selected once, more than once, or not at all.

Questions 298 Through 300

For each cancer chemotherapeutic agent listed below, select the adverse reaction with which it is most commonly associated.

(A) pulmonary fibrosis in 5% of patients

(B) alopecia and hemorrhagic cystitis

(C) cardiac toxicity at cumulative doses > 500 mg/m^2

(D) megaloblastic changes in bone marrow prevented by folinic acid

(E) areflexia, peripheral neuritis, and paralytic ileus

298. Methotrexate

299. Doxorubicin hydrochloride (Adriamycin)

300. Cyclophosphamide

Questions 301 Through 303

For each of the abnormalities listed below, choose the set of serum electrolytes with which it is usually associated.

(A) Na$^+$ 132, K$^+$ 5.8, Cl$^-$ 82, CO$_2$ 18

(B) Na$^+$ 100, K$^+$ 10, Cl$^-$ 10, CO$_2$ 86

(C) Na$^+$ 106, K$^+$ 3.4, Cl$^-$ 84, CO$_2$ 26

(D) Na$^+$ 139, K$^+$ 4.0, Cl$^-$ 102, CO$_2$ 26

(E) Na$^+$ 170, K$^+$ 5.4, Cl$^-$ 120, CO$_2$ 26

301. Diabetes insipidus

302. Uncontrolled diabetes mellitus with glucose of 400

303. SIADH

Questions 304 Through 306

For each disease listed below, select the circulating antibodies with which it is most closely associated.

(A) antibodies to acetylcholine receptors

(B) antibodies to native deoxyribonucleic acid (DNA)

(C) antibodies to smooth muscle cells

(D) antibodies to mitochondria

(E) antibodies to parietal cells

304. Primary biliary cirrhosis

305. Myasthenia gravis

306. Systemic lupus erythematosus

Questions 307 and 308

For each clinical setting described below, select the set of arterial blood gas (ABG) determinations with which it is most likely to be associated.

	pH	PaO_2	$Paco_2$
(A)	7.23	64	80
(B)	7.39	88	40
(C)	7.22	74	33
(D)	7.54	75	24
(E)	7.37	67	52

307. A 60-year-old man with long-standing obstructive pulmonary disease

308. A 30-year-old female with an acute pulmonary embolus

Questions 309 Through 311

For each antihypertensive agent listed below, select the set of undesirable side effects with which it is most commonly associated.

(A) cough, hyperkalemia, renal failure

(B) positive Coombs' test, hemolytic anemia, hepatitis

(C) hypokalemia, hyperuricemia, hyperglycemia

(D) sodium retention, heart failure, increased body hair

(E) increased angina, tachycardia, systemic lupus erythematosus (SLE)

309. Hydrochlorothiazide

310. Hydralazine

311. Captropril

DIRECTIONS (Questions 312 through 378): Each of the numbered items or incomplete statements in this section is followed by answers or completions of the statement. Select the ONE lettered answer or completion that is BEST in each case.

Questions 312 Through 314

312. In a 34-year-old patient with a thyroid nodule, which of the following raises the index of suspicion for carcinoma?

(A) a hyperfunctioning nodule

(B) a family history of childhood irradiation to the neck

(C) a prior history of childhood irradiation to the neck

(D) a cystic nodule

(E) a family history of Graves' disease

313. This young woman's fine-needle aspiration of the thyroid is positive for cancer. What histologic cell type is the most common?

(A) medullary

(B) papillary

(C) follicular

(D) lymphoma

(E) anaplastic

314. Her serum calcitonin level is normal. Which cell type is associated with elevated levels?

(A) medullary

(B) papillary

(C) follicular

(D) lymphoma

(E) anaplastic

Questions 315 and 316

315. A previously healthy 19-year-old woman has the sudden onset of headache, profound myalgias, profuse vomiting, and diarrhea. The woman is near the end of her menstrual period and is using tampons. She appears to be suffering from toxic shock syndrome (TSS). What is the most likely skin finding?

(A) papular rash on the trunk

(B) scaly rash on the face

(C) pustular rash on the extremities

(D) macular erythroderma

(E) heliotrope facial rash

316. What else is a common finding and part of the case definition?

(A) hypertension: systolic BP > 160 mm Hg

(B) hyperreflexia

(C) fever with temperature ≥ 102°F

(D) elevated platelet count > 400,000

(E) hypercalcemia

317. A 15-year-old boy is brought by his mother for evaluation of fever. Which of the following is a major criterion for the diagnosis of acute rheumatic fever?

(A) leukocytosis

(B) migratory polyarthritis

(C) fever

(D) elevated sedimentation rate

(E) shortened PR interval on ECG

318. A 24-year-old woman presents for evaluation of headaches, amenorrhea, and galactorrhea. The serum prolactin level is 850 ng/mL (normal = 0 to 25). CT scan of the pituitary demonstrates a 7-mm sellar lesion most consistent with a microadenoma. Besides pituitary adenomas, which of the following can also raise prolactin levels above normal?

(A) cocaine

(B) bromocriptine

(C) oral contraceptives

(D) phenothiazines

(E) selective serotonin reuptake inhibitors (SSRIs)

319. A 52-year-old woman has had diabetes mellitus since childhood. She has controlled her glucose well and kept her glycohemoglobin (HgbA1C) below 7% (normal 4 to 7%). Which of the following complications is she still at risk of, despite excellent glucose control?

(A) autonomic dysfunction

(B) coronary heart disease

(C) blindness

(D) peripheral neuropathy

(E) peripheral vascular disease

320. A middle-aged white male presents to your office complaining of arthralgias, diarrhea, abdominal pain, and weight loss. On exam, you note generalized increased skin pigmentation. Which of the following is true regarding Whipple's disease?

(A) Acute renal failure is a common complication.

(B) This disease usually strikes young adults before the third decade.

(C) It is predominantly a disease of women.

(D) Microscopic examination of the small intestine shows infiltration by large macrophages with periodic acid–Schiff (PAS)-positive inclusions.

(E) It is associated with a gram-positive cocci.

321. A 42-year-old patient suffering from alcoholism has advanced liver disease with ascites. He is hospitalized for agitation and bizarre behavior. Which of the following findings is most helpful in making the diagnosis of hepatic encephalopathy?

(A) jaundice

(B) asterixis of the hands

(C) spider angiomas on the face and chest

(D) heme-positive stool

(E) positive fluid wave on abdominal exam

322. In the above patient, his blood ammonia level is twice his baseline. Which of the following is a likely precipitating factor?

(A) bleeding esophageal varices

(B) noncompliance with diuretic therapy

(C) excessive lactulose therapy

(D) insufficient protein ingestion

(E) recent alcohol ingestion

323. Which of the following statements concerning *Campylobacter* gastroenteritis is true?

(A) Affected patients are usually afebrile.

(B) It is the most common cause of travelers' diarrhea.

(C) Most human infections are the result of person-to-person transmission.

(D) Abdominal pain is often the most prominent symptom.

(E) Antibiotics are necessary for recovery from diarrhea.

324. A 67-year-old man has a long history of constipation and recurrent, brief episodes of gripping lower abdominal pain. He is currently asymptomatic; his barium enema x-ray is shown in Figure 3–15. Which of the following is appropriate therapy?

(A) surgical resection

(B) colonoscopy with biopsy

(C) histamine receptor antagonist

(D) corticosteroid rectal enema

(E) bulk-producing colloid, such as bran or psyllium

Questions 325 Through 327

325. A 44-year-old secretary presents with a fever of 103°F, headache, and stiff neck. You entertain a diagnosis of bacterial meningitis and begin antibiotics immediately. With bacterial meningitis, which of the following is a likely finding in the cerebrospinal fluid (CSF)?

(A) leukocytes between 100 and 500/mm

(B) CSF pressure between 100 and 120 mm H_2O

(C) negative Gram stain

(D) glucose > 120 mg/dL

(E) protein levels > 45 mg/dL

326. In this otherwise healthy adult woman, what is the most likely organism?

(A) group B *Streptococcus*

(B) *Staphylococcus aureus*

(C) *Hemophilus influenzae*

(D) *Streptococcus pneumoniae*

(E) *Listeria monocytogenes*

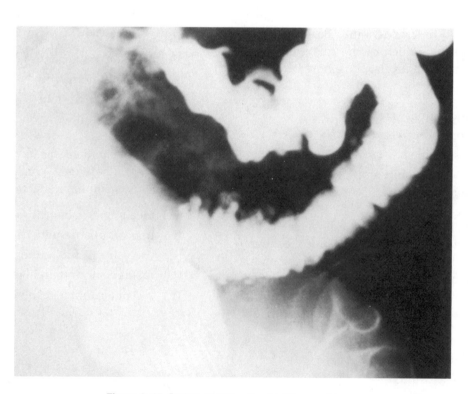

Figure 3–15. Barium enema x-ray of a 67-year-old man.

327. In the adult neutropenic patient, what is the most likely organism to cause bacterial meningitis?

    (A) group B *Streptococcus*
    (B) *Staphylococcus aureus*
    (C) *Hemophilus influenzae*
    (D) *Streptococcus pneumoniae*
    (E) *Listeria monocytogenes*

328. A 50-year-old woman complains of worsening dyspnea of 1 month's duration, but is otherwise asymptomatic. Lung examination is normal; her chest x-ray is shown in Figure 3–16. What is the most likely diagnosis?

    (A) pulmonary tuberculosis
    (B) lung metastases
    (C) sarcoidosis
    (D) mycoplasma pneumonia
    (E) silicosis

329. A 63-year-old man complains of a new cough and of breathlessness after walking up a flight of stairs. Chest examination reveals late inspiratory crackles but no wheezes. There is a mild clubbing of the fingers. His chest x-ray is shown in Figure 3–17. What would be found on pulmonary function testing?

    (A) increased arterial carbon dioxide pressure ($PaCO_2$)
    (B) normal compliance
    (C) decreased carbon monoxide diffusing capacity (DL_{CO})
    (D) increased vital capacity
    (E) increased oxygen saturation with exercise

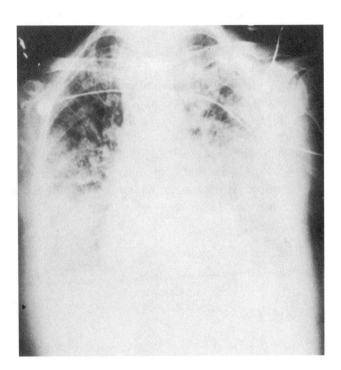

Figure 3–17. Chest x-ray of a 63-year-old man.

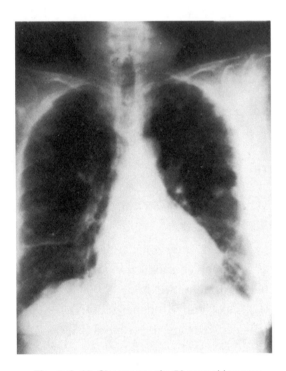

Figure 3–16. Chest x-ray of a 50-year-old woman.

330. Which of the following statements is true concerning the pneumococcal polysaccharide vaccine?

    (A) Healthy adult recipients demonstrate a twofold rise in type-specific antibody in 20 to 30 weeks.
    (B) Very few recipients (< 5%) experience erythema and pain at the injection site.
    (C) Adults with respiratory disorders should receive the vaccine every 2 to 3 years.
    (D) Young adults with sickle cell disease should be vaccinated.
    (E) Recipients will not develop pneumococcal pneumonia because protection is so complete.

331. A 60-year-old man presents with a nonproductive cough for a week and generalized malaise. He also has noted some abdominal pain associated with diarrhea for the past few days. His temperature is 101.5°F, and clinical exam is unremarkable. A chest x-ray shows a left lower lobe infiltrate. His urinalysis shows 50 red blood cells (RBCs), and his BUN (30) and creatinine (1.6) are both mildly elevated. In light of the extrapulmonary symptoms and signs, which of the following is the most likely cause of his pneumonia?

    (A) *Pseudomonas aeruginosa*
    (B) *Staphylococcus aureus*
    (C) *Hemophilus influenzae*
    (D) *Streptococcus pneumoniae*
    (E) *Legionella*

332. A 63-year-old man with chronic bronchitis presents to the emergency department with worsening shortness of breath. He is dyspneic, his respiratory rate is 32/min, and he has peripheral cyanosis. A chest examination reveals increased anteroposterior diameter and scattered rhonchi, but no wheezes or evidence of consolidation. His ABG determinations on room air are pH of 7.36, arterial oxygen pressure (Pao_2) of 40 mm Hg, and $Paco_2$ of 47 mm Hg. He is given oxygen by face mask while awaiting a chest x-ray. His res-

piratory rate falls to 12/min, but his ABGs on oxygen are now pH of 7.31, Pao_2 of 62 mm Hg, and $Paco_2$ of 58 mm Hg. What should the next step be?

    (A) Repeat the ABG.
    (B) Initiate mechanical ventilation.
    (C) Obtain a chest x-ray.
    (D) Check the oxygen delivery system.
    (E) Decrease the fraction of inspired oxygen (Fio_2).

Questions 333 Through 335

333. A 26-year-old man presents with a hard, painless testicular mass. At operation, frozen section reveals testicular cancer. Which of the following is a risk factor?

    (A) family history of testicular cancer
    (B) masturbation
    (C) prior history of radiation exposure
    (D) cryptorchidism
    (E) maternal diethylstilbestrol (DES) during pregnancy

334. What is the most common cell type?

    (A) choriocarcinoma
    (B) embryonal cell
    (C) seminoma
    (D) teratocarcinoma
    (E) endodermal sinus

335. What serum marker can be used to monitor therapy?

    (A) carcinoembryonic antigen (CEA)
    (B) human chorionic gonadotropin (hCG)
    (C) sedimentation rate
    (D) lactic dehydrogenase (LDH)
    (E) prostate-specific antigen (PSA)

336. Which of the following is true concerning aldosterone and its secretion?

    (A) Secretion is regulated by the renin–angiotensin mechanism.
    (B) Increased aldosterone secretion reduces blood volume.

(C) Aldosterone secretion stimulates renin release.

(D) Aldosterone secretion causes retention of K^+ and loss of Na^+.

(E) Aldosterone secretion causes low diastolic blood pressures.

337. A 25-year-old man has the sudden onset of chest pain on the right side and dyspnea. On chest x-ray his trachea is deviated to the left. Which of the following would be anticipated on examination?

(A) rales on the left

(B) rales on the right

(C) hyperresonance on the left

(D) distant breath sounds on the right

(E) pleural friction rub on the left

338. What is the distinguishing feature of left ventricular failure?

(A) elevated liver enzymes

(B) pulmonary edema

(C) ascites

(D) peripheral edema

(E) jugular venous distension

339. A 42-year-old man admitted with a high fever and leukocytosis is transferred to the intensive care unit in shock. What is a common finding in septic shock in early stages?

(A) reduced cardiac output

(B) bradycardia

(C) decreased systemic vascular resistance (SVR)

(D) hypertension

(E) metabolic alkalosis

340. Which of the following statements concerning transmission of viral hepatitis B is true?

(A) Children are at considerably more risk for hepatitis B infection than spouses of infected individuals.

(B) Hepatitis B is rarely transmitted through sexual contact.

(C) Vertical transmission results most often from transplacental infection.

(D) In developing countries, vertical transmission (mother to child) is the major route of transmission.

(E) Most cases of hepatitis B have a history of exposure.

341. Which of the following arrhythmias is most likely to respond to adenosine infusion?

(A) ventricular tachycardia

(B) atrial fibrillation

(C) atrial flutter

(D) paroxysmal supraventricular tachycardia

(E) ventricular fibrillation

342. A 48-year-old man complains of fatigue and shortness of breath. His hematocrit is 32%, and hemoglobin is 10.3 g/100 mL. Peripheral blood smear reveals macrocytosis. His serum vitamin B_{12} level is 90 pg/mL (normal, 170 to 940); serum folate level is 6 ng/mL (normal, 2 to 14). What is the most likely cause?

(A) poor dietary habits

(B) colonic diverticulosis

(C) regional enteritis

(D) chronic constipation

(E) vagotomy

343. What is the single most important prognostic factor in a patient with epidural spinal cord compression secondary to malignancy?

(A) the level at which compression occurs

(B) the patient's level of neurologic function at the beginning of therapy

(C) whether the compression is due to a primary malignancy or a metastatic lesion

(D) the type of primary malignancy if the lesion is metastatic

(E) the patient's cardiovascular status

344. A 33-year-old woman complains of generalized, throbbing headache that is worse in the morning and with coughing. She occasionally feels dizzy and nauseated. Examination is significant only for obesity and bilateral papilledema. A CT scan of the head is normal. At lumbar puncture, the opening pressure is 220 mm H_2O; CSF is clear, with protein of 12 mg/100 mL (normal, 15 to 45), glucose of 68 mg/100 mL (normal, 45 to 80), and no cells are seen. What is the most likely diagnosis?

   (A) migraine headache
   (B) multiple sclerosis
   (C) malignant carcinomatosis
   (D) pseudotumor cerebri
   (E) glaucoma

345. Which of the following is true regarding pulmonary embolism?

   (A) The most common type of embolism begins as a thrombus in a leg or pelvic vein.
   (B) Amniotic fluid and fat emboli are common types of pulmonary embolism.
   (C) Pulmonary embolism often leads to left ventricular failure and shock.
   (D) Resultant hypoxemia is due to left heart failure.
   (E) Examination of the lungs usually reveals decreased breath sounds.

346. A 24-year-old man is found to be seropositive for HIV on a military induction screening test. Which of the following is the opportunistic infection that is most likely to develop in this patient?

   (A) *Pneumocystis carinii* pneumonia
   (B) *Candida albicans* fungemia
   (C) disseminated *Mycobacterium avium-intracellulare* infection
   (D) cryptococcal meningitis
   (E) cytomegalovirus retinitis

347. A 56-year-old man complains of fatigue, dyspnea on exertion, and palpitations. He has had a murmur since childhood. Examination reveals a lift at the left sternal border, split S_1, and fixed splitting of S_2. There is a grade 3/6 midsystolic pulmonic murmur and a 1/6 middiastolic tricuspid murmur at the lower left sternal border. Chest x-ray shows right ventricular enlargement and prominent pulmonary arteries. An ECG demonstrates atrial fibrillation with a right bundle branch block. What is the most likely diagnosis?

   (A) coarctation of the aorta
   (B) atrial septal defect (ASD)
   (C) patent ductus arteriosus
   (D) tetralogy of Fallot
   (E) VSD

348. Which of the folowing causes of pericardial effusion are most likely to lead to cardiac tamponade?

   (A) pneumopericardium
   (B) SLE
   (C) malignancy
   (D) uremia
   (E) pericarditis

349. A 52-year-old executive comes to your office for a routine annual examination as a benefit of his employment. He has never smoked and has no history of colorectal carcinoma or polyps in his personal or family history. A sigmoidoscopy is provided as part of the assessment. Which of the following is true regarding this procedure?

   (A) A stool hemoccult test is just as good as sigmoidoscopy for screening.
   (B) The risk of colonic perforation with sigmoidoscopy is approximately 10%.
   (C) The possibility of significant bleeding is a contraindication to sigmoidoscopy.
   (D) A barium enema would be just as good as sigmoidoscopy and carries no risk.
   (E) Screening sigmoidoscopy of people over 50 decreases mortality of colorectal cancer.

350. A 37-year-old alcoholic patient is found in his apartment by a neighbor and brought to the emergency department in an obtunded state.

Arterial pH is 7.15, serum HCO_3 is 8, glucose is 75, creatinine is 0.9, and the anion gap is determined to be 22 mEq/L (normal, 10 to 14 mEq/L). What is a likely cause of this disorder?

(A) ammonium chloride ingestion

(B) renal failure

(C) diabetic ketoacidosis

(D) alcoholic ketoacidosis

(E) liver failure

351. Five days after a total hip replacement, a 72-year-old woman becomes acutely short of breath, diaphoretic, and hypotensive. Both lung fields are clear to auscultation and percussion, but examination of the neck reveals mild jugular venous distension with prominent A waves. Heart sounds are normal. An ECG shows sinus tachycardia and minor nonspecific ST-T wave changes. What is the most likely diagnosis?

(A) aspiration pneumonia

(B) acute myocardial infarction

(C) aortic dissection

(D) pulmonary embolism

(E) pericarditis

352. What is the most appropriate treatment for the patient described above?

(A) clindamycin

(B) streptokinase

(C) urgent cardiac surgery

(D) heparin

(E) indomethacin

353. A 92-year-old man is referred from his nursing home for evaluation of lethargy. Examination is unrevealing, but laboratory results are significant for a serum sodium level of 118 mEq/L (normal, 135 to 148). Serum osmolality is 260, urine osmolality is 450, and urine sodium is 80. What is the most likely cause?

(A) hyperglycemia

(B) hyperlipidemia

(C) hyperproteinemia

(D) SIADH

(E) diabetes insipidus

354. Which of the following is a "postrenal" cause of acute renal failure?

(A) cardiac failure

(B) septicemia

(C) calculi

(D) rhabdomyolysis

(E) acute glomerulonephritis

355. Which of the following is the most common cause of nephrotic syndrome?

(A) diabetes mellitus

(B) Hodgkin's lymphoma

(C) heroin abuse

(D) malignant hypertension

(E) renal failure

Questions 356 and 357

356. A 33-year-old woman experiences visions of flashing lights followed by throbbing left-sided temporal pain and nausea. What is the most likely diagnosis?

(A) tension headache

(B) transient ischemic attack (TIA)

(C) temporal arteritis

(D) migraine headache

(E) cluster headache

357. This patient is most likely to benefit from acute treatment with which of the following substances?

(A) propranolol

(B) prednisone

(C) sumatriptan

(D) heparin

(E) oxygen

358. A 27-year-old college freshman complains of dysuria and urinary frequency. Urinalysis reveals 8 to 10 white blood cells (WBCs) per high-power field and numerous gram-negative bacteria. Which of the following statements concerning this disease is true?

(A) A single dose of an antibiotic may be sufficient treatment.

(B) Pregnant women with bacteriuria should not be treated if asymptomatic.

(C) Patients with flank pain or fever should be hospitalized.

(D) Hematuria indicates renal involvement.

(E) Urologic investigation is indicated after the treatment course is completed.

359. What is the most common organism in uncomplicated urinary tract infection?

(A) *Klebsiella*

(B) *Chlamydia*

(C) *Escherichia coli*

(D) *Pseudomonas*

(E) *Candida*

360. Which of the following is true in regard to the empty-sella syndrome?

(A) Most patients presenting with this disorder are male.

(B) Most patients presenting with this disorder are thin.

(C) Pituitary function in these patients is usually normal.

(D) On skull x-rays, the sella turcica is found to be decreased in size.

(E) Visual disorders are common.

Questions 361 and 362

361. A 28-year-old man has the acute onset of colicky pain in the left costovertebral angle radiating into the groin, as well as gross hematuria. Abdominal x-ray discloses a stone in the left ureter. Which of the following is true concerning this disease?

(A) The majority of renal stones are radiolucent.

(B) Radiolucent stones are usually composed of uric acid.

(C) Staghorn calculi are associated with acid urine.

(D) Radiopaque stones usually contain cystine.

(E) Urate stones are associated with alkaline urine.

362. The patient spontaneously passes the stone, which is found to contain calcium oxalate. What is the most likely cause of this stone?

(A) chronic urinary tract infection

(B) vitamin D excess

(C) primary hyperparathyroidism

(D) idiopathic hypercalciuria

(E) renal tubular acidosis

363. Which of the following is seen in Addison's disease?

(A) high serum Na^+

(B) high serum K^+

(C) low BUN

(D) dilute urine

(E) elevated hematocrit

364. A 54-year-old man complains of cough, shortness of breath, and pleuritic left-sided chest pain. Examination and chest x-ray are compatible with a large left-sided pleural effusion. At thoracentesis, the pleural fluid is straw colored and slightly turbid, with a WBC count of 53,000/mL, RBC count of 1200/mL, glucose of 42 mg/100 mL, total protein of 5 g/100 mL, LDH of 418 IU/L, and pH of 7.2. Simultaneous serum total protein is 8 g/100 mL (normal, 6 to 8 g/100 mL), and serum LDH level is 497 IU/L (normal, 52 to 149 IU/L). Gram stain is positive for gram-negative rods. What is the most likely cause of his pleural effusion?

(A) parapneumonic effusion

(B) congestive heart failure

(C) malignant effusion

(D) trauma

(E) nephrotic syndrome

365. Which of the following will result from hypersecretion of aldosterone, usually due to an adenoma?

(A) hyponatremia

(B) hypochlorhydria

(C) hyperkalemia

(D) metabolic alkalosis

(E) metabolic acidosis

366. A 52-year-old woman complains of gaining weight and bruising easily. Examination shows truncal obesity, rounded facies, hirsutism, and abdominal striae. She has proximal muscle weakness and atrophy. Her plasma cortisol level at 8:00 AM is 49 mg/100 mL (normal, < 30). What is the next step in evaluation?

(A) plasma adrenocorticotropic hormone (ACTH) determination

(B) metyrapone stimulation test

(C) ACTH stimulation test

(D) dexamethasone suppression test

(E) sella turcica CT

Questions 367 and 368

A 17-year-old girl notes an enlarging lump in her neck. On examination, her thyroid gland is twice the normal size, firm to rubbery, multilobular, nontender, and freely mobile. There is no adenopathy. Family history is positive for both hypo- and hyperthyroidism. Her serum triiodothyronine (T_3) and thyroxine (T_4) levels are low normal, and serum thyroid-stimulating hormone (TSH) is high normal. Technetium scan shows nonuniform uptake. Serum and antithyroglobulin titer is strongly positive.

367. What will thyroid biopsy of this patient most likely disclose?

(A) giant cell granulomas and necrosis

(B) polymorphonuclear cells and bacteria

(C) diffuse fibrous replacement

(D) lymphocytic infiltration

(E) parafollicular cells

368. What is appropriate treatment for this patient?

(A) corticosteroids

(B) antibiotics

(C) thyroid hormone

(D) radioactive iodine

(E) surgery

369. An obese 21-year-old woman complains of increased growth of coarse hair on her lip, chin, chest, and abdomen. She also notes menstrual irregularity with periods of amenorrhea. What is the most likely cause?

(A) polycystic ovary disease

(B) an ovarian tumor

(C) an adrenal tumor

(D) Cushing's disease

(E) familial hirsutism

370. A 71-year-old woman is receiving parenteral methicillin for leg cellulitis. Over 2 days, she develops macroscopic hematuria, oliguria, and marked deterioration in renal functioning. Which of the following is suggestive of methicillin-induced acute interstitial nephritis?

(A) protein in the urine

(B) eosinophils in the urine

(C) RBC casts in the urine

(D) hyaline casts in the urine

(E) myoglobin in the urine

371. A 52-year-old man is receiving a preoperative evaluation prior to elective surgery. He is asymptomatic and has a normal exam, but is noted to have a hemoglobin of 10.8, hematocrit of 33, with a mean corpuscular volume of 70 (normal, 82 to 92), and 6.1 million RBCs (normal, 4.5 to 5.0). What is the most likely diagnosis?

(A) sickle cell anemia

(B) iron-deficiency anemia

(C) alpha-thalassemia major

(D) beta-thalassemia minor

(E) anemia of chronic disease

372. A 27-year-old woman presents with bloody stools. She is found to have multiple, irregular dark brown macules on her lips, buccal mucosa, hands, and feet. What is the most likely cause of her gastrointestinal bleeding?

(A) esophageal carcinoma

(B) jejunal hamartomas

(C) gastric telangiectasia

(D) intestinal neurofibromas

(E) colonic hemangioma

373. A 39-year-old woman presents with induration and atrophy of the fingertips and is diagnosed as having systemic sclerosis (scleroderma). Which of the following complications is the most common cause of death?

(A) esophageal hypomotility

(B) restrictive lung disease

(C) congestive heart failure

(D) intestinal sclerosis

(E) renovascular hypertension

374. A 68-year-old man complains of aching pain around his left hip and right knee; it is worse after exertion and is relieved with rest. Both joints are tender and swollen, with pain and crepitus on passive motion. Tests for rheumatoid factor and ESR are normal. What is an x-ray of the knee likely to reveal?

(A) joint space enlargement

(B) osteoporosis

(C) osteophytes

(D) periosteal lifting

(E) subchondral erosions

375. At a routine company physical examination, an asymptomatic 46-year-old man is found to have a BP of 150/110 mm Hg, but no other abnormalities are present. What do you do next?

(A) Reassure the patient and repeat the physical examination in 12 months.

(B) Order an ECG.

(C) Initiate antihypertensive therapy.

(D) Obtain repeated BP recordings in your office and/or the patient's home or work site.

(E) Counsel the patient on dietary sodium reduction.

376. A 58-year-old man carries the diagnosis of pseudogout (chondrocalcinosis). Which of the following is a common feature?

(A) uric acid deposits within joints

(B) episodic attacks of pain

(C) small joints affected more often than large joints

(D) predilection for women

(E) predilection for young people

377. A 25-year-old man presents with a large malignant melanoma on his back. There is no apparent lymphadenopathy (clinical stage 1). What is the most important prognostic factor?

(A) tumor thickness

(B) tumor diameter

(C) tumor location

(D) the patient's gender

(E) mitotic rate

378. A 62-year-old woman experiences frequent episodes of ptosis, diplopia, and generalized fatigue. The only abnormality on physical examination is an oculomotor nerve palsy, which transiently corrects with the administration of edrophonium. Which of the following medications is used to treat this disorder?

(A) curare

(B) neostigmine

(C) quinidine

(D) ether

(E) succinylcholine

Answers and Explanations

235–237. **(235-A, 236-B, 237-E)** The heliotrope, purple periorbital rash is seen with dermatomyositis and may even precede the muscle involvement. On exam, these patients will usually show proximal muscle weakness and may complain of difficulty getting up from a chair, climbing stairs, and raising the arms over the head. Ataxia may be present with cerebellar lesions. Deep tendon reflexes should be normal and there is no joint inflammation. Polymyalgia rheumatica also occurs in older people but is not associated with muscle weakness. Spinocerebellar degeneration, vasculitis, and rheumatoid arthritis are not associated with this rash. Creatine phosphokinase is usually markedly elevated, and muscle biopsy will confirm the diagnosis. Serum creatinine, sodium, and potassium should be normal, and rheumatoid factor should not be elevated. *(Schumacher, pp 127–131)*

238. **(A)** Ciprofloxacin is the drug of choice in a dose of 500 mg b.i.d. for 1 to 3 days since most cases of travelers' diarrhea are *Escherichia coli*. Erythromycin and tetracycline are effective for *Vibrio*. Cephalexin is not effective against *E coli* or gram-negative organisms. Metronidazole is used for *Clostridium difficile* enteritis. *(Hogan, pp 673–692)*

239. **(D)** Basal cell carcinoma is the most common form of skin cancer and can present as an isolated papule or nodule or with ulceration. Although locally aggressive and destructive, they rarely metastasize. The photo shows a large ulcer with a rodent-like appearance with nodules at the border. Squamous cell carcinoma would be in the differential, but it does not ulcerate as often and is characterized by being hard nodules. Malignant melanomas are usually nodular and pigmented. It would be highly unusual for a benign nevus to ulcerate and have this appearance. A hemangioma is a red vascular lesion. *(Fitzpatrick et al, pp 214–215)*

240–243. **(240-C, 241-A, 242-B, 243-E)** Patients at high risk include those with prior endocarditis, prosthetic heart valves, valvular heart disease, and congenital heart lesions. Too many women have mitral valve prolapse to make it cost-effective for prophylaxis. Congestive heart failure, an S_4 gallop, and diabetes do not increase risk. Recommended antibiotic coverage for high-risk patients prior to dental procedures is amoxicillin 2 gm PO 1 hour before. *Streptococcus* causes about 55% of cases of native valve endocarditis, *Staphylococcus* causes 30% of cases, and *Enterococcus* causes about 6% of cases. In drug abusers, *Staphylococcus aureus* is responsible for more than 50% of cases, and *Candida* and *Pseudomonas* for about 6% each. Penicillin-allergic patients should receive vancomycin and erythromycin. Patients with prior endocarditis are at high risk. Bacterial endocarditis carries a mortality rate of about 25%, and prevention is of paramount importance. As many as 40% of cases occur without underlying heart disease. Ventricular septal defect, patent ductus arteriosus, and tetralogy of Fallot are most commonly associated, whereas atrial septal defect is rarely a predisposing factor. *(Fauci et al, pp 785–791; Dajani, pp 1794–1801)*

244–246. (244-B, 245-D, 246-E) Marfan syndrome is an inherited disorder of connective tissue, but at least one fourth of patients do not have an affected parent. Abnormal metabolism of collagen or elastin is suspected as the cause. Clinical features involve the eyes (upward subluxation of the lenses, myopia), cardiovascular system (aortic dilation, regurgitation, and aneurysms; mitral valve prolapse), and the skeleton (arachnodactyly, pectus deformity, joint laxity). Mental retardation and malar rash are not associated with Marfan. A frequent finding is increased length of the limbs as compared with the trunk. Aortic root dilatation is a serious complication that can lead to aortic regurgitation, dissection, and even rupture. Mitral valve prolapse is also seen, but pulmonary stenosis, VSD, pulmonary hypertension, and CAD are not increased with Marfan. Echocardiography should be performed to follow the course of the heart. The other tests will not reveal aortic root dilatation or aneurysm formation. *(Fauci et al, pp 2192–2193)*

247. (A) After ileostomy, there is a predisposition to gallstone formation because of interference with the enterohepatic circulation of the bile acids. The most common metabolic consequence of ileostomy is salt and water depletion due to loss in the ileal fluid. Hyperkalemia and hypocalcemia do not occur. There is no increased risk for hepatitis or pancreatitis. There is an increased risk of developing stones, so patients need to be encouraged to drink more water. *(Yamada et al, p 799)*

248. (B) Constipation may be the initial manifestation of a variety of illnesses. Colonic tumors, polyps, and strictures may cause mechanical obstruction, but diverticulosis should not worsen constipation. Various medications, such as codeine, anticholinergics, and oral iron therapy may cause constipation. Antacids that contain magnesium decrease constipation. Systemic illnesses, including diabetes mellitus with autonomic neuropathy, Parkinson's disease, depression, and hypothyroidism may be uncovered. Thyrotoxicosis, however, is usually characterized by diarrhea. High dietary fiber intake should decrease constipation. Other causes to search for include painful abnormalities of the anal canal, physical inactivity, and inadequate hydration. *(Goroll et al, pp 369–372)*

249. (E) The x-ray in Figure 3–3 shows a large, pleural-based tumor in the left upper chest; this is most likely a mesothelioma. The tumor is locally invasive, so there are no signs of extrathoracic disease. Direct exposure or contact with asbestos is not required—tumors have occurred in families of asbestos workers. The exposure may be brief and mild, and there is typically a long latent period before appearance of the tumor, about 20 to 40 years. Surgery is curative in local cases. Diffuse malignant mesothelioma responds poorly to all treatments (surgery, radiotherapy, and chemotherapy). *(Goroll et al, pp 240–241)*

250. (A) Mitral valve prolapse can be diagnosed by auscultation and echocardiogram in as much as 10% of the population. They may be asymptomatic or complain of atypical chest pain, palpitation, shortness of breath, or weakness. An increasing number of complications are being recognized. Although they occur infrequently, they may be life threatening and demand careful evaluation of individuals at risk. Both supraventricular and ventricular arrhythmias occur, as may sudden death. Mitral insufficiency, if present, is usually insignificant but may progress and require valve replacement. There is an increased risk of infective endocarditis. Intra-atrial thrombus formation may occur, predisposing to cerebral and peripheral embolism. Because the clot originates in the left atrium, however, pulmonary embolism does not occur more frequently in these patients. *(Fauci et al, pp 1316–1317)*

251. (A) The autopsy specimen illustrated in Figure 3–4 contains a large, multicolored, irregular tumor invading the left hemisphere. There is hemorrhage, necrosis, and surrounding edema. The clinical and pathologic findings are most compatible with a diagnosis of malignant glioma (astrocytoma). Glioma is a highly malignant tumor of astrocytic cells and is the most common primary brain tumor. It infiltrates widely, often involving multiple lobes, as well as the opposite hemisphere via the corpus callosum. Prognosis is poor, with an average survival time of 6 months after diagnosis. Meningiomas are benign primary brain tumors that are usually slow growing and occur outside of the hemispheres, where they are well encapsulated and compress but do not invade brain tissue. Craniopharyngiomas arise from remnants of Rathke's pouch (the craniopharyngeal anlage). They are usually benign, well encapsulated, and found in or near the sella turcica. Acoustic neuromas arise from the root of the eighth cranial nerve in the cerebellopontine angle. Like meningiomas, they are encapsulated and compress rather than invade brain substance. *(Fauci et al, pp 2398–2404)*

252. **(D)** The history of severe, self-induced weight loss with an abnormal attitude toward food, weight, and body image in an adolescent female strongly suggests anorexia nervosa. Common symptoms are amenorrhea, not menorrhagia or metrorrhagia, constipation, and cold intolerance. Examination frequently reveals cachexia, hypothermia, bradycardia, hypotension, hypercarotenemic skin, and increased lanugo-like body hair. Decreased thyroid and pituitary function are evident on laboratory tests, but thrombocytopenia and anemia are not common. *(Goroll et al, pp 1073–1076)*

253–254. **(253-D, 254-B)** Hypercalcemia is a common complication of malignancy. Mechanisms include bone metastases, humoral secretion (eg, osteoclast-activating factor), prostaglandin, or ectopic parathormone production and immobilization. Hypercalcemia is often manifested by confusion and lethargy. The other metabolic abnormalities usually are not associated with confusion. Therapy is directed at increasing renal calcium clearance and inhibiting further bone resorption. Saline infusion raises the glomerular filtration rate and decreases calcium reabsorption in the proximal tubule. Under life-threatening circumstances, the infusion may need to be aggressive, as much as 6 L of sa-

line daily plus furosemide. Radiotherapy will do nothing for the calcium. Tamoxifen is an antiestrogen used in the treatment of breast carcinoma and other malignancies. When used in the presence of bone metastases, it may contribute to hypercalcemia. Chemotherapy will not decrease the calcium levels. Glucocorticoids have an antitumor effect and reduce tumor production of humoral mediators, but act slowly. *(Fauci et al, pp 2233–2240)*

255. **(C)** He should avoid alcohol and spicy foods because these along with the heat, emotional stress, and hot temperature foods can aggravate rosacea. Hydralazine is a vasodilator and could worsen his nasal erythema. Smoking vasoconstricts rather than dilates blood vessels. Metronidazole gel is an effective topical therapy. Laser therapy is usually done after the other interventions have been tried. *(Fitzpatrick et al, pp 14–15)*

256. **(E)** Hypertriglyceridemia has not been proved to be an independent risk factor for the development of premature CAD. Because low HDL levels are associated with premature CAD, hypertriglyceridemia is at least indirectly a risk factor for CAD. Severely elevated triglycerides (> 1000 mg/100 mL) are a recognized risk factor for attacks of acute pancreatitis, and control of the triglycerides can prevent these attacks. Diet alone is usually not sufficient at these high levels. A National Institutes of Health Consensus Conference has recommended that treatment be initiated in all patients with triglycerides greater than 500 mg/100 mL to prevent acute pancreatitis. Skin lesions are not present with hypertriglyceridemia. *(Second report of the National Cholesterol Education Program Expert Panel on Detection, Evaluation and Treatment of High Blood Cholesterol in Adults, pp IV–7)*

257. **(B)** Many drugs require dosage modifications in chronic renal insufficiency. Bioavailability, distribution, action, and elimination of drugs all may be altered. The aminoglycosides, vancomycin, ampicillin, most cephalosporins, methicillin, penicillin G, sulfonamides, and trimethoprim all should be given in reduced dosage to patients with chronic

renal failure. The small group of antibiotics not needing dosage modification includes chloramphenicol, erythromycin, and the isoxazolyl penicillins (nafcillin and oxacillin). *(Fauci et al, pp 415–416)*

258. **(C)** Chronic renal failure treated with hemodialysis results in predictable metabolic abnormalities. The kidneys fail to excrete phosphate, leading to hyperphosphatemia, and fail to synthesize $1,25(OH)_2D_3$. Vitamin D deficiency causes impaired intestinal calcium absorption. Phosphate retention, defective intestinal absorption, and skeletal resistance to parathyroid hormone all result in hypocalcemia. Hypocalcemia causes secondary hyperparathyroidism, and the excess parathyroid hormone production worsens the hyperphosphatemia by increasing phosphorus release from bone. These derangements impair collagen synthesis and maturation, resulting in skeletal abnormalities collectively referred to as renal osteodystrophy. Osteomalacia, osteosclerosis, and osteitis fibrosa cystica may all be seen. *(Fauci et al, pp 1516–1519)*

259. **(E)** Transdermal estrogen avoids the first-pass hepatic metabolism and may attenuate the increase in triglycerides. Risk of the other complications probably is not affected by route of administration. The most serious complication of estrogen replacement is endometrial cancer associated with endometrial hyperplasia. This is ameliorated by concomitant use of progesterone. Estrogen use may also increase the risk of developing breast cancer. Estrogen stimulates hepatic synthesis of renin substrate, resulting in elevated levels of angiotensin I and aldosterone. The hypertension that results is usually reversible if the drug is discontinued. *(Fauci et al, p 2113)*

260. **(A)** Diabetes insipidus, a deficiency of pituitary antidiuretic hormone (ADH) (arginine vasopressin), causes water loss due to failure to facilitate reabsorption of water in the distal tubules and collecting ducts of the kidneys. In central diabetes insipidus, there is impaired production of vasopressin, and in nephrogenic diabetes insipidus, the distal re-

nal tubules are refractory to vasopressin. In central diabetes insipidus, urine osmolality remains unchanged. If water intoxication were present, stopping IV fluids should have increased urine osmolality. With solute overload, serum osmolality would have been higher. In SIADH, urine osmolality is usually higher than serum osmolality. *(Fauci et al, pp 2004–2007)*

261. **(C)** Persons with the type A behavior pattern constantly strive to achieve or do more and more in less time and are often involved in interpersonal conflicts. Their personality traits include competitiveness, aggressiveness, ambition, and impatience coupled with a strong sense of time urgency. Although some studies have suggested that type A behavior is a risk factor for CAD, many others have not. The National Cholesterol Education Program has defined LDL cholesterol levels above 160 mg/100 mL as high risk and HDL cholesterol levels below 35 mg/100 mL as a risk factor. This program has also defined as risk factors a family history of CAD before the age of 55 years in father or other first-degree relative. Type O blood has no correlation with CAD. *(Second report of the National Cholesterol Education Program Expert Panel on Detection, Evaluation and Treatment of High Blood Cholesterol in Adults, pp I 9–13)*

262. **(D)** Postmenopausal estrogen replacement therapy has many proven benefits. It alleviates hot flashes and decreases vaginal dryness, leading to less vaginal infection. It retards bone loss but does not actually increase bone density. However, its use without adding a progestin is definitely attended by an estimated two- to eightfold increase in endometrial cancer. If anything, it decreases stroke risk. Although still controversial, there is probably a slight increase in breast cancer with long-term use. *(Goroll et al, pp 623–625)*

263. **(A)** Viral (follicular) conjunctivitis most often presents with minimal discharge and itching as compared to the moderate to profuse discharge of bacterial conjunctivitis. While mild pain and photophobia may be noted in viral, bacterial, fungal, and allergic conjunctivitis,

preauricular adenopathy is common in viral and fungal conjunctivitis only. Allergic conjunctivitis presents with minimal discharge and marked itching. The patient's young age and normal eye pressure (tonometry) helps to rule out glaucoma. *(Goroll et al, pp 956–957)*

264. **(C)** The clinical features of the patient described in the question are most compatible with ankylosing spondylitis, an inflammatory arthritis that occurs most often in young men. Early findings of low back pain and stiffness may progress to involve the entire spine with straightening (poker spine). The most common extraskeletal manifestation is acute anterior iridocyclitis, occurring in 25 to 30% of patients. Additional manifestations, which occur rarely, include heart block, aortitis with aortic insufficiency, and upper-lobe pulmonary fibrosis. Splenomegaly is associated with rheumatoid arthritis (Felty syndrome) but is not a feature of ankylosing spondylitis, nor are cataracts. *(Schumacher, pp 154–156)*

265–266. **(265-D, 266-D)** This ECG reveals ST segment elevation in II, III, and AVF, indicating acute injury of the inferior wall of the myocardium. Inferior wall ischemia can be perceived as pain in the epigastric area. Anterolateral myocardial infarction would show loss of R wave progression in V_4 through V_6. Although his symptoms could suggest gastroesophageal reflux or gastroenteritis, this ECG shows this a cardiac event. Costochondritis is not present by exam. When ST segment elevation is present, a patient should be considered a candidate for reperfusion therapy. If no contraindications are present, thrombolytic therapy should ideally be initiated within 30 minutes, right in the emergency department. The goal of thrombolysis is prompt restoration of coronary arterial patency. Thrombolytic therapy can reduce the risk of in-hospital death by up to 50% when administered within the first hour of symptoms, so time is of the essence. Arranging for a bed may waste time for limiting infarct size. Catheterization can be performed later when the patient is stable. The ECG would obviously preclude the other two options:

immediate trial of antacid or reassurance and arranging outpatient follow-up. *(Fauci et al, pp 1356–1357)*

267. **(D)** Altered mental status is a poor prognostic sign in community-acquired pneumonia. Other patient factors include age greater than 65 years, systolic BP less than 90 or diastolic pressure less than 60 mm Hg, temperature greater than 38.3°C, and leukocytosis greater than 30,000/mm or less than 4000/mm. *Streptococcus pneumoniae, Legionella*, and *Staphylococcus aureus* are the pathogens associated with poor prognosis, not *Mycoplasma*. *(Bartlett and Mundy, pp 1618–1624)*

268. **(E)** Up to 30% of cases of acquired vitiligo are associated with thyroid disease, especially Hashimoto's thyroiditis. It also may occur with pernicious anemia, diabetes, and other autoimmune disorders. Vitiligo has not been reported with AIDS. Addison's disease, lymphoma, and biliary cirrhosis can be associated with hyperpigmentation. *(Goroll et al, p 894)*

269. **(B)** Adenocarcinoma of the pancreas arises from ductal epithelium. Because of fibrous tissue formation, the terminal bile duct occludes, causing jaundice. Typically, in the early stages, the patient is free of pain. With invasion of retroperitoneal structures, the patient may sometimes have severe and constant pain. Often, patients have a history of weight loss and present with unexplained diabetes. Because of gradual obstruction, the gallbladder distends, unless it has lost its distensibility due to previous scarring. Malignant biliary stricture, choledocholithiasis, and cirrhosis of the liver are ruled out by the appearance of the CT. Pancreatitis is rarely associated with jaundice and would be painful. *(Goroll et al, pp 438–439)*

270. **(A)** The spectrum of infection with *Legionella* organisms ranges from asymptomatic seroconversion to Pontiac fever (a flu-like illness) to full-blown pneumonia. Cough is usually nonproductive initially. Malaise, myalgia, and headache are common. The diagnosis of *Legionella* infection is suggested by extrapulmo-

nary signs and symptoms, including diarrhea, abdominal pain, azotemia, and hematuria. *(Fauci et al, pp 928–931)*

271. **(A)** The causes of lower gastrointestinal (GI) bleeding include hemorrhoids and anal fissure diverticulosis, carcinoma, vascular ectasia, colitis, and polyps. Carcinoma of the colon usually causes chronic GI bleeding, resulting in anemia. Diverticulosis and vascular ectasia are common causes of massive GI bleeding in the elderly. Inflammatory bowel disease can also cause massive GI bleeding but is more frequent in younger-age-group patients. Most of the patients with ischemic colitis will be quite sick and will have had symptoms prior to the onset of bleeding. *(Fauci et al, p 247)*

272. **(C)** The clinical features of the patient described in the question are characteristic of rhabdomyolysis with myoglobinuria. Skeletal muscle injury releases large amounts of myoglobin into the circulation, and myoglobinuria produces a positive ortho-toluidine reaction. Because myoglobin is quickly cleared from serum by the kidneys, the serum does not turn pink, as it does with hemoglobinemia. Muscle damage leads to elevated creatine phosphokinase levels and hyperkalemia. Myoglobin does not bind to haptoglobin as does hemoglobin, so serum haptoglobin levels are normal. The major complication of rhabdomyolysis is acute renal failure. *(Fauci et al, pp 1510, 1517)*

273. **(B)** Heart sounds and murmurs can often be accentuated by various physiologic and pharmacologic maneuvers. These maneuvers aid in the differentiation of multiple valvular and other organic lesions from ordinary sounds. Mitral stenosis is a diastolic murmur that grows louder with increased flow across the stenotic valve, as in exercise. A VSD may be small; its murmur will fade with maneuvers favoring forward flow, such as vasodilatation with amyl nitrate. The murmur of aortic stenosis will grow louder with increased flow across the valve, as with amyl nitrate; it will diminish with maneuvers that decrease flow across the valve, as in stage

two of the Valsalva maneuver. *(Hurst, pp 175–242)*

274–275. **(274-D, 275-E)** *H pylori* infection is present in nearly 100% of uncomplicated duodenal ulcers. Studies show that its eradication effects a cure and reduces recurrence from 80% to 10% in one year. Nonsteroidal use contributes to gastric, not duodenal ulcer. Stress probably plays a minor role in the pathogenesis of ulcer. There are increased gastrin levels with *H pylori* infection, but gastrin-secreting tumors are quite rare. *C difficile* is an antibiotic-related enterocolitis. Eradication of *H pylori* requires antibiotic treatment in combination with a proton pump inhibitor. Clarithromycin is probably most effective, although metronidazole and tetracycline are alternatives. Amoxicillin has unacceptably low success rates and should not be the first line. Antacids and H_2 blockers alone are not as effective for preventing recurrence. *(Laine et al, pp 2106–2112)*

276. **(C)** The CT scan shown in Figure 3–9 demonstrates a smooth, biconvex lens–shaped mass in the periphery of the right temporoparietal region. This picture is characteristic of a subdural hematoma that is a result of laceration of veins bridging the subdural space. Unlike an epidural hematoma, which ex- pands quickly and progresses rapidly to coma, a subdural hematoma is initially limited in size by increased intracranial pressure and expands slowly. Symptoms may follow the inciting trauma by several weeks. Altered mental status is often more prominent than focal signs and may progress from confusion to stupor to coma. Treatment consists of evacuation of the clot via burr holes. Antibiotics and antifungal agents have no role, and fibrinolytic therapy or delay in treatment could be harmful. *(Fauci et al, pp 2392–2393)*

277. **(C)** The history and physical examination of the patient described in the question suggest either an intracerebral hemorrhage or a completed ischemic stroke. The CT scan that accompanies the question demonstrates a large hemorrhage in the region of the right basal ganglia with a surrounding zone of edema

and narrowing of the ventricle. Patients with intracerebral hemorrhage often have a preceding history of hypertension. Carotid occlusion, malignancy, arteriovenous malformation, and coagulopathy all are much less likely causes of this disorder. In general, only cerebellar hemorrhages and cerebral hemorrhages that are easily reached are surgically evacuated. Most intracerebral hemorrhages are managed with general supportive care. *(Fauci et al, pp 2342–2344)*

278. **(B)** The new Joint National Committee on Prevention, Detection, Evaluation, and Treatment of High Blood Pressure guidelines recommend initiating drug therapy for pressure as low as 130/85 for patients with diabetes, heart failure, or renal insufficiency. Family history of heart disease is not included. Weight loss for obesity, high cholesterol reduction, and smoking cessation would be part of the recommended lifestyle changes. *(Joint National Committee)*

279. **(B)** The arteriograms in Figure 3–11 demonstrate a large aneurysm arising from the basilar artery. Intracranial aneurysms occasionally present with new onset or worsening of headaches or may be asymptomatic and found coincidentally during evaluation of an unrelated disorder. Frequently, they leak or rupture, resulting in a subarachnoid hemorrhage with sudden onset of severe headache and meningeal symptoms and signs (eg, nuchal rigidity, photophobia). Rapid progression to stroke, coma, or death may follow. Intracranial aneurysms are not usually associated with hypercalcemia, hypopituitarism, or chronic meningitis and rarely cause tentorial herniation without rupturing. Surgical approaches to intracranial aneurysms include excision and ligation. *(Fauci et al, pp 2345–2347)*

280–282. **(280-A, 281-C, 282-E)** Sleep disturbance is a characteristic symptom associated with fibromyalgia. Patients awaken feeling tired. The exam, other than tenderness in 14 specific, symmetrical points, is usually normal. Fever, rash on the extremities, muscle weakness, and migratory joint inflammation point

to Lyme disease or other rheumatologic disorders. A sedimentation rate should be normal. If elevated, it may point to another diagnosis. Lyme titers are not indicated unless the patient has symptoms or history suggestive of the disease. Electromyelography and spine radiographs are typically normal and unnecessary for help in establishing the diagnosis. Depression can be associated with pain, but screening for it early on does not make sense and might offend the patient. Low-dose antidepressants often help to correct the sleep pattern and result in relief of pain. Nonsteroidal anti-inflammatory agents can also be used as needed; low-dose steroid is not indicated. Exercise is also helpful, and patients should be encouraged to stay physically active. Amoxicillin is not used for fibromyalgia. Benzodiazepines have addictive potential and lose their effectiveness for sleep after a few weeks. *(Goroll et al, pp 799–801)*

283. **(B)** The cerebral arteriogram shown in Figure 3–12 reveals severe stenosis of the common carotid artery proximal to its bifurcation, as well as small lesions in the more distal vessels. Common manifestations are transient monocular blindness (amaurosis fugax), hemiparesis, hemisensory loss, aphasia, and homonymous visual field defects. Ataxia would be an unusual feature of carotid disease and, if present, would suggest involvement of the vertebrobasilar arteries, which results in dysarthria, diplopia, and vertigo. *(Fauci et al, pp 2230–2232)*

284–285. **(284-E, 285-C)** The new case definition for AIDS in 1993 added pulmonary tuberculosis, invasive cervical cancer, and recurrent pneumonia. This Centers for Disease Control and Prevention (CDC) classification system is divided into three categories: category A is symptomatic infection with HIV and includes acute illness and persistent lymphadenopathy; category B includes conditions attributed to HIV infection, such as oral thrush, herpes zoster, and peripheral neuropathy; category C is the AIDS surveillance cases. Anergy to common skin test antigens is a common finding with HIV infection. There is a decline in CD4 cell numbers, a relative increase in the number of T_8 cells, which results in a decreased T_4/T_8 ratio of less than 1. Functional abnormalities occur in both B cells and natural killer cells, which accounts for the increase in certain bacterial infections seen in advanced HIV disease. Elevation of $beta_2$ sub-microglobulin, a serologic finding reflecting immunologic dysfunction, is a fairly reliable marker of progressive immunologic decline and the subsequent development of AIDS. *(Fauci et al, pp 1808–1813)*

286. **(C)** This man has multiple seborrheic keratoses, which are very common, benign pigmented tumors that occur after age 30, especially on the trunk and face. Melanocytic nevi are usually small, circumscribed, pigmented macules or papules, rather than large "stuck-on" nodules. Actinic keratoses are red, scaly (not dark) lesions on the face and arms that are from sun-induced damage. Seborrheic dermatitis is a red, scaly rash along the scalp, eyebrows, and nasolabial folds. Malignant melanoma would be in the differential if it were a single lesion. *(Fitzpatrick et al, pp 168–169)*

287–288. **(287-B, 288-B)** The wide notched R waves in V_5 and V_6 are characteristic for LBBB. In RBBB, there is an rSR' complex in V_1 and qRS pattern in V_6. Accelerated junctional rhythm would not have p waves. Partial blocks, such as left anterior fascicular block, generally do not prolong the QRS duration substantially, but are associated with shifts in the frontal plane QRS axis (left axis deviation). With intraventricular conduction delay, the QRS is between 100 and 120 msec. LBBB is a marker of one of four conditions; severe aortic valve disease, ischemic heart disease, long-standing hypertension, and cardiomyopathy. RBBB is seen more commonly than LBBB in patients without structural heart disease, although RBBB also occurs with congenital heart disease and atrial septal defect or valvular heart disease. Hyper- but not hypokalemia may cause intraventricular conduction delay. Myocarditis does not usually lead to LBBB. *(Fauci et al, pp 1241–1243)*

289. **(A)** Morning stiffness lasting more than 1 hour is characteristic of RA. Bilateral and symmetric metacarpophalangeal (not distal interphalangeal) joint involvement is very common. Some patients experience Raynaud's phenomenon, that is, blanching of the fingers on exposure to cold, but it is not diagnostic of RA. A facial rash in the malar region may be seen with SLE but not RA. Polymorphonuclear leukocytes predominate in synovial fluid from patients with RA. *(Schumacher, pp 90–95)*

290. **(B)** Primary hyperparathyroidism is characterized by hypercalcemia, hypophosphatemia, hyperchloremia, increased urinary calcium excretion, and an increase in serum parathormone level. Multiple myeloma is associated with hypercalcemia when there are many lytic lesions. Chronic ingestion of 50 to 100 times the normal requirement of vitamin D is required to produce hypercalcemia in normal people, so hypervitaminosis D is rare and parathormone levels would be suppressed. With milk alkali syndrome, which is due to excess ingestion of calcium and absorbable antacids, parathormone levels would also be suppressed. In sarcoidosis, about 10% of patients have hypercalcemia due to increased intestinal absorption of calcium and increased production of $1,25(OH)_2D$. *(Fauci et al, pp 2234–2237)*

291. **(B)** Because the symptoms are occurring in the winter, perennial or nonseasonal allergic rhinitis is the most likely cause. Dust mites, along with mold and animal danders, are major allergens in the home. Ragweed grows in late summer. Aerosol spray and cigarette smoke are pollutants that may be more irritating to allergic patients but also cause symptoms in nonatopic people. Houseplants are not a common source of allergy. *(Goroll et al, pp 1013–1015)*

292–293. **(292-C, 293-B)** Acute oliguria is a medical emergency requiring the immediate identification of any correctable cause. Distension of the urinary bladder indicates bladder outlet obstruction. Immediate management should be the passage of a urethral catheter to relieve the obstruction and provide urine for examination. An abdominal flat plate, ultrasonography, or IVP may yield a diagnosis but delay the relief of obstruction. Furosemide may be harmful if given while the bladder is obstructed. Bladder outlet obstruction may be caused by prostatic hypertrophy or prostatitis, stones, clots, malignancy, or urethral stricture; it may also be neurogenic. Posterior urethral valves are a congenital defect that could cause obstruction in children but rarely in adults. Renal carcinoma would not cause outlet obstruction. Renal arterial occlusion can cause acute renal failure but not obstructive uropathy. If urethral catheterization fails to relieve the obstruction, further evaluation, including radiographic or ultrasound studies, is in order. Suprapubic cystostomy may be necessary to empty the bladder. *(Fauci et al, pp 1574–1575)*

294. **(E)** Hashimoto's thyroiditis, an autoimmune condition, is the leading cause of multinodular goiter in the United States. Although not unique to this condition, antimicrosomal antibodies are found in 70 to 95% of patients. Antinuclear antibodies are associated with SLE. Although an autoimmune process, steroids are of no benefit in this condition. One third of patients experience progressive loss of glandular function, and eventually become hypothyroid, but there is no increased incidence of thyroid cancer. *(Goroll et al, p 530)*

295–296. **(295-D, 296-B)** Onset of fatigue, arthralgias, mucosal ulcerations, and facial rash in a young person strongly suggests SLE. Additional features of SLE are low-grade fever, alopecia, pericarditis, arthritis, nephritis, nervous system involvement, and pleural effusions. Women are affected 10 times more often than men. The lupus band test, demonstrating linear IgG and complement deposition at the dermal–epidermal junction, is positive in 90% of cases. However, it is not specific for SLE and may also be seen in bullous pemphigoid, dermatomyositis, and other autoimmune diseases. A positive reaction to the lupus band test on normal-appearing skin is helpful in diagnosis. Serum complement levels decline with disease flares and

are useful in guiding treatment, whereas the ESR often remains elevated during remissions and is an unreliable marker of disease activity. Many autoantibodies are positive in patients with SLE, but anti-Sm is most specific for SLE. Antinuclear antibodies (ANA) are positive in 98% of patients with SLE, so is a sensitive test, but not specific. Anti-RNP is present in 40% of patients and anti-Ro in 30%. Antihistone is positive in 95% of patients with drug-induced lupus. *(Fauci et al, pp 1874–1877)*

297. **(C)** Hypercalcemia associated with malignancy could be the result of bone destruction from metastases (80%) or due to production of parathormone-like substance (20%). Metabolically active tumor secretions cause paraneoplastic syndromes. Hypercalcemia most frequently results from breast, lung, and renal carcinoma. Multiple myeloma is associated with hypercalcemia when there are many lytic lesions. Thiazide ingestion causes a transient increase in serum calcium in normal individuals that persists for about 1 week. Secondary hyperparathyroidism is a consequence of decreased renal function and is characterized by hypocalcemia and hyperphosphatemia, which lead to an increase in serum parathormone level. Prolonged immobilization is a rare cause of hypercalcemia in adults in the absence of underlying disease. *(Fauci et al, pp 2234–2237)*

298–300. **(298-D, 299-C, 300-B)** All of the chemotherapeutic agents listed have adverse effects, some mild and some potentially lethal. Antineoplastic drugs with serious toxicity are used only when the potential benefits outweigh the risks. The alkylating agent cyclophosphamide causes bone marrow depression, alopecia, hemorrhagic cystitis, and bladder tumors. Bleomycin, an antibiotic, causes pulmonary fibrosis in as many as 5% of patients. Another antibiotic, doxorubicin hydrochloride (Adriamycin), has a predictable cumulative cardiac toxicity. The alkaloid vincristine is neurotoxic, and is associated with areflexia, muscle weakness, peripheral neuritis, and paralytic ileus. Methotrexate, an antimetabolite, causes megaloblastic changes in bone marrow that may be prevented ("rescued") by giving folinic acid. *(Fauci et al, pp 527–535)*

301–303. (301-E, 302-E, 303-C) Diabetes insipidus, a deficiency of pituitary ADH (arginine vasopressin), causes water loss due to failure to facilitate reabsorption of water in the distal tubules and collecting ducts of the kidneys. In a water-deprived individual, the plasma osmolarity rises and all electrolytes become uniformly elevated. In the syndrome of inappropriate ADH secretion, which may follow a variety of conditions including head trauma, meningitis, or brain tumor, electrolytes are uniformly depressed. With diabetes and relative insulin deficiency, glucose is an effective osmole and draws water from cells, resulting in hyponatremia. Plasma Na concentration falls by 1.4 mmol/L for every 100 mg/dL rise in plasma glucose. The low CO_2 is from mild acidosis. In salt-losing adrenogenital syndrome, aldosterone production is blocked and there is profound sodium loss due to failure of reabsorption in the distal tubule of the kidney. There is marked potassium retention and chloride loss as well. Electrolytes in choice D are normal. *(Fauci et al, pp 268–271)*

304–306. (304-D, 305-A, 306-B) Many diseases are associated with and perhaps mediated by antibodies produced against normal cell components. SLE is associated with antibodies to several nuclear constituents, including DNA, RNA, histones, and nonhistone proteins. Antibodies to native DNA occur in 50 to 60% of patients. Primary biliary cirrhosis is a chronic progressive disease of middle-aged women and is characterized by cholestasis, jaundice, and xanthomatous eruptions. Antibodies to mitochondria are the hallmark of the disease and are found in 80 to 100% of cases. Myasthenia gravis is characterized by rapid fatigability of muscles. Mild forms may be limited to ocular muscles, whereas severe forms may be generalized. Antibodies to acetylcholine receptors are thought to be the underlying mechanism. Antibodies to parietal cells are found in pernicious anemia and idiopathic atrophic gastritis. Antibodies to smooth mus-

cle cells are found in 10 to 30% of patients with primary biliary cirrhosis, but in as many as 90% of patients with chronic active hepatitis. *(Coffey et al, pp 163–178)*

307–308. (307-E, 308-D) ABG determinations are essential in the diagnosis of respiratory and acid–base disturbances. Extremely obese patients suffer from increased work of breathing, as well as elevation of the diaphragm with decrease in lung volume. The resultant hypoventilation is characterized by carbon dioxide retention leading to chronic respiratory acidosis with metabolic compensation (ABG set E in the question). When associated with somnolence, excessive appetite, and polycythemia, this is known as the pickwickian syndrome. Modest weight loss can lead to dramatic improvement in respiratory functioning. The earliest derangement in salicylate poisoning is hyperventilation, resulting in decreased Pa_{CO_2} and increased arterial pH (ABG set D). Eventually, there is central nervous system (CNS) depression with somnolence and hypoventilation resulting in respiratory acidosis. ABG set A reflects acute respiratory acidosis (hypoventilation) without metabolic compensation. ABG set B is normal. ABG set C suggests metabolic acidosis with modest respiratory compensation. *(Kelley, pp 575–592)*

309–311. (309-C, 310-E, 311-A) All of the drugs used to treat hypertension can cause adverse reactions, ranging from trivial to life threatening. Thiazide diuretics are associated with hypokalemia, causing arrhythmias; hyperuricemia, causing gout; and hyperglycemia, causing clinical diabetes. The vasodilator hydralazine can cause tachycardia with increased angina, tachycardia, and a lupus-like syndrome. As many as 10% of patients on an angiotensin-converting enzyme (ACE) inhibitor develop an annoying dry cough. Because they block aldosterone, they can lead to hyperkalemia. Renal failure has been noted with underlying kidney disease, such as bilateral renal artery stenosis. Coombs'-positive hemolytic anemia and hepatitis are idiosyncratic reactions to the central adrenergic stimulant methyldopa. *(Goroll et al, pp 128–133)*

312–314. (312-C, 313-B, 314-A) There is no known association between a family history of Hashimoto's thyroiditis, or a personal or family history of Graves' disease and thyroid carcinoma. A hyperfunctioning nodule is rarely malignant. Cystic nodules are less likely to be malignant than solid nodules. Childhood neck or head irradiation clearly predisposes to thyroid malignancies. Papillary is the most common type of thyroid carcinoma, accounting for about 70% of all tumors. It has a bimodal frequency with peaks in the second and third decades and then later in life. Follicular carcinomas comprise 15% of all carcinomas, and anaplastic are the least common, about 5% of tumors. Lymphoma also constitutes about 5% of all thyroid malignancies. Medullary carcinomas occur in less than 0.5% of thyroid nodules. Eighty percent of medullary carcinomas are sporadic, but 20% are familial and may be part of the multiple endocrine neoplasia (MEN) syndrome. Calcitonin levels correlate with tumor burden and serve as a marker for residual disease after treatment. *(Fauci et al, pp 2030–2031)*

315–316. (315-D, 316-C) Toxin-producing *Staphylococcus aureus* organisms have been implicated in the pathogenesis of toxic shock syndrome (TSS) and are frequently cultured from the vagina and cervix of affected women. There is no diagnostic laboratory test, and diagnosis is based on the typical clinical findings. Diffuse macular erythroderma (sunburn-like rash) occurs in the first few days of illness, followed by desquamation, usually of the palms and soles 1 to 2 weeks later. Fever, hypotension, and multiorgan-system involvement (GI, CNS, muscular, renal, hepatic, hematologic) are also part of the case definition. Platelet counts are usually reduced below 100,000. Disorientation may occur but without focal neurologic signs like hyperreflexia. Complications include shock, arrhythmias, renal failure, respiratory failure, and coagulopathy. Hypercalcemia is not a part of the picture. *(Fauci et al, pp 877–879)*

317. (B) Rheumatic fever is diagnosed on the basis of its typical clinical features. Major criteria include polyarthritis, carditis, subcutaneous nodules, a characteristic rash (erythema marginatum), and involuntary movements (Sydenham's chorea). Minor criteria are fever, arthralgia, previous rheumatic fever, elevated sedimentation rate, prolonged PR interval on ECG, and leukocytosis. Evidence of recent streptococcal infection is required. Elevated serum antistreptolysin, hyaluronidase, and DNase B titers can be found in 95% of cases. A positive throat culture or history of scarlet fever may also be obtained. *(Fink and Fauci, pp 2716–2721)*

318. (D) Any medication that inhibits dopamine synthesis, release, or action may give rise to hyperprolactinemia, although usually not at levels above 100 μg/L. Dopamine probably functions as a hypothalamic inhibitory factor for prolactin secretion. Bromocriptine, a dopamine agonist, would decrease prolactin levels and is used to treat microadenomas. A common culprit for hyperprolactinemia are the phenothiazines. SSRIs primarily affect serotonin and do not inhibit dopamine. Although high doses of estrogen can cause hyperprolactinemia, oral contraceptives with low estrogen doses do not. *(Fauci et al, pp 1974–1978)*

319. (B) Diabetes mellitus is associated with hyperglycemia, disease of the microvasculature (retinopathy, nephropathy, neuropathy) and large-vessel disease. Severe peripheral vascular disease is also common. The Diabetes Control and Complications Trial demonstrated that tight control can decrease complications of microvascular disease significantly, but does not appear to affect coronary artery disease. *(Diabetes Control and Complications Trial Research Group, pp 977–986)*

320. (D) Whipple's disease is a systemic illness characterized by arthralgias, diarrhea, abdominal pain, and weight loss. The usual patient is a middle-aged white male. Reported in 1907 by George Whipple, it has been associated with a bacillus, which has only recently been identified. The disease can affect nearly every organ system, although it usually involves the GI tract, heart, and CNS. Renal failure is not a common complication. *(Relman et al, pp 293–301)*

321–322. (321-B, 322-A) Hepatic encephalopathy is a syndrome of declining intellectual function, altered state of consciousness, and neurologic abnormalities in the setting of advanced liver disease. Other findings include hyperactivity, delirium, agitation, and personality changes, progressing to confusion, somnolence, and coma. Asterixis (lapses of sustained muscle contraction) or "flapping tremor" is common. Jaundice, spider angiomas, and ascites can be present in alcoholic liver disease without the presence of encephalopathy. Precipitating factors must be looked for and reversed if possible. GI bleeding (due to esophageal varices, gastritis, ulcer, and so forth) increases the nitrogen load in the gut and reduces cerebral perfusion. Excessive diuresis with prerenal azotemia increases extrahepatic circulation of urea and ammonia production, so noncompliance with diuretics would decrease ammonia levels. Lactulose acidifies the stool, traps ammonia and other nitrogenous substances, and decreases their absorption from the gut so excessive lactulose would decrease ammonia levels. Excessive protein intake is a common precipitant. *(Fauci et al, pp 1715–1717)*

323. (D) *Campylobacter jejuni* is now recognized as a very common cause of gastroenteritis, at least as common as *Salmonella* and *Shigella* organisms. Typical features of *Campylobacter* gastroenteritis are fever, diarrhea, abdominal pain, bloody stools, and constitutional symptoms. Laboratory findings, including Gram stain of the stool, are nonspecific. The organism is identified on stool culture. Human infection is most likely caused by improperly prepared or contaminated food. Fewer than half of patients will benefit from antibiotics. The drug of choice is clarithromycin, azithromycin, or erythromycin, with ciprofloxacin as an alternate. The most frequent cause of travelers' diarrhea is enteropathogenic *Escherichia coli. (Fauci et al, pp 960–962)*

324. (E) The barium enema x-ray shown in Figure 3-15 reveals multiple sigmoid diverticuli. Most cases of colonic diverticular disease do not require surgery, even for active GI bleeding. Colonoscopy is not necessary unless the barium enema reveals additional lesions or the diagnosis is in doubt. Histamine H_2 receptor antagonists such as cimetidine and ranitidine are useful for treating peptic ulcer disease but not for diverticulosis. Rectal corticosteroid enemas have a role in inflammatory bowel disease, but not in diverticular disease. Appropriate management of the acute attack consists of bedrest, liquid diet, and perhaps anticholinergics. Thereafter, a high-fiber diet should be prescribed to help prevent further recurrences. Bran, raw vegetables, legumes, and hydrophilic colloids such as psyllium seed derivatives are all useful. *(Fauci et al, pp 1648–1649)*

325. (E) The Gram stain is positive in three fourths of bacterial meningitis cases. Leukocyte counts average between 5,000 and 20,000; CSF pressure is consistently elevated usually above 180 mm H_2O; glucose levels are usually lower than 40 mg/dL, or less than 40% of blood glucose; and protein levels are higher than 45 mg/dL in 90% of cases. *(Fauci et al, pp 2423–2424)*

326. (D) *Streptococcus pneumoniae* is the most common cause of adult meningitis in people over 30 and accounts for about 15% of cases. *Hemophilus influenzae* is the most common cause in children over a month old. Group B *Streptococcus* is an important cause of neonatal meningitis, but is very rare in adults. *Staphylococcus, E coli,* and *Klebsiella* may be seen with penetrating head wounds or postneurosurgical procedures. *(Fauci et al, pp 2420–2421)*

327. (E) Although *Listeria* still represents only a fraction of total cases (about 10%) of meningitis, it is seen in diabetes and cancer patients, alcoholics, the elderly, and the immunocompromised. *(Fauci et al, p 2420)*

328. (B) The chest x-ray shown in Figure 3–16 contains multiple bilateral pulmonary parenchymal nodules varying in size and shape, most compatible with metastatic disease to the lungs. Other possibilities are bronchogenic carcinoma or fungal granulomas (eg, histoplasmosis or coccidiosis). Sarcoidosis usually presents with bilateral hilar adenopathy and rarely with multiple pulmonary nodules. Tuberculosis presents with a cavitating lesion, pleural effusion, or miliary pattern. Typical findings in silicosis are diffuse nodular fibrosis and eggshell calcification of hilar or bronchopulmonary lymph nodes. The chest x-ray of patients with mycoplasma pneumonia usually shows patchy infiltrates involving the lower lobes and spreading from the hila. The finding of metastatic nodules on chest x-ray should prompt a search for the primary tumor. *(Fauci et al, p 1409)*

329. **(C)** The chest x-ray shown in Figure 3–17 shows a diffuse reticulonodular pattern consistent with interstitial lung disease. The hilar nodes are enlarged, suggesting lymphadenopathy. This is a nonspecific picture and may be caused by a large number of diseases. Occupational exposure to dust, gas, or fumes; sarcoidosis; idiopathic pulmonary fibrosis; and lung disease associated with the rheumatic diseases are the more common factors. Despite the diverse causes, there is a common pathogenesis: Injury leads to alveolitis, which progresses to fibrosis. Abnormalities on pulmonary function testing are also similar: restrictive disease characterized by decreased lung volumes (vital capacity, total lung capacity) and decreased compliance. Loss of the alveolar capillary bed leads to decreased carbon monoxide diffusing capacity. Arterial oxygen pressure (PaO_2) may be normal at rest but is decreased with exercise. Arterial carbon dioxide pressure ($PaCO_2$) may be normal or decreased because of hyperventilation, but it is not usually elevated in pure interstitial lung disease. *(Fauci et al, pp 1412–1413)*

330. **(D)** Purified polysaccharide pneumococcal vaccine contains capsular material from 14 types of *Streptococcus pneumoniae*, which account for 68% of bacteremic pneumococcal disease. Adults show an antibody rise in 2 to 3 weeks that lasts at least 3 to 5 years. Erythema and pain at the injection site are common, but severe adverse reactions are extremely rare. On the other hand, second doses commonly result in severe local and systemic reactions and are generally not advisable. Patients at high risk for pneumococcal infection, those with sickle cell disease, myeloma, asplenia, immunosuppression, or major organ system failure should receive the vaccine, although their antibody response may not be as strong as in normal adults. Protection is incomplete, and any vaccine recipient may still develop pneumococcal infection. *(Fauci et al, pp 874–875)*

331. **(E)** The spectrum of infection with *Legionella* organisms ranges from asymptomatic seroconversion to Pontiac fever (a flu-like illness) to full-blown pneumonia. Cough is usually nonproductive initially. Malaise, myalgia, and headache are common. The diagnosis of *Legionella* infection is suggested by extrapulmonary signs and symptoms, including diarrhea, abdominal pain, azotemia, and hematuria. *(Fauci et al, pp 928–931)*

332. **(E)** Patients with advanced chronic obstructive pulmonary disease (COPD) are at risk for development of acute respiratory failure. Common precipitants are infections, increased secretions, and superimposed bronchospasm. Oxygen therapy is effective in reversing the hypoxemia associated with respiratory failure. A risk of such therapy peculiar to patients with COPD is worsening hypercapnia. Affected patients are thought to have lost their respiratory center's sensitivity to hypercapnia, so that their primary stimulus to breathe is hypoxemia. When the hypoxemia is corrected, they may lose their stimulus to breathe and develop carbon dioxide narcosis with worsening acidosis, confusion, stupor, and eventually coma. Because of this, the usual approach is to begin with a low fraction of inspired oxygen (FIO_2) and increase gradually. Serial ABGs are obtained to ensure that as PaO_2 improves, $PaCO_2$ does not increase. In some cases, even the lowest FIO_2 causes carbon dioxide retention, and mechanical ventilation is required. In the

case presented in the question, a lower F_{IO_2} should be used before mechanical ventilation is initiated. *(Fauci et al, pp 1458–1459)*

333–335. (333-D, 334-C, 335-B) Testicular cancer is the most common cancer in men between the ages of 20 and 40. Predisposing factors include cryptorchidism, hernias, and testicular atrophy. Abdominal testes are at higher risk than inguinal cryptorchid testes. Family history of testicular or prostate cancer, radiation exposure, or maternal DES appear to play no role. Testicular cancers are divided into non-seminoma and seminoma subtypes. Seminoma represents about 50% of all tumors and generally follows a more indolent course. The primary tumor is treated by inguinal orchiectomy regardless of cell type. Pure seminomas do not require retroperitoneal lymph node dissection because radiation is usually adequate therapy. Nonseminomatous testicular tumors (embryonal cell, teratocarcinoma, choriocarcinoma, endodermal sinus) are usually treated by retroperitoneal dissection. Serum alpha-fetoprotein (AFP) and hCG levels are markers that are important for diagnosis and as prognostic indicators and are used to monitor therapy. Serum LDH level is often elevated with bulky tumors but is not as specific as either AFP or hCG. CEA is a nonspecific marker elaborated by many adenocarcinomas. PSA is a marker associated with prostate cancer. *(Fauci et al, pp 602–603)*

336. (A) Aldosterone secretion results in retention of Na^+ and loss of K^+. Na^+ is exchanged for K^+ and H^+ in the distal tubule and transferred out of the lumen into the tubular cells. The Na^+ retention leads to an increase in blood volume, causing a reduction in the secretion of renin. Aldosterone is primarily regulated by the renin–angiotensin system. *(Kelley, pp 272–273)*

337. (D) In the patient described in the question, the movement of the trachea to the left suggests a difference between right and left pleural pressures, either a reduction in pressure on the left or a rise in pressure on the right. The acute onset of right-sided chest pain in an otherwise healthy young man sug-

gests a pneumothorax. On the side of the pneumothorax, one would expect increased resonance and distant breath sounds because of the air trapped in the pleural space between the lung and chest wall. No rales or rhonchi would be expected. A pleural friction rub suggests an inflammatory process involving the left chest, a finding not likely on the basis of the patient's presentation. *(Fauci et al, p 1475)*

338. (B) Congestion secondary to left ventricular failure may lead to pulmonary edema. Failure of the right side of the heart results in peripheral edema and jugular venous distension, and liver enzymes may be elevated secondary to liver congestion. *(Fauci et al, p 1288)*

339. (C) The usual early hemodynamic response to sepsis is a hyperdynamic circulation. This includes tachycardia, elevated cardiac output, and decreased systemic resistance. Septic shock may then progress with intractable hypotension, metabolic acidosis, reduced cardiac output, and death. *(Dixon and Parrillo, pp 1197–1214)*

340. (D) Spouses of individuals infected with hepatitis B virus have approximately a 20 to 30% chance of contracting hepatitis B infection presumably transmitted during sexual contact. Children are at much less risk for hepatitis B infection. The major route of transmission in developing countries is vertical transmission. This occurs through contact of the infant with blood of the mother during birth or close postnatal contact. Transplacental infection with the hepatitis B virus does not appear to be the major route of transmission. In half of cases of hepatitis B, there is no history of percutaneous exposure. *(Fauci et al, p 1685)*

341. (D) The majority of paroxysmal supraventricular tachycardias respond to adenosine, as they involve a reentrant circuit including the atrioventricular node. Adenosine is ineffective in the termination of the majority of other atrial or ventricular tachycardias, although it may slow the ventricular response to an atrial tachycardia. *(Rankin et al, pp 655–665)*

342. **(C)** The most common causes of megaloblastic anemia are folate and vitamin B_{12} deficiencies. Vitamin B_{12} deficiency rarely results from inadequate intake, but has been associated with strict vegetarianism. Decreased absorption may be due to insufficient intrinsic factor (as in pernicious anemia and after gastrectomy), malabsorption of the intrinsic factor–vitamin B_{12} complex in the terminal ileum (as in regional enteritis, sprue, pancreatitis, and after ileectomy), or competition for vitamin B_{12} by gut bacteria (as in the blind loop syndrome and *Diphyllobothrium latum* infections). Because diverticulosis and constipation do not interfere with stomach or small-bowel functioning, they are not causes of vitamin B_{12} deficiency. *(Fauci et al, p 2456)*

343. **(B)** Epidural spinal cord compression is a dreaded complication occurring in approximately 5% of patients who die of cancer annually. Untreated, it progresses to paralysis and sensory loss. The most important single factor in determining prognosis is the level of neurologic function at the start of therapy. *(Byrne, pp 614–619)*

344. **(D)** Pseudotumor cerebri is a disorder of increased intracranial pressure that has no obvious cause. The typical patient is an obese young woman who complains of headache and is found to have papilledema. Slight decrease in visual fields and enlargement of blind spots may also be observed. Neurologic examination is otherwise normal, and the patient appears to be healthy. CSF is under increased pressure and may have slightly low protein concentration, but is otherwise normal. CT scan, arteriogram, and other x-ray studies are usually normal. The most serious complication is severe visual loss, which occurs in about 10% of affected persons. Treatment with corticosteroids and serial lumbar punctures usually leads to resolution in weeks to months. *(Fauci et al, p 167)*

345. **(A)** Pulmonary emboli commonly start as thrombi in a leg or pelvic vein. Rarely, amni-

otic fluid and fat may embolize to the lungs. Since the left ventricle follows the lungs in the circulatory pathway, one would not expect an embolus to lead to the left-sided failure in the absence of some other event (eg, a myocardial infarction brought on by the stress of the pulmonary embolus. Hypoxemia is due to right-to-left shunting. *(Kelley, pp 1943–1951)*

346. **(A)** Although thrush and esophagitis due to *Candida albicans* are common manifestations of AIDS-related immunodeficiency, fungal dissemination and sepsis are extremely rare. Although not uncommon, opportunistic infections in these patients, disseminated *Mycobacterium avium-intracellulare*, cryptococcal meningitis, and cytomegalovirus retinitis are less common than *Pneumocystis carinii* pneumonia, which is the presenting infection in 20% of HIV patients and develops in about 50% of all AIDS patients. *(Fauci et al, p 1824)*

347. **(B)** ASD is the second most common form of congenital heart disease in adults, after a bicuspid aortic valve. The murmur heard in childhood is often considered innocent, and symptoms do not appear until adulthood. A left-to-right shunt of blood between the atria causes right ventricular overload and increased pulmonary circulation. These result in the classic findings of a pulmonic systolic ejection murmur, late pulmonic valve closure with wide splitting of S_2, and a tricuspid flow murmur. Chest x-ray has signs of cardiomegaly and pulmonary overcirculation. Characteristic ECG changes are atrial fibrillation and an incomplete or complete RBBB. In the more common ostium secundum type of ASD, there is often right axis deviation, whereas the ostium primum type has a left axis deviation pattern. Coarctation of the aorta, patent ductus arteriosus, and VSDs are not associated with the findings of the patient described in the question, and tetralogy of Fallot would not present in adulthood. *(Hurst, pp 1188–1191)*

348. **(A)** The normal pericardial cavity is a potential space containing about 15 to 50 mL of fluid. A rapid increase in the amount of fluid

secondary to trauma or cardiac rupture leads to a rapid rise in the intrapericardial pressure. Small amounts of fluid can therefore lead to compromise of cardiac function. More gradual increases are better tolerated. Pneumopericardium such as with SLE, malignancy, uremia, or infection, which may be a complication of trauma, is a rare cause of tamponade. *(Ameli and Shah, pp 665–673)*

349. **(E)** Stool hemoccult tests are associated with many false positives and false negatives. Colonic perforation and serious bleeding with routine sigmoidoscopy are rare. A barium enema exposes the patient to much more radiation than a chest x-ray. Two case-control studies suggest that sigmoidoscopy of people over 50 decreases mortality of colorectal cancer. *(Fauci et al, pp 503–504)*

350. **(D)** The anion gap is determined by subtracting the common serum anions (Cl and HCO_3) from the common serum cation (Na^+). Anion gaps greater than 14 indicate the introduction of unmeasured anions. Ammonium chloride administration does not introduce an unmeasured anion, so the anion gap is normal. Several common conditions can cause acidosis with an elevated anion gap. Renal failure is associated with retention of sulfate, phosphate, and organic acid anions. Tissue hypoxia due to hypotension, shock, CHF, or severe anemia can result in lactic acidosis. Ketoacid accumulation in diabetes is another possible cause. Methanol is metabolized into formaldehyde and formic acid. Salicylate, ethylene glycol, and paraldehyde ingestion all can cause an anion gap acidosis. In an alcoholic patient who is not eating, starvation ketosis can result. *(Adrogue and Madias, pp 26–34)*

351–352. **(351-D, 352-D)** A classic presentation of massive pulmonary embolism is described in the question. The jugular venous distension and RBBB are due to acute right-heart failure. A myocardial infarction large enough to cause hypotension would be expected also to cause gross ST-T wave abnormalities. In the absence of abnormalities of the lung examination or chest x-ray, the probability of pneu-

monia is extremely low. Aortic dissection does not ordinarily cause respiratory distress without first causing a myocardial infarction or aortic regurgitation. Because the correct diagnosis of the case described in the question is pulmonary thromboembolism, only streptokinase and heparin are considerations for treatment. Although streptokinase is more effective than heparin in reversing thromboembolism, the patient's recent surgery provides a strong contraindication to fibrinolytic therapy. *(Fauci et al, pp 1469–1472)*

353. **(D)** Hyponatremia is a common metabolic derangement. Facititious hyponatremia is seen with severe hyperlipidemia or hyperproteinemia (which lower plasma water content) and with hyperglycemia due to water movement out of cells. In the absence of these abnormalities, diagnosis is based on an estimation of circulating blood volume (CBV). Decreased CBV and hyponatremia are associated with diuretic use, dehydration, edematous states (congestive heart failure and cirrhosis of the liver), osmotic diuresis (eg, glycosuria), or adrenal insufficiency. Hyponatremia with normal CBV can be due to the SIADH secretion in which urine osmolality and urine sodium are "inappropriately" high. Diabetes insipidus is a cause of hypernatremia. *(Hurst, pp 1414–1418)*

354. **(C)** Acute renal failure is conveniently divided into three classes: prerenal, renal, and postrenal. The first is failure on the basis of inadequate perfusion; the second is failure on the basis of parenchymal pathology; and the third is failure secondary to obstruction. Calculi would fall under the last heading. *(Kelley, pp 875–883)*

355. **(A)** The nephrotic syndrome is characterized by proteinuria of greater than 3 g/day. Hypoalbuminemia, edema, and lipemia are other defining features. The nephrotic syndrome may result from a primary glomerular disease, such as focal glomerulosclerosis. It is associated with many other systemic diseases, such as lymphoma, and the use of drugs such as heroin. In North America, the

most common cause is diabetes mellitus. *(Kelley, pp 853–856)*

356–357. (356-D, 357-C) The typical migraine attack consists of a visual aura with flashes, scintillating scotomata (field loss), or fortification spectra followed by a throbbing unilateral temporal headache. There may be associated vestibular, GI, or neurologic symptoms. Attacks are often precipitated by stress, fatigue, or foods that contain tyramine (eg, cheese, yogurt, nuts) or phenylethylamine (wine, chocolate). Symptoms peak within an hour of onset and persist for hours to days. A positive family history is found in as many as 50% of cases. Tension headaches are more often bilateral and described as band-like or vise-like and are not usually associated with visual auras. TIAs more typically present as transient monocular blindness without aura or headache. Temporal arteritis may present as painless loss of vision without aura, but is usually in older people. Cluster headaches are much more common in men. Sumatriptan is a newer medication that stimulates the serotonin 5-HT receptors to produce cranial vasoconstriction and reduce vascular inflammation. It comes in oral, injectable, and nasal spray form. Ergotamine tartrate, antiemetics, and analgesics may also be used in the acute treatment of migraine headache. Prophylactic medications such as propranolol, dipyridamole, and methysergide are ineffective for acute attacks. Avoidance of known precipitants and control of stress are also important in prevention. *(Giammarco et al, pp 71–85)*

358–359. (358-A, 359-C) Urinary tract infections are extremely common in young women and in debilitated, bedridden patients. For simple infections uncomplicated by fever, chills, or flank pain, a single dose of an antibiotic may be curative. In the presence of symptoms suggesting renal parenchymal infection (ie, pyelonephritis), treatment should continue for as long as 2 weeks, and parenteral antibiotics may be required (eg, ampicillin plus an aminoglycoside). Bacteriuria in pregnant women should be treated regardless of symptoms, whereas bacteriuria in patients with indwelling catheters should probably be treated only in the presence of symptoms. Chronic suppressive antibiotic therapy in the latter group has not been shown to be useful. Radiologic investigation for underlying anatomic abnormalities should be undertaken in girls up to age 6, in all males after their first infection, and in women of any age with recurrent urinary tract infections. The most common pathogen is *E coli*, accounting for greater than 80% of infections. Other organisms frequently encountered include *Klebsiella*, *Proteus*, and *Enterobacter* species. *(Kelley, pp 1757–1763)*

360. (C) In the empty-sella syndrome, the sella turcica is enlarged but has been largely replaced by CSF. Most of the patients are obese, multiparous women with headaches. About 30% have hypertension. Visual field defects have been reported and are possibly due to herniation of the optic chiasm into the sella turcica. Pituitary function in these patients is usually normal. No specific therapy is indicated if hormone levels are normal. *(Fauci et al, pp 1997–1998)*

361–362. (361-B, 362-D) More than 90% of renal stones are visible on a plain abdominal x-ray, and the majority contain calcium oxalate. Staghorn calculi usually contain magnesium ammonium phosphate (triple phosphate or struvite) and are associated with alkaline urine. This is commonly encountered in chronic urinary tract infections with urea-splitting bacteria (especially *Proteus* species). Radiolucent stones often contain urea, which is associated with acidic urine. A small percentage (fewer than 10%) of renal stones contain cystine. The most common cause of calcium stone disease is idiopathic hypercalciuria. Almost half of these patients will excrete more than 4 mg of calcium/kg body weight/24 hours in the absence of hypercalcemia. Causes of hypercalciuria to be ruled out are sarcoidosis, hyperthyroidism, and Paget's disease of bone. Idiopathic hypercalciuria is believed to result from either increased GI absorption of calcium, increased calcium resorption from bone, or excessive renal calcium leakage into the urine. *(Hurst, pp 1374–1377)*

363. **(B)** Addison's disease, or adrenocortical hypofunction, commonly results in a low serum Na^+, a low serum Cl^-, and a high serum K^+. This is secondary to decreased excretion of K^+ and increased secretion of Na^+ and Cl^- in the urine. *(Fauci et al, p 275)*

364. **(A)** Although the differential diagnosis of a pleural effusion is large, the diagnostic possibilities may be narrowed by classifying the fluid as transudative or exudative. Exudates are characterized by a pleural fluid-to-fluid serum protein ratio greater than 0.5, pleural fluid LDH greater than 200 IU/L, or pleural fluid-to-fluid serum LDH ratio greater than 0.6. Other common findings in exudative effusions are a WBC count greater than 1,000/mL, glucose less than 60 mg/100 mL, and grossly hemorrhagic fluid. Causes of transudative effusions include CHF, nephrotic syndrome, cirrhosis with ascites, and myxedema. Causes of exudative fluid are parapneumonic effusion, neoplasm, pulmonary infarction, tuberculosis, viral disease, and fungal infection. A low pleural fluid pH (< 7.30) limits the differential diagnosis to empyema, carcinoma, collagen vascular disease, esophageal rupture, tuberculosis, or hemothorax. Uncomplicated parapneumonic effusions have WBC counts less than 40,000/mL, normal glucose levels, and a pH less than 7.30; a positive Gram stain or culture constitutes a complicated parapneumonic effusion. These tend to loculate and form adhesions, if not immediately and thoroughly drained by chest tube placement. *(Light, pp 832–842)*

365. **(D)** Secretion of aldosterone, which is regulated by the renin–angiotensin system, causes retention of Na^+ and wasting of K^+. Na^+ is transferred across the distal tubular epithelium in exchange for K^+ and H^+, which are lost in the urine. An alkalosis results. *(Fauci et al, pp 2046–2048)*

366. **(D)** The clinical features of the patient described in the question suggest Cushing syndrome. The most common cause is corticosteroid therapy. Other causes may include adrenal or pituitary disease or ectopic hormone production by a tumor. In addition to the features described, patients may have mood and personality changes, supraclavicular fat pads (buffalo hump), cataracts, hypertension, diabetes mellitus, and osteoporosis. Because true Cushing syndrome is a rare disorder, it is important to rule out the diagnosis as easily as possible. Suppression of 8:00 AM plasma cortisol levels by 1 mg of dexamethasone taken at 11:00 PM the evening before virtually eliminates the diagnosis. An abnormal dexamethasone suppression test result (plasma cortisol remains > 5 mg/100 mL) suggests Cushing's disease, especially if urine-free cortisol also remains elevated. ACTH and metyraprone stimulation tests are no longer recommended. Further evaluation would include radiologic tests for pituitary tumor, such as CT. *(Fauci et al, pp 2042–2046)*

367–368. **(367-D, 368-C)** The patient described in the question most likely has Hashimoto's thyroiditis, also called autoimmune or chronic lymphocytic thyroiditis. It is the most common cause of thyroiditis in the United States and is encountered more frequently in women than in men. Patients note progressive thyromegaly but are usually euthyroid at the outset. Hypothyroidism may appear years later, often heralded by an elevated serum TSH level. Diagnosis is based on the history, examination, heterogeneous uptake on thyroid scan, and the presence of antithyroid and antithyroglobulin antibodies. If the diagnosis is still in doubt, needle biopsy will demonstrate lymphocyte infiltration, sometimes in sheets or forming germinal centers. Subacute (de Quervain's, granulomatous) thyroiditis will show polymorphonuclear cells, necrosis, and giant cells. Bacteria may not be present in acute suppurative thyroiditis. Thyroid infiltration and replacement by rock-hard, woody, fibrous tissue is typical of Riedel's struma. C-cell hyperplasia is associated with medullary thyroid carcinoma. Hashimoto's thyroiditis is treated with thyroid hormone. Lower doses (0.10 to 0.15 mg/day) of levothyroxine are used to treat hypothyroidism alone, whereas higher doses (0.15 to 0.30 mg/day) suppress TSH release and diminish goiter size. Partial resection may result in enlargement of the remaining gland. Steroids, antibiotics, and radioiodine have no role in therapy. *(Goroll et al, pp 455–459)*

369. **(A)** As many as 85% of women with hirsutism, obesity, and menstrual irregularities have polycystic ovary disease (Stein–Leventhal syndrome). Excessive luteinizing hormone (LH) response to gonadotropin-releasing hormone is thought by many to be the primary problem, resulting in ovarian theca-cell hyperplasia and hypersecretion of androgens. Others have found deficiencies of the ovarian enzymes involved in estrogen biosynthesis. Diagnosis is based on an elevated LH level, decreased follicle-stimulating hormone (FSH) level, and an LH/FSH ratio greater than 2:5. Combination estrogen–progestin therapy suppresses the androgen production. Less common causes of hirsutism are drug induced (eg, testosterone, anabolic steroids), adrenal tumor or hyperplasia, Cushing's disease, and ovarian tumors. Familial hirsutism is not associated with menstrual abnormalities or obesity. *(Goroll et al, pp 468–471)*

370. **(B)** Drug-induced acute interstitial nephritis is a frequent cause of reversible renal failure. Methicillin, penicillin, diuretics, nonsteroidal anti-inflammatory drugs (NSAIDs), and allopurinol all have been implicated. An immune basis is postulated, and the acute azotemia may be associated with signs of an allergic reaction: fever, arthralgias, rash, and blood and urine eosinophilia. Discontinuing the offending agent may reverse the renal failure, so a high degree of suspicion and early diagnosis is vital. Steroids are commonly given and may further improve renal function. RBC casts in the urine are diagnostic of glomerulonephritis and are not associated with interstitial nephritis. *(Fauci et al, pp 1495–1496)*

371. **(D)** A low hematocrit can be seen with all of the anemias listed, but is usually much lower (low 20s) in sickle cell anemia. A low MCV (microcytic red cell) is associated with iron-deficiency anemia or beta-thalassemia, but a normal or high number of red blood cells is

characteristic of beta-thalassemia minor. In iron deficiency, the red cell count is usually below normal, and there is an elevated red cell distribution width. Cells are usually normocytic normochromic with anemia of chronic disease. Patients with alpha-thalassemia major have moderate to severe hemolytic anemia early in life. *(Hurst, pp 832–833)*

372. **(B)** Several familial skin disorders have associated GI manifestations. The patient described in the question most likely has Peutz–Jeghers syndrome, which is associated with hamartomatous polyps of the GI tract. These occur most frequently in the jejunum but may be found anywhere between the stomach and the rectum. Malignant transformation of the polyps occurs in 2 to 3% of cases. Tylosis (hyperkeratosis of palms and soles) is associated with esophageal carcinoma. Hereditary hemorrhagic telangiectasia (Rendu–Osler–Weber disease) often involves bleeding of the GI tract. The blue rubber bleb nevus syndrome also causes bleeding due to GI hemangiomas. Neurofibromatosis (von Recklinghausen's disease) is characterized by café au lait spots with cutaneous and intestinal neurofibromas. *(Fauci et al, pp 577, 2104)*

373. **(E)** Systemic sclerosis (scleroderma) is a disease of unknown cause associated with diffuse fibrosis, collagen proliferation, and vascular sclerosis. The fingers are usually involved, with induration of the fingertips (acrosclerosis) and atrophy of the digital pulp (poikiloderma). The skin becomes taut, waxy, and hidebound. Visceral involvement is common and causes significant morbidity. Esophageal hypomotility leads to reflux esophagitis, and intestinal sclerosis in systemic sclerosis leads to congestive heart failure and arrhythmias. Pulmonary involvement is demonstrated by diminished gas diffusion and pulmonary function tests showing restrictive disease. Renal sclerosis may cause severe, malignant hypertension and is a frequent cause of death. *(Schumacher, pp 118–120)*

374. **(C)** The clinical features and laboratory results of the patient described in the question

are most compatible with the diagnosis of osteoarthritis (degenerative joint disease). Loss of joint cartilage and bony hypertrophy account for the typical radiographic findings of a narowed joint space. Subchondral bone increases in thickness, becomes sclerotic, and forms osteophytes. Periosteal lifting is seen with osteomyelitis, and subchondral bony erosions are associated with RA. Osteoporosis is not a feature of osteoarthritis. (Schumacher, pp 184–188)

375.   (D) Before any laboratory evaluation or therapy, the presence of hypertension must be carefully documented. When characteristic end-organ changes are not apparent on physical examination, the presence of hypertension can best be documented by demonstrating a persistent elevation of BP. Although a single observation of mildly elevated blood pressure does not justify either an evaluation for secondary causes or initiation of treatment, it should not be ignored. The patient should be rescheduled for additional BP measurements on several occasions within the next few weeks. There is no need to obtain an ECG or begin counseling if this is not true hypertension. (Hurst, pp 1077–1080)

376.   (B) Pseudogout (chondrocalcinosis) is caused by crystalline deposition in the joints of calcium pyrophosphate dihydrate. It afflicts middle-aged and elderly persons, with males affected slightly more often. Asymptomatic periods punctuated by acute attacks are common. Large joints are affected more than the small ones, with the most frequently involved site being the knee. (Schumacher, pp 219–222)

377.   (A) Among patients with clinical stage 1 primary melanoma, tumor thickness has been consistently shown to be the best indicator of prognosis. This is true even when regional lymph node metastases are subsequently discovered (clinical stage 1 but pathological stage 2). Tumors less than 0.85-mm thick are associated with the most favorable prognosis, and those greater than 3.65 mm in thickness are associated with the least favorable. Tumor thickness is also related to the rate at which death occurs. Tumor location, mitotic rate, and the patient's gender are less powerful determinants of prognosis, and tumor diameter is relatively unimportant. (Fauci et al, pp 543–547)

378.   (B) A history of fluctuating oculomotor weakness suggests the diagnosis of myasthenia gravis (MG), which is confirmed by the edrophonium test. MG is an autoimmune disease associated with antibodies to the acetylcholine receptor in striated muscle. The neurotransmitter acetylcholine is unable to bind to the receptor and stimulate muscle contraction. The drugs most commonly used to treat MG, neostigmine and pyridostigmine, inhibit acetylcholinesterase, the enzyme that catabolizes acetylcholine. Thus, there is a greater amount of acetylcholine present to stimulate the antibody-blocked receptors. Many drugs aggravate MG and should be avoided if possible. These include the aminoglycoside antibiotics, quinidine, procaina-mide, lidocaine, ether, curare, and succinylcholine. Respiratory center depressants, such as morphine, may also be hazardous. (Hurst, pp 1754–1758)

REFERENCES

Adrogue HJ, Madias NE. Management of life-threatening acid–base disorders. *New Engl J Med* 1998;338:26–34.

Ameli S, Shah PK. Cardiac tamponade. *Card Clin* 1991;9:665–673.

Byrne TN. Spinal cord compression from epidural metastases. *N Engl J Med* 1992;327:614–619.

Bartlett JG, Mundy LM. Community-acquired pneumonia. *N Engl J Med* 1995;333:1618–1624.

Coffey RL, Zile MR, Luskin AT. Immunologic tests of value in diagnosis. I. Acute phase reactants and autoantibodies. *Postgrad Med* 1981;70:163–178.

Dajani AS, Taubert KA, Wilson W, et al. Prevention of bacterial endocarditis: recommendations by the American Heart Association. *JAMA* 1997;277:1794–1801.

Diabetes Control and Complications Trial Research Group. The effect of intensive treatment of diabetes on the development and progression of long-term complications in insulin-dependent diabetes mellitus. *N Engl J Med* 1993;329:977–986.

Dixon AC, Parrillo JE. Managing the cardiovascular effects of sepsis and shock. *J Crit Illness* 1991; 6:1197–1214.

Fauci A, Braunwald E, Isselbacher KJ, et al. *Harrison's Principles of Internal Medicine,* 14th ed. New York: McGraw-Hill International Book Co; 1998.

Fink JN, Fauci A. Immunological aspects of cardiovascular disease. *JAMA* 1982;248:2716–2721.

Fitzpatrick TB, Johnson RA, Polano MK, Suurmond DS. *Color Atlas and Synopsis of Clinical Dermatology,* 2nd ed. New York: McGraw-Hill; 1994.

Giammarco R, Edmeads J, Dodick D. *Critical Decisions in Headache Management.* Hamilton, Ontario: BC Decker, Inc; 1998.

Goroll AH, Lawrence AM, Mulley AG. *Primary Care Medicine,* 3rd ed. Philadelphia: JB Lippincott; 1995.

Hogan DE. The emergency department approach to diarrhea. *Emerg Clin North Am* 1996;14:673–692.

Hurst JW. *Medicine for the Practicing Physician.* Stamford, CT: Appleton & Lange; 1996.

Joint National Committee on Prevention, Detection, Evaluation, and Treatment of High Blood Pressure. The sixth report. *Arch Intern Med* 1997; 157:2413–2446.

Kelley WN. *Textbook of Internal Medicine,* 2nd ed. New York: JB Lippincott Co; 1992.

Laine L, Suchower L, Connors A, Neil G. Twice-daily, 10-day triple therapy with omeprazole, amoxicillin, and clarithromycin for *Helicobacter pylori* eradication in duodenal ulcer disease: results of three multicenter, double-blind, United States trials. *Am J Gastroenterol* 1998;93:2106–2112.

Light RW. Parapneumonic effusions and empyema: current management strategies. *J Crit Illness* 1995;10:832–842.

Rankin AC, Brooks R, Ruskin JN, McGovern BA et al. Adenosine and the treatment of supraventricular tachycardia. *Am J Med* 1992; 92:655–664.

Relman DA, Schmidt TM, MacDermott RP, Falkow S, et al. Identification of the uncultured bacillus of Whipple's disease. *N Engl J Med* 1992; 327:293–301.

Schumacher HR, ed. *Primer on the Rheumatic Diseases,* 10th ed. Atlanta: Arthritis Foundation; 1993.

Second Report of the National Cholesterol Education Program Expert Panel on Detection, Evaluation and Treatment of High Blood Cholesterol in Adults. NIH Publication No. 93-3095; 1993.

Yamada T, Alpers D, Owyang C, et al. *Textbook of Gastroenterology.* Philadelphia: JB Lippincott; 1991.

Subspecialty List: Internal Medicine

Question Number and Subspecialty

235. Rheumatology
236. Rheumatology
237. Rheumatology
238. Infectious disease
239. Dermatology
240. Infectious disease
241. Infectious disease
242. Infectious disease
243. Infectious disease
244. Endocrine; Nutrition; Metabolism
245. Endocrine; Nutrition; Metabolism
246. Endocrine; Nutrition; Metabolism
247. Gastroenterology
248. Gastroenterology
249. Pulmonary
250. Cardiovascular
251. Neurology
252. Endocrine; Nutrition; Metabolism
253. Oncology
254. Oncology
255. Dermatology
256. Preventive medicine
257. Renal; Acid–Base
258. Renal; Acid–Base
259. Pharmacology
260. Renal; Acid–Base
261. Cardiovascular
262. Preventive medicine
263. Infectious disease; Dermatology
264. Rheumatology
265. Cardiovascular
266. Cardiovascular
267. Pulmonary
268. Dermatology
269. Gastroenterology
270. Pulmonary
271. Gastroenterology
272. Renal; Acid–Base
273. Cardiovascular
274. Gastroenterology
275. Gastroenterology
276. Neurology
277. Neurology
278. Cardiovascular
279. Neurology
280. Rheumatology
281. Rheumatology
282. Rheumatology
283. Neurology
284. Infectious disease
285. Infectious disease
286. Dermatology
287. Cardiovascular
288. Cardiovascular
289. Rheumatology
290. Endocrine; Nutrition; Metabolism
291. Allergy; Immunology
292. Renal; Acid–Base
293. Renal; Acid–Base
294. Endocrine; Nutrition; Metabolism
295. Rheumatology
296. Rheumatology
297. Oncology
298. Oncology
299. Oncology
300. Oncology
301. Renal; Acid–Base
302. Renal; Acid–Base
303. Renal; Acid–Base
304. Allergy; Immunology
305. Allergy; Immunology
306. Allergy; Immunology
307. Pulmonary
308. Pulmonary

309. Pharmacology
310. Pharmacology
311. Pharmacology
312. Oncology
313. Oncology
314. Oncology
315. Infectious disease
316. Infectious disease
317. Infectious disease
318. Endocrine; Nutrition; Metabolism
319. Endocrine; Nutrition; Metabolism
320. Gastroenterology
321. Gastroenterology
322. Gastroenterology
323. Infectious disease
324. Gastroenterology
325. Infectious disease
326. Infectious disease
327. Infectious disease
328. Pulmonary medicine
329. Pulmonary medicine
330. Infectious disease
331. Pulmonary medicine
332. Pulmonary medicine
333. Oncology
334. Oncology
335. Oncology
336. Renal; Acid–Base
337. Pulmonary
338. Cardiovascular
339. Infectious disease
340. Gastroenterology
341. Cardiovascular
342. Hematology
343. Oncology
344. Neurology
345. Pulmonary
346. Infectious disease
347. Cardiovascular
348. Cardiovascular
349. Preventive medicine
350. Renal; Acid–Base
351. Pulmonary
352. Pulmonary
353. Renal; Acid–Base
354. Renal; Acid–Base
355. Renal; Acid–Base
356. Neurology
357. Neurology
358. Renal; Acid–Base
359. Renal; Acid–Base
360. Neurology
361. Renal; Acid–Base
362. Renal; Acid–Base
363. Endocrine; Nutrition; Metabolism
364. Pulmonary
365. Renal; Acid–Base
366. Endocrine; Nutrition; Metabolism
367. Endocrine; Nutrition; Metabolism
368. Endocrine; Nutrition; Metabolism
369. Endocrine; Nutrition; Metabolism
370. Renal; Acid–Base
371. Hematology
372. Gastroenterology
373. Rheumatology
374. Rheumatology
375. Cardiovascular
376. Rheumatology
377. Dermatology
378. Endocrine; Nutrition; Metabolism

CHAPTER 4

Surgery
Questions

Philip N. Redlich, MD, PhD, and Andrea L. Winthrop, MD

DIRECTIONS (Questions 379 through 399): Each of the numbered items or incomplete statements in this section is followed by answers or by completions of the statement. Select the ONE lettered answer or completion that is BEST in each case.

Questions 379 Through 382

A 5-week-old infant presents with a 1-week history of progressive nonbilious emesis, associated with a 24-hour history of decreased urine output. The infant continues to be active and eager to feed. On exam, the infant has a sunken fontanelle and decreased skin turgor. The abdomen is scaphoid, and with a test feed, there is a visible peristaltic wave in the epigastrium.

379. The most probable clinical diagnosis is

infant
nonbilious emesis
↓ output/dehyd
peristaltic λ in epigastrium

 (A) viral gastroenteritis
 (B) gastroesophageal reflux
 (C) urinary tract sepsis
 (D) pyloric stenosis ∅ mass
 (E) milk protein allergy F

380. The diagnosis is best confirmed by

 (A) abdominal ultrasound
 (B) careful clinical examination with palpation of an epigastric mass
 (C) upper gastrointestinal contrast study
 (D) surgical exploration
 (E) endoscopy

381. Electrolytes and a urinalysis are evaluated. The most likely laboratory findings are

 (A) Na 145, K 3.0, Cl 110, CO_2 17, urine pH 8.0
 (B) Na 130, K 3.0, Cl 80, CO_2 36, urine pH 4.0
 (C) Na 135, K 4.0, Cl 104, CO_2 23, urine pH 7.0
 (D) Na 140, K 5.2, Cl 100, CO_2 16, urine pH 4.0
 (E) Na 132, K 3.2, Cl 96, CO_2 25, urine pH 7.0

382. The next steps in management of this infant are

 (A) immediate surgical exploration
 (B) send the child home with an oral electrolyte rehydration solution
 (C) change the infant's formula and feeding regimen
 (D) intravenous (IV) fluid resuscitation, followed by surgical intervention
 (E) initiate therapy with a prokinetic agent

Questions 383 and 384

A 40-year-old previously healthy man presents with sudden onset of severe abdominal pain that radiates from the right loin (flank) to groin. This pain is associated with nausea, sweating, and urinary urgency. He is distressed and restless, but an abdominal exam is normal.

383. The most likely diagnosis is

(A) torsion of the right testicle

(B) pyelonephritis

(C) appendicitis

(D) right ureteral calculus

(E) acute urinary retention

384. Which of the following are the most appropriate next steps in management?

(A) insertion of a urethral catheter

(B) IV fluid hydration, IV analgesics, and intravenous pyelography (IVP)

(C) IV fluid hydration, IV analgesics, and arrangements for lithotripsy

(D) cystoscopy and retrograde pyelogram

(E) urine culture, followed by initiation of antibiotic therapy

Question 385

A 25-year-old woman was involved in a motor vehicle crash and sustained a significant closed head injury, a pulmonary contusion, and a pelvic fracture. She is unresponsive and is ventilated in the intensive care unit (ICU).

385. The best initial approach to the management of this patient's nutritional needs is

(A) insertion of a subclavian venous catheter and initiation of central IV hyperalimentation

(B) wait for extubation and improvement of neurologic status, allowing institution of an oral caloric intake

(C) early institution of nasogastric or nasojejunal tube feeding with an elemental formulation

(D) wait for resolution of the associated gastrointestinal ileus, followed by delayed initiation of nasogastric tube feeding with a complex hypercaloric formulation

(E) peripheral IV hyperalimentation

Questions 386 and 387

A 3-day-old term infant male presents with progressive vomiting and abdominal distension. On questioning the nursery staff, they report that the child passed meconium at 48 hours but only after receiving a glycerin suppository. He has not tolerated oral feeds, and urine output has decreased over the preceding 12 hours.

386. Which of the following diagnostic and/or therapeutic interventions are essential prior to transporting the child to the regional pediatric hospital?

(A) nasogastric tube decompression and IV fluid resuscitation

(B) blood and urine cultures, followed by initiation of broad-spectrum antibiotics

(C) barium enema

(D) plain abdominal radiographs

(E) sweat chloride determination

387. On arrival at the receiving pediatric hospital, the most appropriate approach to establishing the diagnosis would be

(A) anorectal manometry

(B) abdominal ultrasound

(C) plain radiographs, followed by a barium enema and subsequent rectal biopsy if indicated

(D) plain radiographs, followed by an upper gastrointestinal (UGI) contrast study

(E) rectal biopsy

Question 388

A 26-year-old previously healthy man was pinned under a crane at a construction site. After prolonged extrication, he was brought to the emergency department, immobilized on a back board and receiving 100% oxygen by mask. He is alert and complaining of chest pain with respiratory effort. On exam, he is found to have an oxygen saturation of 90% by pulse oximetry, shallow respirations at a respiratory rate of 35/min, heart rate of 120 beats/min, and a blood pressure of 85/60. The trachea is deviated to the right. There is tenderness and crepitation over the left chest wall, asymmetric chest wall movement, and decreased air entry over the left lung field.

388. The next appropriate step in the initial evaluation and management of this patient is

(A) sit the patient upright to assist respiratory effort, and provide IV analgesics to alleviate the associated discomfort

(B) immediate intubation and assisted ventilation

(C) portable chest x-ray

(D) needle decompression of the left chest, followed by insertion of a chest tube

(E) emergency department thoracotomy

Questions 389 Through 391

A 4-year-old previously healthy girl presents to the emergency department with a 24-hour history of rectal bleeding and dizziness. She has no other gastrointestinal symptoms. On exam, she appears pale. Her heart rate is 140/min, and she has a 20 mm Hg postural drop in systolic blood pressure. The child's abdomen is nondistended and nontender, and there is fresh blood and clots in the rectal vault on rectal exam.

389. The most likely diagnosis is

(A) a bleeding Meckel's diverticulum

(B) juvenile rectal polyp

(C) hemorrhoids

(D) an anal fissure

(E) intussusception

390. In this patient, the most appropriate diagnostic study is

(A) colonoscopy

(B) barium enema

(C) technetium scan

(D) UGI contrast study with small bowel follow-through

(E) laparoscopy

391. Definitive management of this child should include

(A) immediate exploratory laparotomy

(B) IV fluid resuscitation, transfusion with blood products as indicated, followed by a laparotomy and Meckel's diverticulectomy

(C) IV fluid resuscitation, followed by a colonoscopic polypectomy

(D) hemorrhoidectomy

(E) stool softeners and topical steroids

Question 392

An unfortunate 45-year-old truck driver is involved in a multivehicle crash, resulting in a significant closed head injury. He is intubated in the field and transported to a Level 1 trauma center. On arrival, he is oxygenating well with assisted ventilation and has a normal blood pressure and moderate tachycardia. His Glasgow Coma score is 7, and his pupils are equal and sluggishly reactive. After stabilization in the emergency department, the patient undergoes a computed tomography (CT) scan of the head that demonstrates a small amount of subarachnoid blood and a right frontal lobe contusion. CT scan of the abdomen is normal. The patient is transferred to the ICU.

392. The optimal initial management of this patient's intracranial pressure would be

(A) fluid restriction, hyperventilation, and IV steroids

(B) fluid restriction, hyperventilation, and ventriculostomy

(C) fluid restriction and osmotic diuresis

(D) normovolemia, normocarbia, and ventriculostomy

(E) craniectomy

Questions 393 and 394

A 55-year-old woman presents with a 6-month history of weight loss, abdominal cramps, and intermittent nonbloody diarrhea. On exam, her abdomen is mildly distended, and there is a palpable mass is the right lower quadrant. Stool cultures yield normal fecal flora. CT scan with oral contrast demonstrates an inflammatory mass in the right lower quadrant, with thickening of the terminal ileum and proximal right colon.

393. The most probable diagnosis is

 (A) ulcerative colitis
 (B) appendicitis
 (C) Crohn's disease
 (D) irritable bowel syndrome
 (E) lactose intolerance

394. Initial management would include

 (A) antibiotics and IV fluids, followed by exploratory laparotomy
 (B) lactose-free diet
 (C) antispasmodics
 (D) nutritional supplementation and systemic steroids
 (E) colectomy

Question 395

A 14-year-old boy is brought to the emergency department at midnight with a 4-hour history of left scrotal pain that was sudden in onset and associated with nausea and one episode of vomiting. On examination, he is in obvious distress. He has mild left-lower-quadrant tenderness, and a high-riding, tender left testis. Complete blood count and urinalysis are normal.

395. The most appropriate next step in management is

 (A) analgesics and a scrotal support
 (B) antibiotic therapy
 (C) urgent surgical exploration

 (D) admit the patient to the hospital, place him on bedrest, and arrange for a testicular isotope scan in the morning
 (E) elective left inguinal hernia repair

396. A 70-year-old man presents with back pain and increasing difficulty with initiating a urinary stream. On rectal exam, he is found to have a hard, irregularly enlarged prostate. He has an elevated prostate-specific antigen (PSA), and osteoblastic lesions in the vertebral column and bones of the pelvis. A needle biopsy of the prostate shows well-differentiated adenocarcinoma. The treatment of choice is

 (A) radical prostatectomy
 (B) transurethral prostatectomy
 (C) cytotoxic chemotherapy
 (D) hormonal manipulation
 (E) radiotherapy

397. A 25-year-old previously healthy man is scheduled for elective inguinal hernia repair under general anesthesia. After induction of anesthesia and initial inguinal incision, the patient develops tachycardia, muscle rigidity, fever of 38.5°C, and elevated end-tidal carbon dioxide. The most likely diagnosis is

 (A) pneumonia
 (B) atelectasis
 (C) urinary tract infection
 (D) myocardial infarction
 (E) malignant hyperthermia

Question 398

A previously healthy 19-year-old man presents to the emergency department with a penetrating wound to the right neck. There were reports of bleeding at the scene. The patient is talking, complaining of pain at the injury site and pain with swallowing. On examination, he has a normal respiratory rate, clear air entry on ausculation, blood pressure of 120/70, and heart rate of 95/min. There is a penetrating right neck wound in Zone 2 (between the clavicle and the lower part of the mandible), with a surrounding hematoma. On probing, there is violation of the platysma.

398. The next step in the management of this patient is

(A) intubation and observation in the ICU

(B) admission to the ICU for close observation without intubation

(C) observation in the ICU only if carotid angiogram is normal

(D) observation in the ICU only if carotid angiogram, contrast esophagram, and bronchoscopy are normal

(E) neck exploration

Question 399

A 45-year-old man is brought to the emergency department after being involved in an automobile crash. He is alert and oriented, with a normal neurologic exam. His respiratory rate is 20/min, with clear lungs, pulse rate of 120/min, and blood pressure of 60/0 mm Hg. On exam, he is noted to have a distended abdomen, with decreased bowel sounds, and a fracture of the right ankle. Intravenous access is established, and the patient receives a rapid infusion of 2 L of saline, without changes to pulse rate or blood pressure.

399. The most appropriate next step in his management is

(A) cervical spine x-ray

(B) insertion of a Swan–Ganz catheter

(C) exploratory laparotomy

(D) abdominal CT scan

(E) diagnostic peritoneal lavage

DIRECTIONS (Questions 400 through 415): Each set of matching questions in this section consists of a list of 5 to 11 lettered options followed by several numbered items. For each item, select the ONE best lettered option that is most closely associated with it. Each lettered heading may be selected once, more than once, or not at all.

Questions 400 and 401

Select the most likely diagnosis for each of the patients with polyuria.

(A) central diabetes insipidus

(B) nephrogenic diabetes insipidus

(C) water intoxication

(D) solute overload

(E) diabetes mellitus

400. A 25-year-old man was admitted to the ICU with severe head injury with a basal skull fracture. Eighteen hours after the injury, he developed polyuria. Urine osmolality was 150 mOsm/L, and serum osmolality was 350 mOsm/L. Intravenous fluids were stopped, and 1 hour later urine output and urine osmolality remained unchanged. Five units of vasopressin were administered intravenously, and urine osmolality increased to 300 mOsm/L.

401. A 70-year-old man was admitted to the ICU with severe pancreatitis. During his ICU course, he underwent several CT scans with intravenous contrast, and was also treated with an aminoglycoside for a urinary tract infection. The patient required a prolonged course of total parenteral nutrition (TPN), and developed *Candida* sepsis treated with amphotericin. He subsequently developed polyuria with urine osmolality of 250 mOsm/L and serum osmolality of 350 mOsm/L. After receiving 5 units of vasopressin intravenously, there is no change in urine osmolality or urine output.

Questions 402 and 403

For each patient with abdominal pain, select the most likely diagnosis.

   (A) gastroenteritis
   (B) regional enteritis
   (C) acute appendicitis
   (D) perforated peptic ulcer
   (E) sigmoid diverticulitis
   (F) acute pancreatitis
   (G) acute cholecystitis
   (H) superior mesenteric artery embolism
   (I) ruptured abdominal aortic aneurysm
   (J) ruptured ovarian cyst
   (K) cecal volvulus

402. A 21-year-old previously healthy woman presents with abdominal pain of 48 hours' duration. The pain was initially periumbilical, and on progression became localized in the right lower quadrant. The woman had nausea, and a decreased appetite. She denied dysuria. Her last menstrual period was 2 weeks earlier. On exam, the woman was febrile (temperature 38.2°C), and was found to have localized tenderness in the right lower quadrant with guarding. Rectal examination was normal. Laboratory exam demonstrated mild leukocytosis.

403. A 40-year-old man with a history of alcohol abuse presents after an episode of binge drinking. He is complaining of epigastric pain, radiating to the back, associated with nausea and vomiting. On exam, he has marked tenderness in the epigastrium, with guarding, decreased bowel sounds, and moderate abdominal distension. Laboratory findings include leukocytosis and increased serum amylase and lipase. Abdominal roentgenograms demonstrate several dilated bowel loops in the upper abdomen.

Questions 404 Through 410

For each patient with a neck mass, select the most likely diagnosis.

   (A) thyroglossal duct cyst
   (B) cystic hygroma
   (C) acute suppurative lymphadenitis
   (D) thyroid carcinoma
   (E) lipoma
   (F) carotid artery aneurysm
   (G) mixed parotid tumor (pleomorphic adenoma)
   (H) laryngeal carcinoma
   (I) parathyroid adenoma
   (J) tuberculosis
   (K) hemangioma

404. A 5-year-old boy presents to the physician's office with an asymptomatic neck mass located in the midline, just below the level of the thyroid cartilage. The mass moves with deglutition and on protrusion of the tongue.

405. A 6-year-old boy presents to the emergency department with a cough, sore throat, and malaise of 4 days' duration. Exam reveals a temperature of 101.5°F, erythematous pharynx, and a left neck mass with overlying erythema.

406. A 2-year-old girl is brought to the physician's office for evaluation of a slowly enlarging left neck mass. Exam reveals a 4-cm soft, nontender, fluctuant, and multiloculated mass in the left lateral neck.

407. A 45-year-old man presents to the physician's office for evaluation of a posterior neck mass. The mass has been present for years, but has slowly enlarged over the last 2 years. Exam reveals a subcutaneous mass that is soft, nontender, and movable.

408. A 50-year-old woman presents to the physician's office for evaluation of a right neck mass. The mass has been present for 3 years and is painless. On exam, a nontender, firm,

2.5-cm mass is noted slightly below and posterior to the angle of the mandible on the right.

409. A 35-year-old woman presents to the physician's office for evaluation of a left neck mass discovered 1 month ago on a routine physical exam. On exam, the mass measures 2 cm and is located anterolateral to the larynx and trachea. It is nontender and moves with swallowing. Past history is pertinent for a 15-pack year smoking history and occasional alcohol intake.

410. A 55-year-old man presents to the physician's office with complaints of hoarseness and left neck fullness for the past month. On exam, a firm, movable, left submandibular mass is noted. Past history is pertinent for a 30-pack year smoking history with occasional alcohol intake.

Questions 411 Through 415

For each patient with jaundice, select the most likely diagnosis.

(A) hepatitis A
(B) hemolysis
(C) choledocholithiasis
(D) biliary stricture
(E) choledochal cyst
(F) pancreatic carcinoma
(G) liver metastases
(H) cirrhosis
(I) pancreatitis

411. A 50-year-old man presents to the emergency department for increasing abdominal distension and jaundice over the last 4 to 6 weeks. Exam reveals mild jaundice, spider angiomas, and ascites. Enlarged veins are noted around the umbilicus.

412. A 75-year-old man is brought to the emergency department by his family for evaluation of jaundice. He complains of pruritus of 2 weeks' duration and a recent 10-pound weight loss. On exam, he is deeply jaundiced and has a nontender, globular mass in the right upper quadrant of the abdomen that moves with respiration.

413. A 75-year-old woman is brought to the emergency department from the nursing home for jaundice and mental confusion. The nursing home notes state that she has become less responsive and has developed jaundice over the last 2 weeks. Past history is pertinent for hypertension, diabetes, and prior colon resection for cancer at age 55. Exam reveals mild jaundice with vital signs of temperature 101.5°F, pulse 110, and BP 100/60. She does not respond to verbal commands, but withdraws to pain. Abdominal exam reveals tenderness in the epigastrium and right upper quadrant.

414. A 65-year-old man presents to the physician's office with complaints of abdominal discomfort and jaundice for the past 3 weeks. Past history is pertinent for 30-pack year smoking history, occasional alcohol intake, and a 5.5-mm ulcerating melanoma removed from his back 2½ years ago. Exam reveals a mildly jaundiced patient with normal vital signs and a slightly distended abdomen with mild right-upper-quadrant tenderness and significant hepatomegaly.

415. A 54-year-old man presents to the emergency department upon transfer from another hospital at the request of the family. He was admitted to the outside hospital 2 weeks ago with abdominal pain, nausea, vomiting, and fever. He was treated with antibiotics, nasogastric tube decompression, and TPN without significant improvement. He developed jaundice 2 days ago. His past history is pertinent for a 40-pack year smoking history, chronic alcohol abuse, and diabetes. Exam reveals a mildly jaundiced patient with vital signs of temperature 100°F, pulse 95, and BP 110/60. Cardiac exam is unremarkable, lung exam reveals decreased breath sounds at the bases bilaterally, and abdominal exam reveals a fullness in the epigastrium with tenderness and voluntary guarding.

DIRECTIONS (Questions 416 through 474): Each of the numbered items or incomplete statements in this section is followed by answers or by completions of the statement. Select the ONE lettered answer or completion that is BEST in each case.

Question 416

A 56-year-old woman presents to the physician's office with complaints of a new left breast mass. She denies any pain, nipple discharge, or skin dimpling. She has a prior history of breast cysts 5 years ago, treated by aspiration at that time. Her last mammogram was at age 53. Past history is pertinent for a 30-pack year smoking history, prior total abdominal hysterectomy–bilateral salpingo-oophorectomy (TAH-BSO) at age 54 for leiomyomas, and current use of hormone replacement therapy (HRT). Family history is negative for breast disease. Exam reveals a firm, well-defined, mobile, 1.5-cm nodule in the upper outer quadrant of the left breast without any regional lymphadenopathy.

416. Which of the following is the most appropriate next step in management?

(A) fine-needle aspiration biopsy
(B) discontinuation of HRT and re-exam in 4 to 6 weeks
(C) breast imaging
(D) open surgical biopsy
(E) core needle biopsy

Question 417

A 56-year-old woman presents to the clinic for routine health screening. Her concern is the development of breast cancer. She has no current breast-related complaints. Past history is pertinent for fibrocystic changes with atypical ductal hyperplasia and a single fibroadenoma, both diagnosed by open biopsy 5 years ago. She smokes one pack per day and drinks one can of beer daily. Family history is positive for breast cancer in her mother, diagnosed at the age of 85. Current medications include a cholesterol-lowering agent, an antihypertensive, and HRT, which she has taken for 5 years. Physical exam is unremarkable. Mammograms show dense breasts, decreasing the accuracy of the study, but no suspicious findings were noted.

417. Which of the following risk factors in this patient are identifiable in most patients with breast cancer?

(A) fibrocystic changes with atypical ductal hyperplasia
(B) alcohol consumption
(C) positive family history
(D) HRT
(E) none of the above

Question 418

A 42-year-old woman returns to the clinic following an uneventful biopsy for a well-defined, mobile mass. The pathology report describes the mass as a fibroadenoma, but lobular carcinoma in situ (LCIS) is identified in the breast parenchyma adjacent to the fibroadenoma and extending to the margin of resection. She has no current illnesses, is on no medications, and her family history is negative for breast cancer. Breast imaging studies show fatty breasts with no abnormal findings except for the fibroadenoma.

418. Which of the following is the most appropriate management option?

(A) re-excision of the biopsy cavity to gain negative margins of resection
(B) ipsilateral mastectomy
(C) contralateral breast biopsy
(D) observation including exams and mammography
(E) bilateral total mastectomies

Question 419

A 60-year-old woman presents to the physician's office for a second opinion on the management options for recently diagnosed breast cancer. She presents with a 2.5-cm mass in the upper outer quadrant of the left breast associated with palpable axillary nodes suspicious for metastatic disease. The remainder of her exam is normal. Mammography demonstrates the cancer and shows no other suspicious lesions in either breast. Chest x-ray, bone scan, and blood test panel, including liver function tests, are normal. Family history is positive for breast cancer diagnosed in her sister at age

65. Past history is unremarkable. The first physician recommended modified radical mastectomy.

419. Which of the following is the most appropriate management option for locoregional control yielding results equally effective as mastectomy?

(A) radical mastectomy

(B) lumpectomy, irradiation, and axillary node dissection

(C) lumpectomy and axillary node dissection

(D) irradiation of the breast and axilla

(E) quadrantectomy, irradiation, and axillary node dissection

Questions 420 and 421

A 62-year-old woman presents to the physician's office for evaluation of an abnormal mammogram. She denies any breast masses, nipple discharge, or skin changes. Past history is pertinent for hypertension. Family history is negative for breast cancer. Bilateral mammograms show an abnormality on the left. The mediolateral oblique (MLO) view is shown in Figure 4–1. On exam, she has a 5-cm fullness in the left breast without any regional adenopathy. The remainder of her exam is unremarkable.

420. Which of the following is the most likely diagnosis?

(A) cystosarcoma phyllodes

(B) LCIS with or without an invasive component

(C) ductal carcinoma in situ (DCIS) with or without an invasive component

(D) degenerating fibroadenoma

(E) milk of calcium

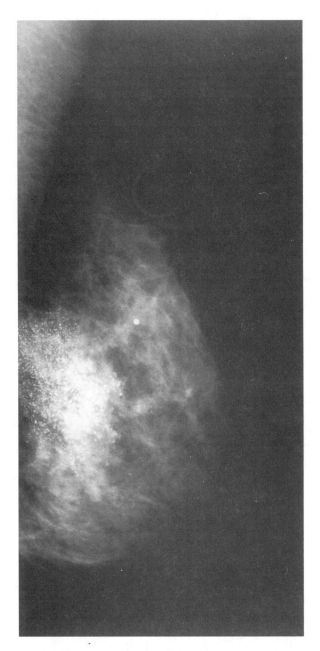

Figure 4–1. Left MLO mammogram of a 62-year-old woman.

421. Which of the following is the most appropriate next step in management?

(A) radical mastectomy

(B) modified radical mastectomy

(C) total mastectomy

(D) lumpectomy with negative margins

(E) biopsy

Questions 422 and 423

A 67-year-old woman presents to the physician's office with a new left breast mass noted 1 month ago. There is no associated pain or nipple discharge. Past history is pertinent for diabetes and hypertension. Family history is positive for breast cancer in her mother, diagnosed at age 70. Exam reveals a 2-cm firm mass in the left lateral breast without any regional adenopathy. The remainder of her exam is unremarkable. Bilateral mammograms show an abnormality on the left. The left craniocaudal (CC) projection is shown in Figure 4–2. Chest x-ray and blood tests are normal.

422. Which of the following is the most likely diagnosis?

   (A) DCIS
   (B) LCIS
   (C) invasive ductal carcinoma
   (D) cystosarcoma phyllodes
   (E) papilloma

423. Which of the following is the most appropriate next step in management?

   (A) radical mastectomy
   (B) biopsy
   (C) modified radical mastectomy
   (D) lumpectomy, axillary dissection, and irradiation
   (E) irradiation

Questions 424 and 425

A 65-year-old woman presents to the physician's office with a 6-month history of epigastric discomfort, poor appetite, and 10-pound weight loss. Past history is pertinent for hypertension, diabetes, a 30-pack year smoking history, and occasional alcohol intake. Exam is unremarkable except for mild epigastric tenderness to deep palpation. An abdominal ultrasound reveals cholelithiasis, and one view of a UGI x-ray series is shown in Figure 4–3.

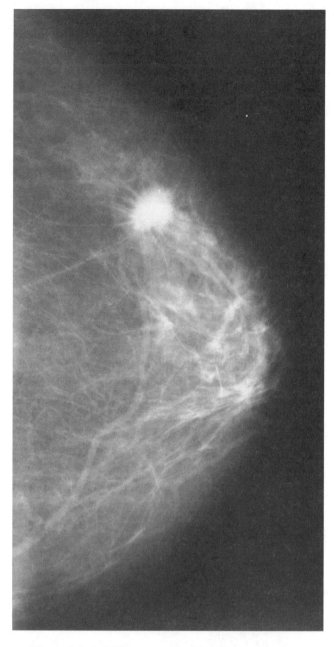

Figure 4–2. Left CC mammogram of a 67-year-old woman.

424. Which of the following is the most likely diagnosis?

   (A) cholecystoenteric fistula
   (B) duodenal ulcer
   (C) gastric ulcer
   (D) gastric diverticulum
   (E) duodenal diverticulum

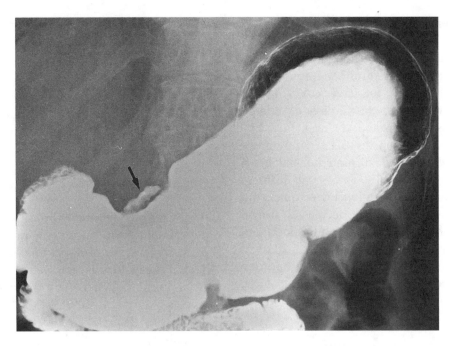

Figure 4–3. UGI of a 65-year-old woman. Arrow indicates abnormality. *(Reprinted with permission from Zinner MJ.* Maingot's Abdominal Operations, *10th ed., vol. 1. Stamford, CT: Appleton & Lange, 1997.)*

425. Which of the following is the most appropriate next step in management?

(A) H₂ blockers with re-evaluation by UGI in 6 months
(B) vagotomy and pyloroplasty
(C) total gastrectomy
(D) endoscopy
(E) CT scan

Question 426

A 55-year-old man presents to the physician's office for his yearly physical exam. He is asymptomatic. Past history is pertinent for hypertension. Family history is positive for breast cancer in his mother at age 70 and colon cancer in his father at age 65. His exam is unremarkable except for hematest-positive stool. Barium enema shows a sigmoid colon polyp. Colonoscopy confirms a 3-cm pedunculated polyp in the sigmoid colon, and snare polypectomy is performed. Pathologic exam reveals an adenomatous polyp with a focus of inva-sive carcinoma in the head, with a 4-mm resection margin and no tumor noted in the stalk.

426. Which of the following is the most appropriate next step in management?

(A) CT scan
(B) magnetic resonance imaging (MRI) scan
(C) surgical resection of sigmoid
(D) observation
(E) regular use of nonsteroidal anti-inflammatory drugs (NSAIDs)

Questions 427 Through 429

A 55-year-old man presents to the emergency department with left-lower-quadrant abdominal pain. The pain has been present for 1 week, but has increased in intensity over the last 2 days associated with nausea, constipation, and dysuria. Past history is unremarkable. Exam reveals a temperature of 101°F, pulse 95, BP 130/70, and normal heart and lung exams. Abdominal exam reveals fullness and marked tenderness in the left lower quadrant, with voluntary guarding and decreased bowel sounds. Laboratory tests reveal a white blood cell (WBC) count of 18,000 with a left shift and 20 to 50 WBCs in the urinalysis. A CT scan of the abdomen reveals a thickened sigmoid colon with pericolonic inflammation. He is admitted to the hospital for treatment.

427. Which of the following is the most likely diagnosis?

    (A) colon cancer with contained perforation
    (B) ischemic colitis
    (C) pseudomembranous colitis
    (D) diverticulitis
    (E) pyelonephritis

428. Which of the following tests should be obtained?

    (A) air contrast barium enema
    (B) colonoscopy
    (C) IVP
    (D) mesenteric angiogram
    (E) none

429. Which of the following is the most appropriate management of this patient?

    (A) NPO, IV fluids, and IV antibiotics for gram-negative and anaerobic coverage
    (B) NPO, IV fluid hydration, followed by immediate sigmoid colon resection
    (C) NPO, IV fluids, and anticoagulation

    (D) NPO, IV fluids, evaluation of stool for *Clostridium difficile* toxin, and either metronidazole or vancomycin antibiotic therapy
    (E) NPO, IV fluids, initiation of bowel preparation for elective sigmoid colon resection during the current hospitalization

Questions 430 and 431

A 75-year-old woman is brought to the emergency department from a nursing home for abdominal pain, distension, and obstipation over the last 2 days. Past history is pertinent for stroke, diabetes, atrial fibrillation, and chronic constipation. Exam reveals a temperature of 98.6°F, pulse 90 and irregularly irregular, and BP 160/90. Heart exam reveals irregularly irregular rhythm with no murmurs, lung exam reveals few bibasilar rales, and abdominal exam reveals a distended, tympanic abdomen with mild tenderness and no rebound tenderness. Plain abdominal x-rays reveal dilated loops of bowel, and a barium enema is obtained and shown in Figure 4-4.

430. Which of the following is the most likely diagnosis?

    (A) ischemic colitis with stricture
    (B) diverticulitis with obstruction
    (C) cecal volvulus
    (D) sigmoid volvulus
    (E) colon cancer with obstruction

431. Which of the following is the most appropriate next step in management following nasogastric tube decompression and resuscitation?

    (A) urgent sigmoid resection
    (B) nonoperative reduction with proctoscopy and rectal tube
    (C) proximal colostomy
    (D) urgent operative detorsion
    (E) nonoperative reduction with passage of well-lubricated rectal tube

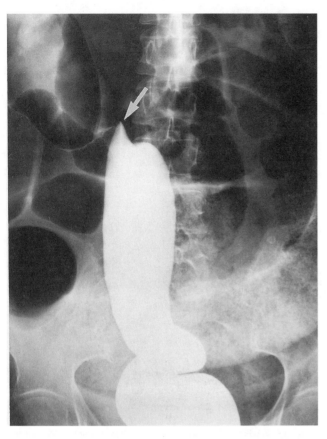

Figure 4–4. Barium enema. *(Reprinted with permission from Zinner MJ.* Maingot's Abdominal Operations, *10th ed., vol. 1. Appleton & Lange, 1997.)*

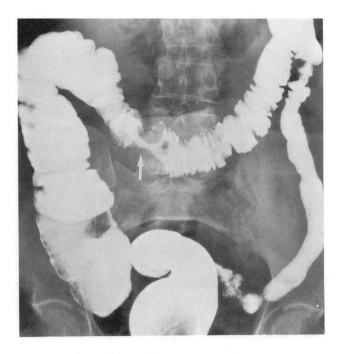

Figure 4–5. Barium enema. *(Reprinted with permission from Zinner MJ.* Maingot's Abdominal Operations, *10th ed., vol. 1. Appleton & Lange, 1997.)*

Questions 432 and 433

A 65-year-old man presents to the physician's office for his yearly physical. His only complaints relate to early fatigue while playing golf. Past history is pertinent for mild hypertension. Exam is unremarkable except for trace hematest-positive stool. Blood tests are normal except for a hematocrit of 32. A UGI series is performed and is normal. A barium enema is performed, and one view is shown in Figure 4–5.

432. Which of the following is the most likely diagnosis?

(A) diverticular disease
(B) colon cancer
(C) lymphoma
(D) ischemia with stricture
(E) Crohn's colitis with stricture

433. Which of the following is the most appropriate therapy?

(A) proximal colostomy with mucous fistula
(B) radiation therapy
(C) chemotherapy
(D) surgical resection and primary anastamosis
(E) surgical bypass (colocolostomy)

Questions 434 and 435

A 54-year-old woman presents to her physician for an opinion regarding additional therapy following curative resection of recently diagnosed colon cancer. She underwent uncomplicated sigmoid resection for invasive colon cancer 4 weeks ago. The pathology revealed carcinoma invading into, but not through, the muscularis propria, with one of eight positive mesenteric nodes. There was no evidence of liver metastases at the time of operation. Preoperative chest x-ray and CT scan of the abdomen showed no evidence of distant disease. Preoperative carcinoembryonic antigen (CEA) level was normal. Past history is positive for diabetes and mild hypertension. Exam is unremarkable except for a healing abdominal incision.

434. Which of the following is the correct stage of this patient's colon cancer?

   (A) stage 0
   (B) stage I
   (C) stage II
   (D) stage III
   (E) stage IV

435. Which of the following is the most appropriate recommendation regarding adjuvant therapy?

   (A) no therapy indicated
   (B) 5-fluorouracil chemotherapy
   (C) 5-fluorouracil chemotherapy with levamisole or leucovorin
   (D) doxorubicin (Adriamycin) chemotherapy
   (E) Adriamycin chemotherapy with methotrexate and cytoxan

Question 436

A 62-year-old woman presents to the physician's office with complaints of constipation. She has had constipation for the last 6 months, which has worsened over the last month, associated with mild bloating. She noted that her stool has become "pencil thin" in the last month, with occasional blood, but she continues to have bowel movements daily. Past history is unremarkable. Exam reveals normal vital signs and heart and lung exam. Abdominal exam reveals mild fullness, especially in the lower quadrants. Rectal exam shows no rectal masses but the stool is hematest positive. A barium x-ray is obtained, and one view is shown in Figure 4–6.

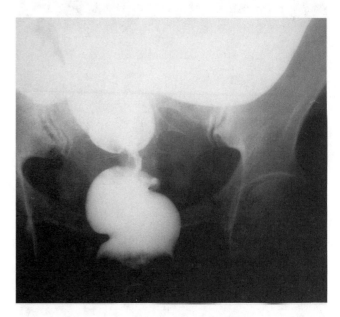

Figure 4–6. Barium x-ray. *(Reprinted with permission from Zinner MJ.* Maingot's Abdominal Operations, *10th ed., vol. 2. Appleton & Lange, 1996.)*

436. Which of the following is the most likely diagnosis?

   (A) Crohn's disease
   (B) ischemia with stricture
   (C) rectal carcinoma
   (D) sigmoid volvulus
   (E) diverticulitis with colovesical fistula

Questions 437 and 438

A 45-year-old man presents to the physician's office for evaluation of a skin lesion on his abdomen. He states that the lesion has been present for 1 year, but has recently enlarged over the last 2 months. The mass is nontender and he is otherwise asymptomatic. Past history is unremarkable. Exam reveals a 3-cm, pigmented, irregular skin lesion located in the left lower quadrant of the abdomen, as

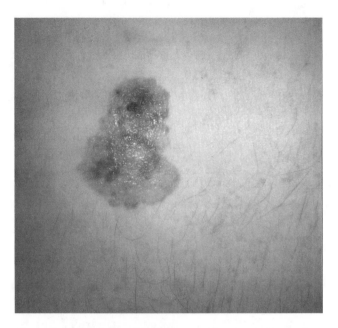

Figure 4–7. Skin lesion of the abdomen. *(Reprinted with permission from Hurwitz RM, Hood AF.* Pathology of the Skin: Atlas of Clinical–Pathological Correlation. *Appleton & Lange, 1998.)*

shown in Figure 4–7. Heart, lung, and abdominal exam is normal. There are no palpable cervical, axillary, or inguinal lymph nodes. Chest x-ray and liver function tests are normal.

437. Which of the following is the most likely diagnosis?

(A) squamous cell carcinoma

(B) basal cell carcinoma

(C) Merkel cell carcinoma

(D) melanoma

(E) keratoacanthoma

438. Which of the following is the most appropriate next step in management?

(A) wide excision with 2-cm margin

(B) wide excision with 2-cm margin and sentinel lymph node mapping

(C) shave biopsy

(D) excisional biopsy with 1- to 2-mm margins

(E) Mohs' surgical excision

Question 439

A 75-year-old woman is admitted to the hospital from a nursing home for abdominal pain and pneumonia. She was noted to be short of breath with increasing cough for 2 days prior to admission. Treatment, consisting of supplemental oxygen, intravenous antibiotics, and pulmonary toilet, is instituted, with improvement within 2 days. On the third hospital day, her abdominal pain worsens. Exam reveals a mildly distended abdomen with bowel sounds but no signs of peritonitis. Remainder of exam reveals a tender bulge in the medial left thigh below the inguinal ligament. Gentle pressure causes more pain but does not change the size or shape of the bulge. Abdominal films show a nonspecific bowel gas pattern. Laboratory analysis shows a WBC of 13,000, decreased from 18,000 at the time of admission.

439. Which of the following is the most likely diagnosis?

(A) incarcerated direct inguinal hernia

(B) lymph node with abscess

(C) femoral artery aneurysm

(D) incarcerated indirect inguinal hernia

(E) incarcerated femoral hernia

Questions 440 and 441

A 65-year-old woman presents to the physician's office for her yearly physical exam. She has no complaints except for a recent 10-pound weight loss. Past history is pertinent for a 40-pack year smoking history, hypertension, asthma, and hypothyroidism. Exam reveals a thin woman with normal vital signs and unremarkable heart and abdominal exams. Lung exam reveals mild wheezing and a few bibasilar rales. A chest x-ray is obtained and is shown in Figure 4–8. A chest x-ray obtained 3 years ago was normal. Yearly laboratory tests including a complete blood count (CBC), electrolytes, and lipid panels are normal.

440. Which of the following is the most likely diagnosis?

   (A) small cell lung cancer
   (B) tuberculosis
   (C) non–small cell lung cancer
   (D) hamartoma
   (E) abscess

441. Which of the following is the most appropriate next diagnostic test?

   (A) percutaneous needle biopsy
   (B) CT scan
   (C) pulmonary function tests
   (D) mediastinoscopy
   (E) bronchoscopy

Questions 442 and 443

A 75-year-old man is brought to the emergency department for severe pain in the left flank and back of 1 hour's duration. He has a prior history of a myocardial infarction and coronary artery bypass grafting 8 years ago. On exam, he is found to have a BP of 80/50, pulse of 110, respiratory rate of 15, and a pulsatile, tender abdominal mass. He has had two large-bore IV lines placed by the paramedics. He is alert and oriented, and gives consent for surgery.

442. Which of the following are the most appropriate next steps in management of this patient?

   (A) immediate consultation with cardiology to assess cardiac risk for surgery, followed by transfer to the operating room
   (B) resuscitation in the emergency department with IV fluids, transfer to radiology for a CT scan to assess for the location and degree of rupture, followed by transfer to the operating room
   (C) resuscitation in the emergency department with IV fluids to achieve a systolic BP greater than 100, followed by transfer to the operating room
   (D) immediate transfer to the operating room with concomitant resuscitation and laparotomy
   (E) resuscitation in the emergency department with IV fluids, transfer to radiology for immediate aortic angiogram for assessment of the location of the rupture, followed by transfer to the operating room

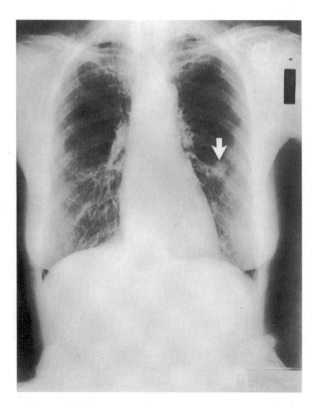

Figure 4–8. Posteroanterior chest x-ray. *(Reprinted with permission from Niederhuber JE. Fundamentals of Surgery. Appleton & Lange, 1998.)*

443. On postop day 3, the patient develops dark-colored diarrhea but remains normotensive, on full mechanical ventilation, and is awake. Laboratory analysis reveals normal electrolytes, blood urea nitrogen (BUN), and creatinine; hematocrit of 30; and WBC of 15,000. Which is the most appropriate next step in management?

(A) stool for *Clostridium difficile* toxin test and institution of metronidazole

(B) sigmoidoscopy

(C) air contrast barium enema

(D) CT scan

(E) abdominal x-rays

Questions 444 Through 446

A 65-year-old man presents to the emergency department with sudden onset of pain and weakness of the left lower extremity of 2 hours' duration. Past history reveals chronic atrial fibrillation following a myocardial infarction 12 months ago. On examination, he is found to have a cool, pale left lower extremity with decreased strength and absent popliteal and pedal pulses. The opposite leg has a normal appearance with palpable pulses.

444. Which of the following is the most appropriate first step in management of this patient?

(A) echocardiography

(B) anticoagulation with heparin

(C) anticoagulation with warfarin

(D) arteriography

(E) alkalinization of the urine with IV sodium bicarbonate

445. Which of the following is the treatment of choice for this patient?

(A) streptokinase infusion following anticoagulation

(B) administration of vasodilators

(C) four-compartment fasciotomy

(D) thromboembolectomy

(E) anticoagulation and close observation

446. Following successful surgery for an embolus to the left femoral artery with no evidence of a reperfusion injury, which of the following long-term treatments would most likely decrease the chance of recurrent embolus?

(A) anticoagulation

(B) exercise program

(C) coronary artery bypass grafting

(D) aortofemoral bypass grafting

(E) placement of a vena cava filter

Questions 447 and 448

A 65-year-old man presents to the emergency department with an abrupt onset of excruciating chest pain 1 hour ago. The pain is localized to the anterior chest, but radiates to the back and neck. On exam, the patient is afebrile, with a BP of 210/110, pulse of 95, and a respiratory rate of 12. He appears pale and sweaty. Unequal carotid, radial, and femoral pulses are noted. An electrocardiogram (ECG) shows nonspecific ST-T segment changes. Chest x-ray shows a slightly widened mediastinum and normal lung fields.

447. Which of the following is the preferred modality in establishing the diagnosis?

(A) transcutaneous echocardiography

(B) transesophageal echocardiography

(C) CT scan

(D) coronary angiography

(E) aortography

448. Which of the following is the first step in management of this patient?

(A) treatment with thrombolytic agents

(B) systemic anticoagulation

(C) control of hypertension

(D) placement of an intra-aortic balloon pump

(E) immediate operation

Questions 449 and 450

A 39-year-old woman presents to the physician's office for evaluation of a palpable nodule in the neck of 2 years' duration. Her past history is pertinent for Hashimoto's disease diagnosed 5 years ago, for which she takes thyroid hormone. She has a history of low-dose chest irradiation for an enlarged thymus gland during infancy. On exam, a 2.5-cm nodule is palpable in the left lobe of the thyroid and is firm and nontender.

449. Which of the following portions of her history increases the risk for thyroid cancer?

   (A) age group of 20 to 40 years
   (B) female gender
   (C) low-dose irradiation during infancy
   (D) chronicity of the nodule
   (E) past history of Hashimoto's disease

450. Which of the following is the most appropriate next step in her management?

   (A) ultrasound of the neck
   (B) thyroid scintiscan
   (C) MRI of the neck
   (D) CT scan of the neck and chest
   (E) fine-needle aspiration of the nodule

Questions 451 and 452

A 45-year-old man presents to the physician's office complaining of dysphagia and retrosternal pressure and pain of 2 years' duration. The symptoms have worsened over the last 3 months. He has a 30-pack year smoking history and drinks beer on weekends. Vital signs include a BP of 150/90, pulse 90, and respiratory rate 12, with a normal temperature. Exam reveals a thin man with a normal heart, lung, and abdomen exam. An esophagogram reveals a 6-cm, smooth, concave defect in the mid-esophagus with sharp borders. Esphagoscopy reveals intact overlying mucosa and a mobile tumor.

451. Which of the following is the most likely diagnosis?

   (A) esophageal carcinoma
   (B) bronchogenic carcinoma with invasion of the esophagus

   (C) benign esophageal polyp
   (D) leiomyoma
   (E) lymphoma

452. Which of the following is the most appropriate next step?

   (A) repeat esophagoscopy with biopsy
   (B) thoracotomy with extramucosal resection
   (C) thoracotomy with esophageal resection
   (D) radiation therapy
   (E) chemotherapy

Questions 453 and 454

A 49-year-old woman presents to her physician with dysphagia, regurgitation of undigested food eaten hours earlier, and coughing over the last 6 months. She was hospitalized 1 month ago for aspiration pneumonia and successfully treated with antibiotics. Exam reveals a thin-appearing woman with normal vital signs and unremarkable chest, heart, and abdominal exam. A UGI contrast study is performed and reveals a pharyngoesophageal (Zenker's) diverticulum.

453. Which of the following statements is true regarding Zenker's diverticula?

   (A) Cervical dysphagia is related to the size of the diverticulum.
   (B) Pharyngoesophageal diverticula are of the pulsion type.
   (C) Pharyngoesophageal diverticula are true diverticula.
   (D) Pharyngoesophageal diverticula are congenital in origin.
   (E) Upper esophageal sphincter function is usually normal.

454. Which of the following is the most important aspect of treatment?

   (A) resection of the diverticulum
   (B) cricopharyngeal muscle myotomy
   (C) H_2 blockers
   (D) elevation of the head of the bed
   (E) diverticulopexy

Question 455

A 55-year-old man presents to the emergency department at 5 AM complaining of vomiting blood. After binge drinking last night, the patient began to vomit repeatedly. After a number of episodes, the patient noted blood in the vomitus, followed by a melanotic stool 5 hours later. His past history is pertinent for ethanol abuse and a 40-pack year smoking history. Vital signs reveal a BP of 100/60, pulse 95, respiratory rate 12, and temperature of 97°F. Exam reveals a thin man with normal chest, cardiac, and abdominal findings. Rectal exam reveals heme-positive stool. Laboratory data show normal electrolytes and a hematocrit of 30. A chest x-ray is unremarkable. Volume resuscitation, gastric lavage, and nasogastric tube decompression are initiated.

455. Which of the following is the most appropriate diagnostic test?

(A) barium esophagogram
(B) water-soluble contrast esophagogram
(C) esophagoscopy
(D) CT scan
(E) angiogram

Questions 456 and 457

A 68-year-old man presents to the physician's office complaining of progressive dysphagia over the last 3 months associated with mild chest discomfort. He reports a 15-pound weight loss, a 30-pack year smoking history, and occasional alcohol intake. The physical exam, including vital signs, is unremarkable. A chest x-ray was normal, and a barium esophagogram shows an irregular filling defect in the distal third of the esophagus with distortion and narrowing of the lumen.

456. Which of the following is the most likely diagnosis?

(A) esophagitis with stricture
(B) esophageal carcinoma
(C) lung carcinoma with invasion into the esophagus
(D) lymphoma
(E) achalasia

457. Which of the following is the most appropriate next step in management?

(A) CT scan
(B) esophagoscopy
(C) MRI scan
(D) surgical resection
(E) bronchoscopy

Questions 458 Through 460

A 30-year-old man presents to the emergency department with sudden onset of severe epigastric pain and vomiting 3 hours ago. He reports a 6-month history of chronic epigastric pain occurring nearly every day and relieved by antacids. On exam, he appears sweaty and avoids movement. Vital signs reveal a temperature of 100°F, BP 100/60, pulse 110, and respiratory rate of 12. The remainder of his exam reveals diminished bowel sounds and a markedly tender and rigid abdomen. A chest x-ray and abdominal films reveal pneumoperitoneum.

458. Which of the following is the most likely diagnosis?

(A) small-bowel obstruction
(B) dead bowel
(C) perforated colon carcinoma
(D) perforated duodenal ulcer
(E) perforated gastric ulcer

459. Which of the following is the most appropriate next diagnostic test?

(A) CT scan
(B) UGI water-soluble contrast study
(C) lower GI water-soluble contrast study
(D) abdominal ultrasound
(E) none of the above

460. Which of the following is the most appropriate next step in management?

(A) immediate laparotomy
(B) nonoperative management with nasogastric decompression and antibiotics
(C) fluid resuscitation
(D) administration of H_2 blockers
(E) placement of a central venous line

Questions 461 and 462

A 55-year-old man presents to the physician's office complaining of upper abdominal pain of 2 months' duration. The pain is described as gnawing, localized to the upper midline, and associated with nausea. The pain is exacerbated by food, and there is an associated 20-pound weight loss over 2 months. His past history is pertinent for a 30-pack year smoking history, occasional alcohol intake, and a prior history of a benign gastric ulcer 5 years ago. Physical exam reveals normal vital signs, mild epigastric pain with deep palpation, and mildly heme-positive stool. An evaluation for recurrence of a gastric ulcer is recommended.

461. Which of the following tests is the most reliable method for diagnosing a gastric ulcer?

   (A) UGI barium x-rays
   (B) fiberoptic upper endoscopy
   (C) CT scan
   (D) endoscopic ultrasound
   (E) MRI

462. In this patient, a benign gastric ulcer was found, and he was placed on a proton pump inhibitor and triple antibiotics for *Helicobacter pylori*. He returns to the physician's office 3 months later with similar complaints and, on re-evaluation, the gastric ulcer was found to persist. Which of the following is the most appropriate next step in management?

   (A) a second trial of proton pump inhibitors with triple antibiotics and re-evaluation in 2 months
   (B) a trial of H_2 blockers with triple antibiotics and re-evaluation in 2 months
   (C) a trial of sucralfate and re-evaluation in 2 months
   (D) surgical management
   (E) a trial of prostaglandins and re-evaluation in 2 months

Questions 463 Through 465

A 65-year-old man presents to the physician's office for his yearly exam. His past history is pertinent for a 40-pack year smoking history and colon cancer 3 years ago for which he underwent a sigmoid colectomy. The most recent colonoscopic follow-up 3 months ago was negative. His physical exam is normal. Lab results show a normal CBC and electrolytes, markedly elevated cholesterol, and a CEA of 12 compared to values of less than 5 obtained every 6 months since colectomy. A repeat CEA 4 weeks later was 15, and liver function tests revealed a minimally elevated alkaline phosphatase, with normal transaminases and bilirubin.

463. Which of the following is the most appropriate next diagnostic test in this patient?

   (A) anti-CEA monoclonal antibody radionuclide scan
   (B) radionuclide liver scan
   (C) ultrasound
   (D) CT scan
   (E) MRI scan

464. The imaging studies demonstrate three lesions in the right hepatic lobe suspicious for metastatic disease, each measuring 3 to 4 cm in diameter. There was no evidence of extrahepatic disease. Which of the following is the most appropriate next step in management?

   (A) systemic chemotherapy
   (B) intra-arterial chemotherapy through the hepatic artery
   (C) surgical resection
   (D) radiation therapy to the liver
   (E) repeat imaging studies in 3 months to determine the growth rate of the disease

465. In your discussion with the patient regarding the risks and benefits of the different management options listed above, which of the following values should you quote regarding the expected 5-year survival rate following curative surgical resection?

   (A) 5 to 10%
   (B) 15 to 20%

(C) 25 to 35%

(D) 40 to 50%

(E) 60 to 70%

Questions 466 and 467

A previously healthy 45-year-old man presents with a 9-month history of a slow-growing, painless right neck mass. He is a nonsmoker and has no significant past medical history. On examination, there is a nontender, discrete, 3-cm mass over the angle of the right mandible. Facial muscle function and sensation are normal. An oropharyngeal exam is normal.

466. The most likely diagnosis in this patient is

(A) metastatic carcinoma

(B) infectious parotitis

(C) pleomorphic adenoma of the parotid

(D) Hodgkin's disease

(E) reactive cervical lymphatic hyperplasia

467. The next step in the management of this patient is

(A) antibiotics

(B) excisional biopsy

(C) observation with re-evaluation in 2 to 4 weeks

(D) superficial parotidectomy

(E) chest x-ray

Questions 468 and 469

A 10-month-old infant presents to the emergency department with a 24-hour history of low-grade fever and anorexia. The parents report several episodes in which the child has been suddenly inconsolable and crying, followed by periods of lethargy. He has had nonbilious vomiting and several loose stools. On exam, the infant is pale and mildly dehydrated. His abdomen is soft and nondistended, with fullness to palpation in the right upper quadrant. The child passed another stool in the emergency department (Figure 4–9).

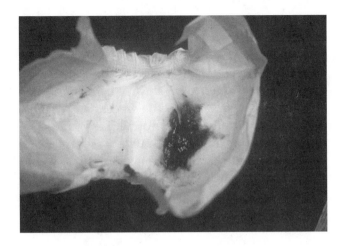

Figure 4–9. Stool from a 10-month-old infant.

468. The most probable diagnosis is

(A) gastroenteritis

(B) intussusception

(C) midgut volvulus

(D) Meckel's diverticulum

(E) juvenile rectal polyp

469. The most appropriate steps in the diagnostic evaluation and management include

(A) proctoscopy

(B) oral rehydration and stool cultures

(C) IV fluid rehydration and a hydrostatic barium enema

(D) technetium scan

(E) IV fluid rehydration, nasogastric decompression, and a UGI contrast study

Question 470

A 65-year-old diabetic man presents to the emergency department with a history of a penetrating wound to his buttock by a wooden stump while working in his garden 24 hours earlier. On examination, he is febrile, the tissue around the wound is violaceous in color, and several bullae and crepitus are noted in the buttock. The drainage from the wound is foul smelling, watery, and grayish in appearance.

470. The optimal treatment for this patient would include

(A) high-dose IV penicillin G

(B) high-dose IV penicillin G and local wound care with unroofing of bullae and culture of wound drainage

(C) high-dose IV penicillin G with surgical debridement only if and when there is no improvement with antibiotics

(D) radical surgical debridement

(E) high-dose IV penicillin G, radical surgical debridement, and hyperbaric oxygen therapy

Question 471

A 23-year-old man presents to the emergency department with a soft-tissue injury to the left lower extremity. The injury was sustained 8 hours earlier in a motorcycle accident on a gravel road. On examination, the patient has a 7-cm-deep laceration to the calf, with visible road debris. He had full tetanus immunization as a child and a tetanus booster immunization at age 15.

471. Appropriate management of this injury would include

(A) irrigation and debridement of the wound

(B) irrigation and debridement of the wound; tetanus toxoid and tetanus immune globulin

(C) irrigation and debridement of the wound; tetanus toxoid

(D) irrigation and debridement of the wound; IV antibiotics

(E) tetanus toxoid and IV antibiotics

Question 472

A 6-year-old boy presents to the emergency department with a painful, markedly swollen elbow. While ice skating, he fell with his arm outstretched. Radiographs of the elbow demonstrate a displaced, supracondylar fracture of the humerus. On examination, there is pain on passive flexion at the wrist and a decreased radial pulse, with diminished capillary refill in the hand.

472. Appropriate management of this injury would be

(A) admission to hospital for close observation, with immobilization of the elbow at 90 degrees of flexion

(B) closed reduction with percutaneous pinning under general anesthesia

(C) open reduction and pinning under general anesthesia

(D) open reduction with pinning, and exploration of the brachial artery

(E) open reduction with pinning, exploration of the brachial artery, and decompression fasciotomy of the forearm fascial compartments

Questions 473 and 474

A 35-year-old woman is involved in a motor vehicle crash, sustaining a severe pelvic fracture, with disruption of the pelvic ring. In the trauma resuscitation room, she is confused and tachypneic, with a blood pressure of 90 mm Hg systolic and a heart rate of 130/min. Laboratory investigations include serum electrolyte analysis, revealing a sodium of 139, a chloride of 103, and a bicarbonate of 14 mEq/L.

473. This patient demonstrates a

(A) nonanion gap metabolic acidosis

(B) anion gap metabolic acidosis

(C) metabolic alkalosis

(D) respiratory acidosis

(E) normal serum electrolytes

474. Appropriate management of this acid–base derangement would be

(A) administration of sodium bicarbonate to correct the base deficit

(B) restoration of blood volume with aggressive IV fluid resuscitation

(C) IV hydrochloric acid

(D) intubation and hyperventilation

(E) this patient has no acid–base abnormality

DIRECTIONS (Questions 475 through 477): For each item, select the ONE best lettered option that is most closely associated with it. Each lettered heading may be selected once, more than once, or not at all.

For each newborn with vomiting and illustrated radiographs, select the most likely diagnosis.

(A) congenital hypertrophic pyloric stenosis

(B) annular pancreas

(C) duodenal atresia

(D) midgut volvulus

(E) intussusception

(F) imperforate anus

(G) Meckel's diverticulum

(H) meconium ileus

(I) Hirschprung's disease

(J) jejunal atresia

475. A 10-day-old infant presenting with bilious vomiting, paucity of gas on plain radiographs, and duodenal obstruction on UGI contrast study (Figures 4–10 and 4–11)

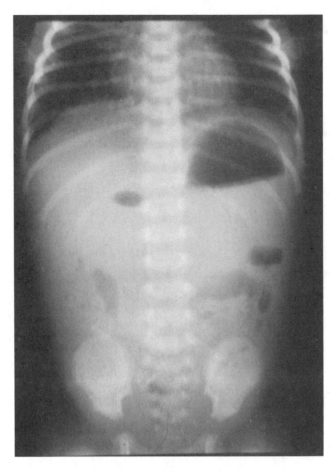

Figure 4–10. Abdominal x-ray of infant.

476. A neonate with bile-stained vomiting, abdominal distension, dilated loops of bowel on plain radiographs, and a small-caliber colon on contrast enema (Figure 4–12)

477. A 1-day-old infant with Down syndrome, feeding intolerance, bilious vomiting, and a double bubble on plain radiographs (Figure 4–13)

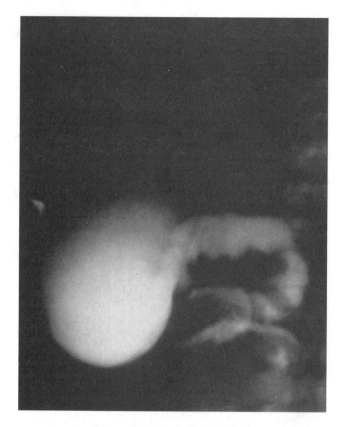

Figure 4–11. UGI study of infant.

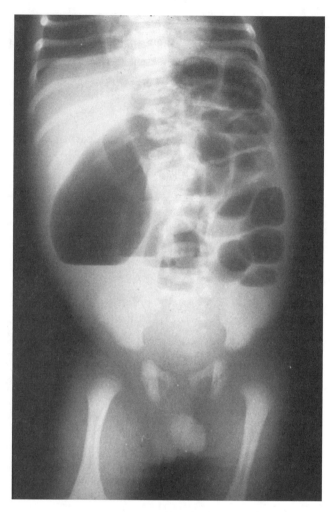

Figure 4–12. Abdominal x-ray of neonate.

DIRECTIONS (Questions 478 through 502): Each of the numbered items or incomplete statements in this section is followed by answers or by completions of the statement. Select the ONE lettered answer that is BEST in each case.

Questions 478 and 479

A 36-year-old man with a past history of bilateral orchiopexy for cryptorchidism presents with a painless, unilateral right scrotal enlargement. On examination, there is a palpable right testicular mass. Scrotal ultrasonography demonstrates heterogeneity of the testis, with an associated hydrocele. A CT scan of the abdomen, pelvis, and chest is normal.

478. The next step to confirm the diagnosis should be

(A) trans-scrotal aspiration of the hydrocele for cytology

(B) trans-scrotal exploration with orchiectomy

(C) trans-scrotal needle biopsy

(D) radical orchiectomy through an inguinal incision

(E) laparotomy with pelvic and retroperitoneal node dissection

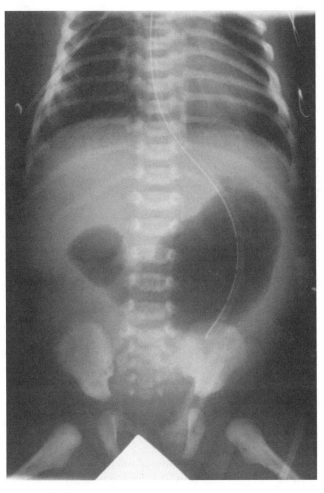

Figure 4–13. Abdominal x-ray of 1-day-old infant.

479. Staging workup and surgery reveal a seminoma of the testicle, with negative inguinal and retroperitoneal nodes. Therapeutic management for this patient is

(A) external beam radiotherapy

(B) multidrug combination chemotherapy

(C) combination radiotherapy and multidrug chemotherapy

(D) laparotomy with pelvic and retroperitoneal node dissection

(E) clinical surveillance

Questions 480 and 481

A 6-month-old previously healthy male infant presents with a 4-hour history of irritability. He has had one episode of nonbilious vomiting and has refused to breast feed. In the emergency department, the infant appears inconsolable. He is afebrile, and his abdomen is mildly distended but soft. An abnormality is revealed on removal of the child's diaper, as illustrated in Figure 4–14. There is no previous documentation of this finding, according to the parent's history.

480. The most likely clinical diagnosis is

(A) testicular torsion

(B) inguinal adenitis

(C) undescended testicle

(D) incarcerated inguinal hernia

(E) noncommunicating hydrocele

481. The next most appropriate step in management is

(A) urgent surgical exploration

(B) systemic antibiotics

(C) elective surgical repair

(D) sedation with manual reduction and arrangements for elective surgical repair

(E) sedation with manual reduction, rehydration, and surgical repair within 24 hours

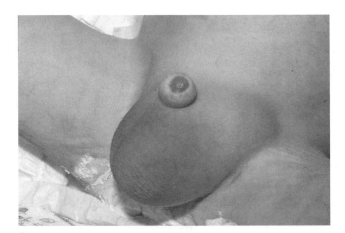

Figure 4–14. Photo of groin of 6-month-old infant.

Questions 482 and 483

A 70-year-old man with a 50-pack year history of smoking presents with a 6-week history of intermittent, painless, gross hematuria and urinary frequency. There are no masses palpable on abdominal exam, and rectal examination is normal. Urinalysis confirms the presence of hematuria, and urine culture is negative.

482. The initial diagnostic evaluation of this patient should be

   (A) plain abdominal radiographs and an IVP
   (B) voiding cystourethrogram
   (C) cystourethroscopy
   (D) abdominal ultrasound
   (E) urine for cytology

483. The initial diagnostic evaluation does not reveal any abnormalities. The next step in the diagnostic workup is

   (A) an abdominal CT scan
   (B) cystourethroscopy and urinary cytology
   (C) a transrectal ultrasound
   (D) exploratory laparoscopy
   (E) re-evaluation in 2 to 4 weeks, with repeat urinalysis and urine culture

Question 484

A 7-week-old, breast-fed, term infant presents with increasing jaundice, abdominal distension, and abnormal stools (Figure 4–15). Liver function tests demonstrate a conjugated hyperbilirubinemia, mildly elevated transaminases, and an elevated gamma-glutamyl transpeptidase. TORCH (congenital infection complex, including toxoplasmosis, rubella, cytomegalovirus, and hepatitis) serology and screening for inborn errors of metabolism are negative.

484. As part of the diagnostic evaluation, the most sensitive imaging study in this clinical setting would be

   (A) radioisotope scanning
   (B) radioisotope scanning with preimaging phenobarbital administration
   (C) abdominal ultrasound

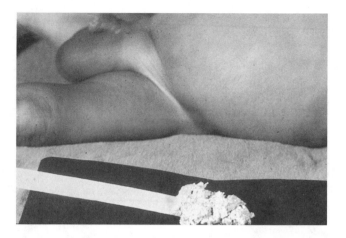

Figure 4–15. Stool from jaundiced 7-week-old infant.

   (D) CT scan of the abdomen
   (E) MRI scan of the abdomen

Questions 485 and 486

During diagnostic evaluation, a 14-year-old girl with menorrhagia, frequent nosebleeds, and iron-deficiency anemia is found to have a low platelet count with a normal coagulation profile. Bone marrow biopsy reveals abundant megakaryocytes. On abdominal examination, no organomegaly is noted.

485. Appropriate initial therapy for this patient would be

   (A) splenectomy
   (B) platelet transfusion when peripheral platelet count drops below 50,000/µL
   (C) systemic steroids
   (D) chemotherapy
   (E) expectant, with intervention only if the patient develops significant clinical bleeding

The patient has a satisfactory response to the initial therapeutic intervention, but over 6 to 12 months' time, the response is less dramatic and shorter in duration. There are signs and symptoms of increasing side effects from therapy.

486. The next step in management would be to recommend

   (A) partial splenectomy
   (B) splenectomy

(C) increase in steroid dose and frequency

(D) bone marrow transplant

(E) plasmapheresis

Question 487

A 50-year-old man is admitted to the hospital with a UGI bleed from acute erosive gastritis, secondary to chronic nonsteroidal anti-inflammatory use. His hematocrit is 28%. With fluid resuscitation, his blood pressure normalizes, but he has a persistent hyperdynamic precordium, tachycardia, and flow murmur on auscultation. He complains of shortness of breath on ambulation. An ECG shows depressed ST-T segments.

487. The next appropriate step in management is

   (A) initiation of iron supplementation therapy

   (B) supplemental oxygen

   (C) continued intravenous fluid resuscitation

   (D) initiation of a calcium channel blocker

   (E) blood transfusion

Question 488

A previously healthy 28-year-old woman develops significant postpartum hemorrhage, with a rapid drop in hematocrit to 18%. Despite aggressive IV fluid resuscitation, the patient has a persistent tachycardia, labile systolic blood pressure and poor urine output. Ongoing resuscitation includes emergency transfusion with 2 units of O-negative packed red blood cells. During transfusion of the second unit, the patient develops chills, fever, vomiting, and hypertension.

488. These symptoms are most likely the result of

   (A) a febrile nonhemolytic transfusion reaction

   (B) an anaphylactic transfusion reaction

   (C) ABO incompatability with acute hemolytic transfusion reaction

   (D) delayed hemolytic transfusion reaction

   (E) acute bacterial infection transmitted in the blood product

Question 489

A 22-year-old professional basketball player falls on his outstretched hand during a scrimmage game. He has mild swelling at the wrist and tenderness to palpation in the anatomic snuffbox. No fracture is visible on multiple radiographs of the wrist and hand.

489. The appropriate management of this patient is

   (A) anti-inflammatory medication and application of ice

   (B) elastic wrist support, analgesics, and restricted activity for 1 to 2 weeks

   (C) presumptive diagnosis of a scaphoid fracture, with application of a wrist splint, and repeat x-rays in 10 to 14 days

   (D) presumptive diagnosis of a scaphoid fracture, with application of a short-arm cast including the thumb

   (E) presumptive diagnosis of a scaphoid fracture, application of a short-arm cast including the thumb, and removal of the cast, with repeat x-rays in 10 to 14 days

Question 490

A previously healthy 45-year-old woman is involved in a motor vehicle crash, sustaining multiple rib fractures, a complex duodenal injury, and a fractured pelvis. She is ventilated in the ICU. Because of a persistent high-output duodenal fistula, the patient has required prolonged parenteral alimentation. During her ICU course, the patient develops diarrhea, mental depression, alopecia, and perioral and periorbital dermatitis.

490. Administration of which of the following trace elements is most likely to reverse these complications?

   (A) iodine

   (B) zinc

   (C) selenium

   (D) silicon

   (E) tin

Questions 491 and 492

A 70-year-old man is admitted to the ICU after repair of an abdominal aortic aneurysm. He has a prior history of hypertension and mild congestive heart failure, which were adequately controlled with digoxin and diuretics. To facilitate perioperative management, a Swan–Ganz (multilumen pulmonary artery) catheter was inserted in the operating room. During the first few hours postoperatively, the patient is noted to have a blood pressure of 140/70 mm Hg, heart rate of 110/min, flat neck veins, a pulmonary arterial wedge pressure of 9 mm Hg, and poor urine output.

491. The next appropriate step in management of this patient would be

(A) IV furosemide
(B) a bolus of IV crystalloid
(C) a dopamine infusion
(D) a nitroprusside infusion
(E) IV digoxin administration

Several hours after this intervention, the patient is reassessed. The blood pressure is 150/85 mm Hg, heart rate is 90/min, neck veins are distended, and the pulmonary arterial wedge pressure is 17 mm Hg. Urine output is still low in volume.

492. At this point, management should be

(A) IV furosemide
(B) a bolus of IV crystalloid
(C) a dopamine infusion
(D) a nitroprusside infusion
(E) IV digoxin administration

Question 493

A 19-year-old previously healthy man is an unbelted driver of a motor vehicle involved in a front-end collision. On arrival in the emergency department, the patient is noted to have stridor, with marked respiratory distress, and an oxygen saturation of 88% despite 100% oxygen by mask. He has obvious extensive facial injuries, a flail chest, and poor chest expansion. Bag–mask–valve ventilation is ineffective.

493. The most appropriate next step in management is

(A) orotracheal intubation
(B) nasotracheal intubation
(C) cricothyroidotomy
(D) tracheostomy
(E) placement of bilateral chest tubes

494. A 40-year-old alcoholic is brought to the emergency department with frostbite to both lower extremities. His core body temperature is 36°C. The most appropriate initial treatment for the patient's thermal injury is

(A) sympathectomy without any delay
(B) debridement of devitalized tissues
(C) slow rewarming at room temperature
(D) slow rewarming with dry heat
(E) rapid rewarming in warm water

Questions 495 Through 497

A 50-year-old woman with a history of essential hypertension presents to the emergency department with a severe headache, nausea and vomiting, and photophobia. On examination, her BP is 160/100 mm Hg. She is mildly confused and has nuchal rigidity, without focal neurologic signs.

495. The most likely diagnosis is

(A) hemorrhagic stroke
(B) ruptured cerebral aneurysm
(C) meningitis
(D) ischemic cerebrovascular accident
(E) transient ischemic attack

496. The diagnosis is best confirmed with

(A) lumbar puncture
(B) Doppler ultrasonography of the carotid arteries
(C) cerebral MRI scan
(D) head CT scan, followed by cerebral angiography
(E) electroencephalogram (EEG)

497. Once the diagnosis has been confirmed, the next most important step in patient management is

(A) urgent surgical intervention with aneurysm clipping

(B) admission to the ICU, close monitoring, and aggressive treatment of hypertension

(C) admission to the ICU, close monitoring, and intravenous antibiotics

(D) anticoagulation and antiplatelet therapy

(E) serial lumbar punctures to drain cerebrospinal fluid (CSF)

498. During an elective laparoscopic cholecystectomy, the anesthesiologist reports that the patient has developed a sudden drop in systolic blood pressure, arterial desaturation, and an increase in ventilatory pressure. The most appropriate step in management is

(A) an IV fluid bolus

(B) decompression of the pneumoperitoneum

(C) insertion of a chest tube

(D) re-evaluating the position of the endotracheal tube and obtaining a portable chest x-ray

(E) aborting the procedure and converting to an open cholecystectomy

Questions 499 Through 501

A 55-year-old man with a history of diverticulosis presents with a 2-week history of dysuria, urgency, and pneumaturia. Furthermore, he has a 3-month history of vague, intermittent, left-lower-quadrant abdominal pain and irregular bowel habits. On examination, he has fullness on palpation in the left lower quadrant, and urine culture demonstrates a polymicrobial infection. A CT scan demonstrates an inflammatory mass in the left pelvis.

499. The investigation most likely to aid in diagnosis is

(A) voiding cystourethrogram

(B) cystoscopy

(C) air contrast barium enema

(D) colonoscopy

(E) laparoscopy

500. After confirming the diagnosis, the most appropriate initial steps in management of this patient include

(A) broad-spectrum antibiotics and insertion of an indwelling bladder catheter

(B) outpatient oral antibiotics and stool softeners

(C) clear fluids, magnesium citrate, and oral antibiotics

(D) urgent exploratory laparotomy

(E) proximal defunctioning colostomy

501. Optimal definitive surgical management for this patient would be

(A) a proximal defunctioning loop colostomy

(B) sigmoid colon resection with primary anastomosis

(C) sigmoid colon resection with Hartmann's procedure

(D) abdominoperineal resection and permanent colostomy

(E) total abdominal colectomy and ileorectal anastomosis

Question 502

An 80-year-old female resident of a nursing home presents to the emergency department with a history of sudden onset of crampy abdominal pain, vomiting, and abdominal distension. Her last bowel movement was 4 days prior to presentation, and she has not passed flatus since the onset of her symptoms. On examination, the patient is mildly dehydrated and afebrile, with a markedly distended but nontender abdomen. Barium enema is shown (Figure 4–16). The patient receives intravenous resuscitation and nasogastric tube decompression.

502. The next step in management of this patient is

(A) urgent laparotomy

(B) admission to the hospital and serial abdominal examinations

(C) placement of a rectal decompression tube in the emergency department

(D) rigid proctoscopy and directed placement of a colonic decompression tube

(E) colonic enemas

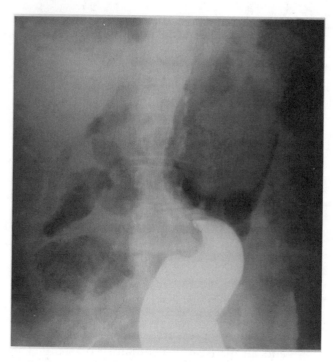

Figure 4–16. Barium enema of an 80-year-old female. *(Reprinted with permission from Zinner MJ. Maingot's Abdominal Operations, 10th ed., vol. 2. Appleton & Lange, 1996.)*

Answers and Explanations

379–382. (379-D, 380-B, 381-B, 382-D) Infants with pyloric stenosis usually present after the third week of life with symptoms of progressive pyloric outlet obstruction secondary to increasing hypertrophy of the pyloric muscle. There are often clinical signs of dehydration, but the infant usually appears well and is eager to feed. Viral gastroenteritis and urinary tract sepsis may be associated with signs of systemic illness such as lethargy, poor feeding, and, in some cases, fever. Gastroesophageal reflux more typically presents with a history of regurgitation since birth. Milk protein allergy is often associated with colicky abdominal pain and diarrhea. The pathognomonic sign on clinical exam is a palpable "olive" in the epigastrium or right upper quadrant. Abdominal ultrasound is operator dependent, but with expertise in interpretation of the study, the thickened elongated pyloric channel can be demonstrated. A UGI contrast study may show the classic "shouldering" of the pyloric muscle, with a "string sign"; this also requires expertise in performing the exam, and other causes of pyloric outlet obstruction such as pylorospasm may be misinterpreted as a positive study. Surgical exploration should be reserved for those patients in whom the diagnosis has been confirmed and the infant who has received fluid resuscitation. Infants with gastric outlet obstruction develop a hypo-chloremic, hypokalemic metabolic alkalosis. This is secondary to the loss of chloride in the gastric contents, and the renal reabsorption of sodium in exchange for potassium and hydrogen. Carbonic anhydrase converts carbonic acid to hydrogen and bicarbonate ions, allowing hydrogen to be excreted in the urine, with retention of the bicarbonate. Hence, with the metabolic alkalosis, there is a "paradoxical aciduria." Hypernatremic, hy- perchloremic, hypokalemic metabolic acidosis develops in infants with diarrhea. Infants with gastroesophageal reflux do not usu-ally develop significant electrolyte derangements. Infants with pyloric stenosis will usually require a period of fluid resuscitation to correct hypovolemia as well as electrolyte and acid–base abnormalities. This is followed by a pyloromyotomy. Infants with vomiting and diarrhea from viral gastroenteritis are often successfully managed with oral rehydration. Prokinetic agents have been used in the management of gastroesophageal reflux. Soy formulas or elemental formulas are recommended for the infant with a milk protein allergy. (*Sabiston, pp 100–101, 1251–1252; Greenfield et al, pp 2066–2067*)

383–384. (383-D, 384-B) The clinical signs and symptoms of a ureteral calculus are secondary to sudden obstruction of a hollow viscus, with visceral referred pain from loin to groin. The pain is severe and colicky in nature, with ureteral peristalsis against the obstruction. This is often associated with reflex vomiting mediated by visceral stretch and pain fibers. Typically, the patient is restless and cannot find a position of comfort. Urinary urgency and hematuria are common. Torsion of the testes produces sudden scrotal pain, and may have associated vague lower abdominal pain and vomiting. Pyelonephritis is associated with flank pain and costovertebral angle tenderness that is progressive in severity and constant in nature. Appendicitis will present with vague periumbilical pain, migrating to the right lower quadrant with the development of peritonitis. In the latter stages, the patient will lie quietly, as movement exacerbates the pain from peritoneal irritation. By increasing hydration and adequate analgesia, most patients will pass ureteral stones spontaneously. An IVP should be obtained in all patients presenting with symptoms of urinary calculi. The IVP will identify the location of the stone, size and number of stones, whether there is complete or partial urinary tract obstruction, and the presence or absence of associated urinary tract anomalies. This information assists with planning further management options, including referral for lithotripsy or cystoscopy and retrograde ureteroscopy. (Sabiston, pp 1526, 1533–1536; Greenfield et al, pp 2204–2206)

385.   (C) During the early catabolic phase after injury, nutritional support is essential in the management of the multiply injured patient. Elemental tube feeding can be initiated via the nasogastric route, or via the nasojejunal route if there is delayed gastric emptying. Enteral nutrition will aid in maintaining the integrity of the gastrointestinal mucosal barrier, thereby reducing the risk of bacterial translocation and sepsis. The enteral route is less expensive than parenteral nutrition, and does not subject the patient to the complications associated with an indwelling central venous catheter. (Sabiston, pp 149–150; Greenfield et al, pp 52, 54–55, 58–64)

386–387.   (386-A, 387-C) This infant presents with the clinical picture of a bowel obstruction. Initial management should include IV fluid resuscitation and nasogastric decompression. These interventions are essential prior to safe transport of the child to another center for further diagnostic studies. A septic workup, with initiation of antibiotic therapy, would be indicated only if there were perinatal risk factors for sepsis. Progressive abdominal distension, vomiting, and delayed passage of meconium is suggestive of Hirschprung's disease. This infant presents with a clinical picture

of a distal bowel obstruction. Plain abdominal radiographs will demonstrate multiple dilated bowel loops. A contrast enema is important to exclude other causes of distal bowel obstruction in the neonate. Hirschsprung's disease is then confirmed with rectal biopsy. Anorectal manometry is a useful diagnostic tool in older children, as it requires the subject's cooperation and communication skills. (Sabiston, pp 1243–1244; Greenfield et al, pp 2057–2059)

388.   (D) This patient has a left tension pneumothorax, a diagnosis established based on symptoms and clinical examination. The patient is hypoxic, with respiratory distress, and demonstrates deviation of the mediastinum to the contralateral side, with hypotension from the mediastinal shift that compromises venous return. A chest x-ray is unnecessary and will delay definitive life-saving intervention. The patient requires urgent decompression with a large-bore needle in the second intercostal space anteriorly, followed by insertion of a chest tube. Although assisted ventilation can improve oxygenation, positive pressure may increase the pneumothorax if initiated prior to adequate decompression. (Sabiston, p 308; Greenfield et al, pp 323)

389–391.   (389-A, 390-C, 391-B) Hemorrhage associated with a Meckel's diverticulum classically presents with painless rectal bleeding in the absence of other gastrointestinal symptoms. The amount of hemorrhage may be enough to result in hypovolemia, with pallor, tachycardia, and postural hypotension. Abdominal exam is usually normal. Diagnosis is confirmed by technetium scan, with the isotope concentrated in the gastric mucosa of the diverticulum. Initial management should include IV fluid resuscitation and transfusion as needed, prior to laparotomy and diverticulectomy. Rectal polyps, hemorrhoids, and anal fissures may be associated with rectal bleeding. The bleeding is usually small in amount and often temporally related to defecation, typically on the surface of the stool or after defecation. Colonoscopy and proctoscopy are useful adjuncts to diagnosis. Bleeding associated with intussusception is described as "currant jelly" and is secondary to mucosal ischemia of the lead point. These children are most commonly between 2 months and 2 years of age, and often have a prodromal viral illness. They present with colicky abdominal pain and dehydration. Management includes hydrostatic reduction. *(Sabiston, pp 254–255; Greenfield et al, pp 2069–2071)*

392. **(D)** The guiding principle of management of closed head injury is to maintain cerebral perfusion and oxygenation, thereby preventing secondary brain insult. Cerebral perfusion pressure (CPP) is dependent on systemic blood pressure, circulating blood volume, and intracranial pressure (ICP) (ie, CPP = mean BP – ICP). Normal CPP requires an adequate circulating blood volume with maintenance of normovolemia. Hypercarbia should be avoided, as it leads to cerebral vasodilatation and increased ICP. Early insertion of a ventriculostomy is beneficial to permit controlled drainage of CSF as required to maintain a normal ICP. Fluid restriction and hyperventilation should be avoided in the early stages of management of a closed head injury. Autoregulation of cerebral blood flow is disrupted in the early phases after head injury. Aggressive hyperventilation with resultant cerebral vasoconstriction may precariously compromise the perfusion to the injured brain and to the surrounding noninjured brain. In patients with deteriorating neurologic status and/or evidence of increasing ICP that is not well controlled with a ventriculostomy, osmotic diuretics and moderate hyperventilation may be useful adjuncts to therapy. The use of steroids in the management of closed head injury is not indicated. *(Greenfield et al, pp 292–295)*

393–394. **(393-C, 394-D)** Crohn's disease is a chronic inflammatory disease of the gastrointestinal tract that presents with intermittent crampy abdominal pain and diarrhea. It most commonly involves the terminal ileum and right colon. Because eating can exacerbate symptoms, oral intake may be decreased, contributing to the associated weight loss. Transmural inflammation leads to bowel wall thickening, and with adjacent mesenteric inflammation, the patient may develop a palpable mass. It may be difficult to differentiate Crohn's disease from ulcerative colitis on the basis of history and clinical exam. However, ulcerative colitis is a mucosal disease that is limited to the colon and nearly always involves the rectum. Diarrhea is usually bloody, and hemorrhage may be significant enough to require transfusion therapy. Complicated appendicitis may present with a right-lower-quadrant mass and diarrhea if there is perforation with abscess formation. The history is that of an acute illness in a previously well patient. Irritable bowel syndrome is associated with intermittent crampy abdominal pain, and diarrhea alternating with constipation. There is no inflammatory process, and weight loss is not a clinical feature. The principle of initial management of Crohn's disease is relief of symptoms, nutritional therapy, and suppression of the inflammatory process. Nutritional supplementation may require TPN in conjunction with bowel rest. Acute exacerbations of the disease are initially treated with systemic steroids. The use of antispasmodics may be effective in the treatment of irritable bowel syndrome. In Crohn's disease, however, antispasmodics may lead to an ileus or toxic bowel dilatation. Surgery in Crohn's disease is indicated for the management of complications, including fistula or abscess formation, stricture with obstruction, and perforation. *(Sabiston, pp 923–928; Greenfield et al, pp 834–841)*

395. **(C)** Testicular torsion presents with acute onset of scrotal pain, reflex vomiting, referred abdominal pain, and an elevated tender testis. If there is a high index of suspicion based on history and clinical exam, the patient should undergo an urgent surgical exploration. Delay in definitive therapy increases the risk of testicular loss secondary to ischemia. Isotope scan may demonstrate absence of testicular blood flow in torsion, and increased flow in orchitis or epididymitis. Although useful in the differential diagnosis, these nuclear medicine studies may not be readily available, and definitive therapy should not be delayed awaiting imaging. Orchitis and epididymitis present with a more

insidious clinical course associated with the progression of the inflammatory process. There may be a concomitant urinary tract infection, and therapy includes analgesics and antibiotics. *(Sabiston, pp 1559–1560; Greenfield et al, p 2110)*

396. **(D)** This elderly patient has metastatic adenocarcinoma of the prostate, and management is therefore aimed at tumor control for palliation of symptoms. This is achieved with hormonal manipulation, either by orchiectomy or exogenous estrogen therapy. Radical prostatectomy is indicated only for patients in whom the malignancy is confined to the prostate gland. Transurethral prostatectomy is used to treat benign prostatic hypertrophy, and is not considered adequate surgical therapy for prostatic malignancy. Cytotoxic chemotherapy may be useful as an adjunct to radical surgical excision of localized disease. Chemotherapy is not indicated for the treatment of metastatic disease. Radiation therapy has been used for the management of localized disease, and there is some evidence that it affords equivalent survival when compared to surgical excision. In patients with bone pain that is not well palliated with hormonal manipulation, radiation therapy may be useful. *(Sabiston, pp 1565–1567; Greenfield et al, pp 2210–2212)*

397. **(E)** Malignant hyperthermia may occur after administration of succinylcholine for muscle relaxation and induction of general anesthesia. This is a result of a genetic defect in calcium release from the sarcoplasm of skeletal muscle. It often occurs within 30 minutes of induction, and in addition to fever, tachycardia, and muscle rigidity, there is a metabolic acidosis and hyperkalemia. The treatment is administration of dantrolene to block calcium release from the sarcoplasm and insulin/bicarbonate/dextrose infusion to treat the hyperkalemia. Diagnosis is confirmed by muscle biopsy. Pneumonia is an infective, inflammatory process; is not associated with muscle rigidity; and is not likely to have a rapid progressive onset after induction of anesthesia in a previously healthy patient. Atelectasis is unlikely under general anesthe-

sia, particularly in patients receiving positive pressure ventilation. Although pyelonephritis may be associated with fever, it is not associated with muscle rigidity or metabolic acidosis and would be unlikely to become symptomatic after induction in an otherwise healthy patient. Myocardial infarction may be associated with tachyarrhythmias but would not account for the muscle rigidity, fever, or metabolic acidosis and, in the absence of risk factors, would be very unlikely in this healthy patient. *(Sabiston, p 343)*

398. **(E)** The anterior triangle of the neck is divided into three zones: zone I at the base of the neck and thoracic inlet, zone II in the midbody of the neck, and zone III above the angle of the mandible. Zone II, the most common area injured with penetrating trauma, encompasses the carotid artery, jugular vein, larynx, trachea, and esophagus. Patients with penetrating injuries to the neck that violate the platysma should be admitted to the hospital for further evaluation. This patient has a penetrating injury through the platysma, in zone II of the anterior triangle. He has signs of significant injury (ie, external bleeding at the scene, odynophagia, and a neck hematoma on exam). This patient should undergo surgical exploration, without prior diagnostic studies. Observation in the ICU, with or without intubation, is not appropriate in a patient with obvious clinical signs of injury. Furthermore, extensive preoperative imaging studies are not necessary for zone II injuries, because surgical exposure of vital structures in this area of the neck is easily achieved. All patients with clinical signs of injury should undergo surgical exploration. However, there is controversy with respect to the management of patients *without* clinical signs of injury. There are two approaches: (1) mandatory surgical exploration, or (2) selective observation with or without imaging studies. *(Sabiston, pp 300–303; Greenfield et al, pp 309–312)*

399. **(C)** This patient has a distended abdomen, with decreased bowel sounds, in the presence of shock that is unresponsive to aggressive fluid resuscitation. Intra-abdominal hemorrhage from solid visceral injury (hepatic, splenic, or renal) is the most likely etiology. The patient should undergo an urgent exploratory laparotomy for control of the bleeding, in conjunction with continued infusion of IV fluids and blood products. If the patient is alert and oriented, the cervical spine can be evaluated clinically. Although hypotension can result from a cervical cord injury, it is unlikely in this case, in the presence of a documented normal neurological exam. A Swan–Ganz catheter is not indicated in the initial evaluation and management of a patient presenting in hypovolemic shock from blunt trauma. Abdominal CT scan is indicated only for evaluation of blunt abdominal trauma in patients who are hemodynamically stable. Diagnostic peritoneal lavage may be indicated in the evaluation of patients with hypotension in which the source of bleeding is unclear. In this patient, however, the presence of a distended abdomen suggests hemoperitoneum, and therefore lavage is not necessary. (*Sabiston, pp 1359–1360*)

400–401. (400-A, 401-B) Diabetes insipidus (DI) is a disorder due to impaired renal conservation of water. DI presents with polyuria and a dilute urine in the presence of an elevated serum osmolality. This is either secondary to impaired production of antidiuretic hormone (ADH) from the posterior pituitary (central DI), or refractoriness of the distal renal tubules to ADH (nephrogenic DI). Central DI may complicate closed head injury, and is considered a poor prognostic sign. These patients will respond to exogenous IV vasopressin, with resultant increase in urine osmolality and decrease in urine volume. Nephrogenic DI may be congenital, familial, or acquired. Acquired nephrogenic DI may occur in the setting of repeated renal tubular insults such as sepsis, IV contrast, and nephrotoxic drug therapy. With administration of vasopressin, these patients will have no change in urine osmolality or urine volume because the renal tubules are unresponsive. DI must be differentiated from other causes of polyuria. Water intoxication results from ingestion of a large volume of fluid, with resultant dilutional hyponatremia. If the

patient has a normal diluting capacity, there will be polyuria, with a proportionally low serum and urine osmolality. Prolonged fluid restriction will result in appropriate rise in urine osmolality. Osmotic diuresis may occur from solute overload when the renal tubules are unable to reabsorb adequate quantities of filtered solutes. This is associated with administration of mannitol or, in the presence of glycosuria, from diabetes mellitus. (*Harrison's, pp 2004–2009*)

402–403. (402-C, 403-F) Acute appendicitis initially presents with periumbilical pain secondary to obstruction of the appendiceal lumen. This is mediated through visceral pain fibers, and because the appendix is from the embryologic midgut, the pain is referred to the umbilicus. With obstruction of a hollow viscus, there may be associated nausea. As the inflammatory process progresses to involve the visceral and parietal peritoneal surfaces, the pain becomes localized directly over the appendix in the right lower quadrant. Fever and leukocytosis are nonspecific signs of an inflammatory process. Gastroenteritis may be associated with nausea, anorexia, and low-grade fever. Periumbilical pain is colicky and secondary to increased peristalsis. Localized pain and signs of peritoneal irritation are uncommon. A ruptured right ovarian cyst may mimic appendicitis. Patients may exhibit right-lower-abdominal peritoneal irritation. However, the onset of pain is usually sudden, and the pain is initially felt in the right lower quadrant. These patients do not have anorexia or other gastrointestinal symptoms. The clinical picture of regional enteritis (Crohn's disease) is one of a chronic illness, often associated with weight loss, intermittent cramps, and diarrhea. Fever, tenderness, and a palpable right-lower-quadrant inflammatory mass may result from complications of ileal involvement. Sigmoid diverticulitis is more common in older patients, often with a prodromal history of irregular bowel habits. There may be left-lower-quadrant pain and tenderness, with a palpable left-sided inflammatory mass. A cecal volvulus presents with sudden onset of colicky abdominal pain and signs and symptoms of a bowel obstruction, including bilious emesis and abdominal distension. Alcohol-related acute pancreatitis presents with pain referred to the epigastrium, with radiation to the back mediated through the celiac ganglia. The patient may develop abdominal distension secondary to the associated paralytic ileus. Hyperamylasemia and an elevated serum lipase, in this clinical setting, are suggestive of pancreatitis. Perforated peptic ulcer and acute cholecystitis may also present with epigastric pain, and elevations of both serum lipase and amylase. Pain from a perforated ulcer, however, is sudden in onset and may be associated with shoulder-tip pain from diaphragmatic irritation. Acute cholecystitis will usually commence after a large meal and initially presents as colicky epigastric pain, progressing to pain localized in the right upper abdomen when transmural inflammation of the gallbladder wall produces peritoneal irritation. Acute mesenteric occlusion presents with sudden onset of severe but poorly localized periumbilical abdominal pain, associated with acidosis. There may be elevation of serum amylase and lipase. A ruptured abdominal aortic aneurysm will present with sudden onset of midabdominal pain, back pain, and hemodynamic instability. (*Sabiston, pp 964–970, 1156–1160; Greenfield et al, pp 877–883, 1246–1256*)

404. **(A)** A thyroglossal duct cyst represents the remnants of the thyroglossal duct tract left over from descent of the thyroid gland from the foramen cecum. It is located in the midline and moves superiorly as the tongue protrudes because the tract communicates with the foramen cecum. (*Greenfield et al, pp 1998–1999*)

405. **(C)** Acute suppurative lymphadenitis is related to bacterial pathogens and most often accompanies an infectious illness, such as an upper respiratory tract infection. The nodes enlarge rapidly, are tender, and demonstrate overlying erythema of the skin. (*Greenfield et al, pp 1999–2000*)

406. **(B)** Cystic hygromas are composed of disorganized, dilated lymphatic channels presenting as lateral neck masses usually by the age of 2. They are generally soft and multiloculated and may result in significant airway compromise. (*Greenfield et al, p 1999*)

407. **(E)** Lipomas present as soft, subcutaneous masses that arise in all areas of the body. They are treated by simple excision. (*Greenfield et al, pp 1236–1237*)

408. **(G)** Most tumors of the salivary glands present in the parotid, the most common of which is the pleomorphic adenoma. These occur most frequently in the fifth decade and present as a solitary painless mass in the superficial lobe of the parotid gland. Surgical treatment is complete excision with negative margins. (*Schwartz et al, pp 650–655*)

409. **(D)** The location of this neck mass and its movement with swallowing is strongly suggestive of a thyroid mass. The most common type of thyroid cancer is papillary carcinoma, which has an excellent prognosis under the age of 40. Needle biopsy should be performed as a diagnostic test, followed by operation. (*Greenfield et al, pp 1301–1303*)

410. **(H)** Laryngeal carcinoma is the most common malignancy of the upper aerodigestive tract in the United States. Presenting symptoms include hoarseness of the voice and, for supraglottic lesions, early metastatic disease to the neck. Risk factors include exposure to tobacco and alcohol. (*Schwartz et al, pp 639–646*)

411. **(H)** Chronic liver disease, such as cirrhosis, may be a cause of jaundice. Clinical features such as spider angiomas, ascites, and varices suggest cirrhosis. (*Schwartz et al, pp 1375–1376*)

412. **(F)** Pancreatic carcinoma occurs in the head of the gland in 75% of cases. About 75% of the patients with carcinoma in the head of the pancreas present with obstructive jaundice, weight loss, and, in the presence of advanced disease, abdominal pain. (*Schwartz et al, p 1421*)

413. **(C)** Common duct stones (choledocholithiasis) may be the cause of acute bile duct obstruction without warning, resulting in jaundice, pain, and sepsis. The sepsis may manifest as fever, hypotension, and altered mental status. *(Schwartz et al, pp 1382–1383)*

414. **(G)** Liver dysfunction resulting in jaundice may be a manifestation of advanced metastatic disease to the liver. In a patient with a known malignancy at high risk for metastases (ie, deeply invasive and ulcerative melanoma), metastatic disease must be considered in the evaluation of the jaundiced patient. Hepatomegaly found on abdominal exam is supportive of advanced metastatic disease. *(Schwartz et al, pp 1375–1376)*

415. **(I)** Pancreatitis may be the cause of jaundice by different mechanisms, resulting in compression of the common bile duct (CBD). Acute pancreatitis may cause edema of the head with resultant compression of the CBD; pancreatitis may lead to a pseudocyst in the head with compression of the duct; and chronic pancreatitis may lead to dense scarring around the duct with a resultant stricture. The clinical scenario of an alcohol abuser with acute abdominal pain; nausea; vomiting; jaundice; and a tender, palpable epigastric mass is most consistent with acute pancreatitis with CBD obstruction due to a pseudocyst. *(Greenfield et al, pp 874–888)*

416. **(C)** A new mass in a woman of this age group must be fully evaluated to rule out carcinoma. Though biopsy by fine needle, core needle, or open biopsy will be required to determine the etiology of the mass, they should not be performed until all necessary breast imaging studies have been performed. Imaging should include diagnostic mammography, and possibly sonography to determine whether the mass is solid or cystic. An appropriate type of biopsy can be chosen (ie, fine-needle aspiration for cystic lesions or core biopsy for solid lesions). Imaging should not be delayed, though the patient should discontinue HRT until the etiology of the mass is determined. *(Niederhuber, pp 446–447)*

417. **(E)** A number of breast cancer risk factors have been identified. These include family history, benign breast disease with atypical epithelial hyperplasia, alcohol consumption, and HRT in some studies. In most patients (70%) with breast cancer, however, no major risk factor can be identified other than increasing age and female gender. *(Niederhuber, pp 447–448)*

418. **(D)** LCIS is considered a marker for susceptibility of the breasts for malignant change. Lobular and ductal elements of both breasts are at risk. The lifetime risk of cancer is thought to be approximately 30%, equally divided between the two breasts. Therefore, re-excision to gain negative margins is not indicated, nor is ipsilateral mastectomy. There is no known added significance to bilateral LCIS; therefore, contralateral breast biopsy is not useful for determining appropriate management. Both breasts should be treated the same. For patients without any other identifiable risk factors, close observation with frequent physician exams, monthly breast self-exam, and yearly mammography may be the best option. However, some patients may prefer bilateral total mastectomies as a personal preference or for situations in which they cannot adhere to close follow-up recommendations, or whose risk for cancer is deemed too high. *(Greenfield et al, pp 1404–1405)*

419. **(B)** Prospective randomized trials have addressed the issue of locoregional control of breast cancer. Conservative management consisting of lumpectomy (with negative margins), irradiation, and axillary node dissection is equally effective as modified radical mastectomy in patients with stage I or II breast carcinoma. Although radical mastectomy yields equivalent survival to modified radical mastectomy, it is disfiguring and disabling and is rarely employed for treatment of primary operable breast cancer. Lumpectomy without irradiation leads to unacceptably high local recurrence rates. Irradiation without surgery is not as effective as surgery in the presence of gross disease. Quadrantectomy removes excessive tissue and leads to an inferior cosmetic result compared to

lumpectomy. If quadrantectomy is thought to be required to gain negative margins, mastectomy with reconstruction should be entertained. *(Greenfield et al, pp 1390–1391)*

420–421. (420-C, 421-E) The mammographic appearance is most consistent with DCIS with or without an invasive component. The calcifications of DCIS are clustered, pleomorphic, irregular, and linear, and may be associated with a mass representing an invasive carcinoma. LCIS does not usually present with calcifications. Cystosarcoma phyllodes presents as a mass, often indistinguishable from a fibroadenoma. A degenerating fibroadenoma often presents as a mass with large, coarse calcifications, indicating its benignity. Milk of calcium will often layer differently in the craniocaudal and mediolateral projections, suggesting fluid with calcium. The next step in management is to obtain a biopsy, preferably a core needle biopsy, for histologic confirmation and to evaluate for invasive disease. Without an invasive component, axillary node dissection is not recommended because the incidence of axillary node metastasis of DCIS is rare (1%). All other choices (ie, radical mastectomy, modified radical mastectomy, or lumpectomy) are not indicated until a diagnosis by biopsy is obtained. *(Sabiston, pp 581–583)*

422–423. (422-C, 423-B) A new mass in an older woman must be evaluated for malignancy. In this case, the mammogram has characteristics of malignancy, which include a density or mass that is stellate or spiculated, irregular in size or sharp, and possessing ill-defined borders. Other features suggestive of malignancy include clustered microcalcifications, asymmetric density, architectural distortion, and skin or nipple retraction. DCIS usually presents as calcifications without a definite mass. LCIS has no specific mammographic features and is often discovered as an incidental finding. Cystosarcoma phyllodes presents much like a fibroadenoma as a well-defined mass with smooth margins. Papillomas are small and not usually palpable or noted by mammography. The next step is biopsy, preferably by core biopsy, so a histologic

diagnosis can be made and options for management (ie, modified radical mastectomy or lumpectomy, axillary dissection, and irradiation) discussed. Neither radical mastectomy nor irradiation alone has any role in the management of the tumor shown in the figure. *(Greenfield et al, pp 1364–1366)*

424–425. (424-C, 425-D) The symptoms of gastric cancer are nonspecific and may mimic those of benign conditions such as benign gastric ulcer. Pain, nausea, anorexia, and weight loss are common nonspecific symptoms. A UGI series shows a gastric ulcer that has characteristics of malignancy, including an intraluminal crater with nodular margins. A gastric diverticulum would extend as a protrusion beyond the gastric lumen. The duodenum is not well visualized in the x-ray, making the diagnosis of duodenal disease difficult. A fistula would be suggested by contrast filling of the gallbladder and biliary tree. Given the x-ray findings suggestive of malignancy, the next step would be to obtain a tissue diagnosis for confirmation by endoscopy. Once malignancy is confirmed, a CT scan would be helpful to evaluate for liver metastasis and extent of disease. Operative intervention may be determined at that time, usually a subtotal or total gastrectomy. Vagotomy and pyloroplasty would not be appropriate for gastric cancer. Medical therapy with H_2 blockers may improve the patient's symptoms but should not delay endoscopy and biopsy. *(Greenfield et al, pp 795–803; Zinner, pp 16–17)*

426.   (D) The prevalence of adenomas without symptoms in patients over the age of 50 ranges between 20 and 40%. Screening studies suggest that 30% of patients without symptoms over the age of 50 who undergo colonoscopy for evaluation of positive fecal occult blood have a polyp detected. Polyps greater than 2 cm have a high potential for malignant degeneration. The polyp should be completely removed, preferably by snare polypectomy. Most studies indicate that polypectomy is adequate for polyps with carcinoma in the head if the margin of resection is 2 mm or greater, especially if the stalk is not invaded. Following adequate polypectomy, observation would be indicated with postpolypectomy colonoscopic surveillance. If cancer is present at or near the margin, then colon resection is indicated. Since the incidence of residual cancer and metastatic disease is very low after successful polypectomy, scanning by CT or MRI is not indicated. The data on NSAID use is promising but insufficient to support a clinical recommendation. *(Greenfield et al, pp 1110–1117)*

427–429. (427-D, 428-E, 429-A) The gradual onset of left-lower-quadrant pain over a number of days with left-lower-quadrant abdominal tenderness and CT scan showing sigmoid colon inflammatory changes is most consistent with diverticulitis. Most patients with ischemic colitis are elderly (over 70 years of age) and have multiple medical problems. A contained perforation, either due to the diverticulitis or colon cancer, should be noted on the CT scan. There is no history of antecedent antibiotic therapy to suggest the diagnosis of pseudomembranous colitis. Though WBCs were present in the urinalysis, a diagnosis of pyelonephritis cannot be made on this basis alone since pericolonic inflammation may be responsible for the WBCs. CT scanning is very accurate in diagnosing diverticulitis, so there is no need for any additional test. Barium enema and colonoscopy should not be performed in patients with suspected acute diverticulitis. The increased intraluminal pressure from either of these exams may lead to free rupture of a contained abscess or phlegmon, leading to emergent surgery. However, either exam, or both, should be performed after complete resolution of diverticulitis (eg, in 6 weeks' time) to evaluate for extent of disease, complications, and carcinoma. IVP and angiography are not indicated for diverticulitis. The appropriate management in this patient with his first episode of diverticulitis is medical management with intravenous antibiotics for gram-negative and anaerobic bacteria. Colon resection, either immediate or elective, should not be undertaken unless the patient's condition deteriorates or recurs. Bowel preparation cannot be performed safely in patients with acute diverticulitis. Anticoagulation has no

role in therapy. Metronidazole or vancomycin therapy would be appropriate for pseudomembranous colitis, but not for diverticulitis. *(Sabiston, pp 987–993)*

430–431. (430-D, 431-B) The diagnosis of sigmoid volvulus is based on the history, exam, and radiographs. Acute onset of abdominal pain, distension, and obstipation is suggestive of volvulus. Barium enema is diagnostic of sigmoid volvulus showing the characteristic tapering to a "bird's beak" pointing to the site of obstruction. Cecal volvulus would show complete filling of the left colon. Stricture as a result of ischemic colitis would show a long, narrowed segment of colon. Diverticulitis would be suggested by a different clinical presentation including fever, sepsis, and pain localized to the left lower quadrant. Obstruction from colon cancer would show an irregular narrowing of the colon segment rather than a smooth tapering. In patients who have no signs of bowel wall ischemia (eg, rebound tenderness, sepsis, etc), nonoperative reduction should be attempted and would be expected to be successful in 70 to 80% of patients. The most widely used method of reduction is proctoscopy and rectal tube placement under direct vision. Blind passage of a rectal tube may lead to perforation and is contraindicated. Operation is indicated if nonoperative reduction is unsuccessful, with operative reduction preferred, followed by delayed resection and primary anastamosis rather than sigmoid resection. Operative reduction by detorsion alone is unacceptable due to the high recurrence rate and is, therefore, combined with sigmoidopexy or sigmoidostomy. Proximal colostomy alone is contraindicated since strangulation of the sigmoid or recurrent volvulus is not prevented. *(Sabiston, pp 1015–1020)*

432–433. (432-B, 433-D) The clinical features of colon cancer are variable depending on the location. On the right, fatigue, as a manifestation of anemia, may be the predominant symptom, whereas obstructive complaints may predominate for lesions on the left. In the figure, an annular or "apple core" lesion is noted, consistent with carcinoma. Radiography of diverticular disease would show numerous protrusions from the lumen, usually localized to the sigmoid colon. Lymphoma may occur in the colon, but this site of disease is rare, and widespread disease can be documented in most cases. Ischemia usually occurs at the splenic flexure, and the resultant stricture would produce a longer segment of narrowing than that usually seen with carcinoma. Patients with Crohn's disease would manifest symptoms of abdominal pain and diarrhea, and barium x-rays would show thickened bowel wall, mucosal ulcerations, and cobblestone appearance. The treatment of colon cancer in this patient would be surgical resection and anastamosis. Colostomy may be appropriate in selected patients with obstruction in an unstable patient in whom resection is not feasible. Surgical bypass would be appropriate only for palliative therapy of unresectable disease. Radiation therapy or chemotherapy without surgical resection and staging is not recommended. *(Sabiston, pp 1024–1031; Zinner, pp 34–36)*

434–435. (434-D, 435-C) The stage of colon cancer is based on the depth of invasion, nodal involvement, and distant metastases. Stage 0 represents carcinoma in situ, stage I invasion of the submucosa or muscularis propria without node involvement, stage II invasion through the muscularis propria or directly invading other organs without nodal involvement, stage III any depth of invasion with nodal metastasis, and stage IV any depth of invasion or nodal status with distant metastases. Adjuvant therapy has been shown to be beneficial in patients with stage III disease in randomized studies. The recommended regimen is 5-fluorouracil–based chemotherapy with levamisole or leucovorin, rather than 5-fluorouracil alone. Adriamycin therapy, either alone or with other agents, has not been shown to be beneficial in patients with colon cancer. No adjuvant therapy would be indicated for patients with stage 0, I, or II disease, although some patients with stage II disease manifesting poor prognostic indicators may be candidates for adjuvant therapy. *(Niederhuber, pp 320–324)*

436. **(C)** The history of decreasing caliber of the stool with evidence of bleeding is highly suggestive of rectal carcinoma. The barium x-ray shows a near-obstructing lesion of the rectum with an "apple core" appearance of cancer. Diverticulitis does not occur in the rectum due to the lack of diverticular disease at this site. Ischemia usually does not involve the rectum due to its more abundant blood supply than the colon. The barium enema findings of sigmoid volvulus would show a smooth, tapering, so-called "bird's beak" at the rectosigmoid junction, rather than an irregular lesion in the midrectum as shown in the figure. Crohn's disease would be expected to show fistulas, either by exam or radiography. *(Sabiston, pp 1024–1031)*

437–438. (437-D, 438-D) A multicolored brown or black pigmented lesion with irregular borders should raise the concern of melanoma. Squamous cell carcinoma usually presents as an erythematous papularnodule. The most common type of basal carcinoma presents as an ulcerative, well-circumscribed nodule, though occasionally they may be pigmented and confused with melanoma. Merkel cell carcinomas appear as red to purple papular nodules. Keratoacanthoma is a well-circumscribed keratotic lesion that may regress without treatment. The most appropriate next step is to perform an excisional biopsy with narrow margins to confirm the diagnosis and determine depth of invasion. Shave biopsy would yield a pathologic diagnosis, but would not allow appropriate staging and is never recommended. The margin of resection and determination of lymph node management would depend on the depth of invasion of the melanoma measured in millimeters. Therefore, wide excision is not recommended until the depth of invasion of the lesion is determined by excisional biopsy with narrow margins. Mohs' surgery should be considered for nonmelanoma tumors but is not recommended for melanoma. *(Greenfield et al, pp 2231–2245)*

439. **(E)** The diagnosis of an incarcerated hernia must be considered in the differential diagnosis of a patient with abdominal symptoms and a nonreducible inguinal bulge. Femoral hernia presents as a bulge below the inguinal ligament medial to the femoral artery. Direct or indirect inguinal hernias would present above the inguinal ligament. An aneurysm of the femoral artery should be pulsatile. If there is concern for an aneurysm, a Doppler ultrasound exam may be diagnostic. A lymph node with abscess may present as a tender, nonreducible mass, but should be accompanied by additional adenopathy and a source of the infection. (*Niederhuber, pp 390–399*)

440–441. (440-C, 441-B) The finding of a new, irregular lesion in a patient with a long smoking history must be considered a lung carcinoma and should be managed accordingly. Non–small cell carcinoma is the most common lung neoplasm. Small cell carcinomas usually grow rapidly and disseminate widely by the time of diagnosis. Tuberculosis would present with systemic symptoms and apical disease on chest x-ray. Likewise, a lung abscess would be accompanied by systemic symptoms and may show air–fluid levels in the abscess cavity. A hamartoma presents as an extremely slowly growing nodule that may contain popcorn calcifications. The most appropriate test following suspicious findings on a chest x-ray would be a CT scan to further evaluate the nodule, evaluate the lymph node status, and triage subsequent diagnostic tests. If enlarged mediastinal nodes are seen, then mediastinoscopy may be indicated. Bronchoscopy may be helpful to assess for endobronchial lesions and to obtain tissue for diagnosis. Pulmonary function tests are necessary once a decision is made to consider operation. Percutaneous needle biopsy may be required to obtain tissue once CT scanning is performed. (*Niederhuber, pp 535–540*)

442–443. (442-D, 443-B) The clinical manifestations of ruptured abdominal aneurysm are back, flank, or abdominal pain; hypotension; and a pulsatile abdominal mass. The treatment should be immediate transfer to the operating room for laparotomy. Additional diagnostic tests, such as CT scan, angiography, or additional consultations delay immediate treatment, thereby putting the patient at risk

for further rupture and death. Following successful treatment, diarrhea may suggest ischemic colitis, and urgent sigmoidoscopy is indicated. A delay in diagnosis of bowel ischemia caused by numerous other diagnostic tests may increase the mortality rate. If bowel ischemia is found, immediate colon resection should be undertaken. (*Greenfield et al, pp 1881–1890*)

444–446. (444-B, 445-D, 446-A) The diagnosis of arterial embolism is suggested when the patient presents with an acute onset of severe pain, pallor, pulselessness, paresthesia, and paralysis (five P's). The presence of atrial fibrillation is strongly suggestive of a cardiac source of the emboli. The first step in management is immediate heparinization to prevent propagation of the clot and maintain patency of collaterals. The cornerstone of treatment is thromboembolectomy. Thrombolytic therapy is reserved for treatment of irretrievable clots in small vessels. Fasciotomy, alkalinization of the urine, and mannitol diuresis are adjuncts to treatment, particularly if there is a delay in operation, increasing the risk of a reperfusion injury. Anticoagulation has been shown to reduce the rate of recurrent embolism. (*Greenfield et al, pp 1621–1630*)

447–448. (447-B, 448-C) The diagnosis of a dissecting aortic aneurysm is strongly suggested by the history of an abrupt onset of excruciating pain in the chest and back with variable radiation patterns, and a hypertensive, ill-appearing patient. A chest x-ray showing a widened mediastinum may be noted, but the radiograph may be normal. The differential diagnosis of an acute myocardial infarction must be entertained and an ECG performed. Though aortography has historically been the definitive diagnostic procedure and may be required in some patients, transesophageal echocardiography has become the preferred diagnostic modality. It can be performed in the emergency department, thus obviating the need to move an extremely ill patient. CT scan may also be helpful in establishing the diagnosis. Immediate drug therapy to control hypertension is mandatory, followed by deitive therapy, depending on the type of issection. Thrombolytic therapy and anticoagulation are not indicated and may precipitate exsanguination. (*Schwartz et al, pp 914–918*)

449–450. (449-C, 450-E) Factors that increase the risk for carcinoma include exposure to low-dose irradiation, age less than 20 or older than 60, male gender (especially over age 40), and recent onset. An increased incidence of thyroid carcinoma in patients with Hashimoto's thyroiditis has not been substantiated. For diagnosis, fine-needle aspiration is highly accurate and has become the preferred diagnostic modality. Fine-needle aspiration is the most important diagnostic test for selecting patients for operation, supplanting all other diagnostic tests. (*Greenfield et al, pp 1299–1301*)

451–452. (451-D, 452-B) Leiomyomas are the most common benign tumors of the esophagus. They are intramural, occur between 20 and 50 years of age, and may be symptomatic when over 5 cm. Symptoms may include dysphagia and retrosternal pressure and pain. Esophagogram shows characteristic features of a smooth concave defect with sharp borders. Esophagoscopy is indicated to rule out carcinoma. These tumors are mobile, with intact overlying mucosa. Biopsy should not be performed so that subsequent extramural resection can be performed without complication. Excision is recommended for symptomatic leiomyomas or those greater than 5 cm. (*Sabiston, pp 744–747*)

453–454. (453-B, 454-B) Pharyngoesophageal (Zenker's) diverticulum is the most common esophageal diverticulum and typically occurs in the 30 to 50 age group and, therefore, believed to be acquired. Its symptoms include cervical dysphagia, regurgitation of undigested food, and recurrent aspiration. It is categorized as a pulsion type, creating protrusion of mucosa, resulting in a false diverticulum. An underlying neuromotor abnormality exists, which is responsible for increased pharyngeal pressure. The most important aspect of treatment is a cricopharyngeal muscle myotomy, which can be

combined with resection or diverticulopexy. (*Sabiston, pp 729–731*)

455. (C) Mallory–Weiss tear involves acute UGI hemorrhage that occurs after retching or vomiting and accounts for 5 to 15% of patients with UGI bleeding. The patient is often an alcoholic who vomits after binge drinking. Hematemesis follows vomiting without blood. After resuscitation, esophagoscopy is required to determine the source of bleeding and may be helpful in nonoperative management. Contrast studies are not helpful, and the use of barium would coat the stomach and preclude a diagnostic endoscopic exam. Most patients with Mallory–Weiss tears stop bleeding spontaneously. Angiography may be helpful in selected patients who continue to bleed and in whom the site of hemorrhage cannot be determined endoscopically. (*Greenfield et al, p 1167*)

456–457. (456-B, 457-B) Progressive dysphagia in an older adult warrants evaluation, especially with associated symptoms of weight loss, chest pain, or hematemesis. A barium esophagogram is the first study that should be obtained. The typical carcinoma demonstrates an irregular, rigid narrowing of the esophageal wall with distortion of the lumen. Achalasia demonstrates a narrow, tapering bird's beak appearance of the distal esophagus. Development of an esophageal stricture causes slowly progressive dysphagia, usually after a long history of gastroesophageal reflux disease (GERD). Esophagoscopy and biopsy are mandatory for evaluation of esophageal stenosis and yield a diagnosis of carcinoma in 95% of patients with malignant strictures. CT scanning is the standard technique for staging, once the diagnosis has been made. Bronchoscopy is helpful in patients with upper and middle third carcinomas to exclude invasion of the trachea or bronchi prior to esophagectomy. (*Niederhuber, pp 284–287*)

458–460. (458-D, 459-E, 460-C) Perforated duodenal ulcer usually presents as a sudden onset of acute abdominal pain. Exam usually reveals severe abdominal tenderness with rigidity of the abdominal musculature (ie, an acute abdomen). With a prior history of abdominal pain relieved by antacids, a chronic ulcer that has now perforated is strongly suggested. Perforated colon cancer occurs in an older age group, as well as gastric ulcer. Following plain radiographs that show pneumoperitoneum, no additional diagnostic tests are required and serve only to delay treatment. The treatment is laparotomy and either patch closure of the perforation or definitive operation, the latter being preferred, depending on operative findings. However, the patient must receive fluid resuscitation prior to laparotomy to avoid hypotension and its consequences. Though nonoperative management for contained perforations has been suggested by some authors, an acute abdomen is an indication for operative management. *(Greenfield et al, p 770)*

461–462. (461-B, 462-D) Gastric ulcers present with symptoms of abdominal pain, aggravated by food, and associated with nausea, vomiting, anorexia, and weight loss. The two principal means of diagnosing a gastric ulcer are UGI radiographs and fiberoptic endoscopy, the latter being the most reliable method. CT scan and endoscopic ultrasound may be helpful in staging gastric cancer, but are not routinely used with benign disease. The failure to respond to 12 weeks of medical management is an indication for surgical therapy to avoid potential complications and to exclude malignancy, despite biopsies obtained by endoscopy that show benign disease. *(Greenfield et al, pp 779–787)*

463–465. (463-D, 464-C, 465-C) In a patient who has undergone surgical resection for colon cancer, elevated CEA and liver function tests must be followed by an evaluation for metastatic disease, including the possibility of extrahepatic disease. The CT scan is the most useful exam to evaluate both intra- and extrahepatic disease. Various CT scans have been advocated for liver tumors, including dynamic and portography scans. Anti-CEA monoclonal scans may be useful in selected patients to detect extrahepatic disease. MRI shows promise as a useful exam, but is not used routinely. Radionuclide liver scans have been supplanted by more accurate scans. Surgical resection, if possible, is the treatment of choice for metastatic colorectal cancer to the liver. Chemotherapy is reserved for patients who are not surgical candidates or refuse surgical treatment. Radiation therapy is not usually utilized in these patients. Observation and repeat imaging delays the treatment for patients who may be resectable. The expected 5-year survival has been shown in multiple studies to be greater than 20%, usually in the range of 25 and 35%. *(Schwartz et al, pp 1339–1340)*

466–467. (466-C, 467-D) The anatomic location of the mass suggests a parotid origin, and the lengthy history and absence of symptoms and signs of inflammation are consistent with a neoplasm of the parotid. The most common salivary gland neoplasm is a benign pleomorphic adenoma. Metastatic carcinoma from a head and neck primary tumor may first present as a neck mass, usually along the anterior or posterior cervical lymph node chain, and often in a patient with risk factors such as a history of smoking. Infectious parotitis may occur in the elderly or diabetic patient, usually presenting with a shorter history, with symptoms and signs of inflammation. Hodgkin's disease can present as a painless neck mass involving the anterior or supraclavicular lymph nodes. Reactive cervical lymphatic hyperplasia is associated with an inflammatory or infectious focus in the head and neck. The optimal management for a pleomorphic adenoma in the lateral lobe of the parotid is a superficial parotidectomy. Intravenous antibiotics are not indicated, in the absence of an inflammatory or infectious process. Although an excisional biopsy may be indicated for a mass arising from cervical lymph nodes, enucleation of a neoplastic parotid mass is insufficient and associated with an increased incidence of local recurrence. Observation and re-evaluation are inappropriate in this patient. A chest x-ray would be indicated in the evaluation of a patient with suspected Hodgkin's disease. *(Sabiston, pp 1322–1324; Niederhuber, p 415)*

468–469. (468-B, 469-C) Intussusception most commonly occurs between 2 months and 2 years of age, often associated with a prodromal viral illness. Children will present with intermittent episodes of abdominal colic, secondary to peristaltic waves of the ileum against the partially obstructing ileocolic lesion. Reflex nonbilious vomiting is secondary to bowel distension and partial obstruction. There may be a palpable, right-sided, "sausage-shaped" mass, but in many patients, the abdominal exam is entirely normal. The classic "currant jelly" stool (Figure 4–9) is a late sign, and is a result of ischemia and mucosal sloughing of the lead point. After the child has received IV fluid resuscitation, the management is hydrostatic reduction, either by contrast enema or air enema. Intussusception may occur during the clinical course of viral gastroenteritis. Bloody stools are more commonly associated with bacterial gastrointestinal infections, with characteristically loose, mucousy stools, and blood mixed with fecal material. Diagnosis is aided by obtaining stool cultures. A midgut volvulus can be associated with passage of a "currant jelly" stool secondary to small-bowel ischemia. However, these children usually present with bilious vomiting. Diagnosis may be confirmed with a UGI contrast study. Rectal bleeding from a Meckel's diverticulum is typically painless, without other associated gastrointestinal symptoms. Technetium scan is useful for diagnosis. Bleeding from a juvenile rectal polyp is usually small in amount and often occurs during normal stool passage. The children are clinically well, without other gastrointestinal symptoms. These polyps may be seen on proctoscopy. (*Sabiston, pp 1253–1254; Greenfield et al, pp 2067–2069*)

470. (E) This patient presents with a rapidly progressive, necrotizing soft-tissue infection. The skin edema, purple hue, bullae, water drainage, and crepitus are classic findings in clostridial infections. Although culture of the wound drainage may be confirmatory, the diagnosis should be suspected on a clinical basis. Antibiotics alone are not sufficient therapy. The mainstay of therapy is radical surgical debridement of devitalized tissues,

in conjunction with high-dose IV antibiotics. Hyperbaric oxygen therapy may facilitate recovery. (*Sabiston, pp 917–919; Niederhuber, pp 300–301*)

471. (C) All traumatic soft-tissue injuries should be managed with aggressive local wound care. Because this injury is greater than 6 hours old, contaminated, and greater than 1 cm in depth, it is a tetanus-prone wound. Therefore, in addition, this patient should receive tetanus toxoid, since it has been more than 5 years since his last immunization. He had full immunization as a child and therefore does not require additional passive immunization with tetanus immune globulin. Prophylactic antibiotics are controversial in the absence of an established wound infection. (*Sabiston, pp 267, 331–332; Niederhuber, pp 163–164*)

472. (E) This child has a displaced supracondylar fracture associated with vascular compromise of the forearm, from associated brachial artery compression, distortion, or vessel injury. Decreased perfusion below the fracture in conjunction with pain on passive wrist flexion are signs of a developing forearm compartment syndrome. Management should include operative exploration of the brachial artery, open reduction and pinning of the fracture, and forearm compartment fasciotomy to limit progression of muscular ischemia. Immobilization of the elbow at 90 degrees is suitable only for undisplaced fractures. For displaced fractures without neurovascular compromise, closed reduction and pinning may be adequate, but if adequate reduction cannot be achieved, open reduction may be required. (*Sabiston, pp 1412, 1422; Niederhuber, p 709*)

473–474. (473-B, 474-B) This patient is acidotic, with a low serum bicarbonate (bicarbonate depletion defined as a serum bicarbonate less than 22 mEq/L). She has hypovolemic shock from trauma and acute blood loss, resulting in decreased tissue perfusion and lactic acidosis. The resultant elevated anion gap (139 − [103 + 14] = 22 mEq/L with a normal anion gap of 8 to 16 mEq/L) is from the increased lactic acid. The tachypnea may be due to the respiratory compensation with decreased P_{CO_2}. Correction of the acidosis should be aimed at improving tissue perfusion with aggressive IV fluid resuscitation. Metabolic alkalosis is associated with serum bicarbonate greater than 26 mEq/L. Respiratory acidosis is related to primary carbon dioxide retention from decreased alveolar ventilation. Administration of sodium bicarbonate is indicated only in severe acidosis (pH < 7.2), and in patients with evidence of myocardial instability or arrhythmias. Hydrochloric acid is indicated only in life-threatening metabolic alkalosis that is not chloride responsive. Respiratory acidosis with alveolar hypoventilation may be corrected with assisted ventilation. (Sabiston, pp 96–101; Niederhuber, pp 210–216)

475–477. (475-D, 476-J, 477-C) Pyloric stenosis presents with nonbilious vomiting and gastric distension. An annular pancreas does not result in obstruction, except when it is associated with an underlying duodenal abnormality. Duodenal atresia is associated with Down syndrome. It results in early onset of bilious vomiting from complete duodenal obstruction distal to the ampulla. There is a "double bubble" sign on plain abdominal radiographs from air in the stomach and proximal duodenum. Midgut volvulus is a life-threatening complication of malrotation. It presents with acute onset of bilious vomiting, usually in infants in the first year of life. There is a paucity of gas on plain radiographs, with evidence of duodenal obstruction. Upper gastrointestinal contrast study will confirm the abnormal position of the duodenal–jejunal junction and may demonstrate a corkscrew of the duodenum from volvulus. Intussusception is uncommon in newborns. Bilious vomiting is unusual at the outset, but may develop if the intussusception has been present for a significant time. Imperforate anus can be excluded by clinical exam. If unrecognized, the infant will develop a clinical picture of a distal bowel obstruction, with dilated small and large bowel. Meckel's diverticulum can present with obstruction secondary to volvulus around a Meckel's band, with a distal small-bowel ob-

struction. Contrast enema will demonstrate a normal-caliber decompressed colon, with proximal dilated small bowel. Meconium ileus is associated with cystic fibrosis. Obstruction occurs from inspissated meconium in the terminal ileum. Plain radiographs may demonstrate a "soap bubble" pattern in the right lower quadrant, with a decompressed colon on contrast enema. Hirschsprung's disease presents with a distal bowel obstruction and delayed passage of meconium. A contrast enema may demonstrate a transition zone, with a narrow distal aganglionic segment, and proximal colonic dilatation. Jejunal atresia is a result of an intrauterine vascular accident. Infants present with bile-stained vomiting and abdominal distension early after birth. The colon is unused, and characteristically, on contrast enema, it is abnormally small in caliber (microcolon). (Sabiston, pp 1239–1247; Niederhuber, pp 791, 792–796)

478–479. (478-D, 479-A) Cryptorchidism increases the risk of developing a testicular malignancy. This patient has a solid testicular mass, which should be presumed to be secondary to a testicular malignancy. Optimal surgical management is inguinal exploration, control of the spermatic cord, biopsy of the mass, and radical orchiectomy if tumor is confirmed. Trans-scrotal aspiration, exploration, or needle biopsy is contraindicated because of risk of tumor spillage, and risk of altering the lymphatic drainage of the scrotum. Laparotomy and retroperitoneal node dissection is not indicated until after confirmation of the diagnosis and excision of the primary tumor. This patient has stage I seminoma with disease limited to the testicle. The tumor is very radiosensitive, and radiotherapy is the primary adjuvant therapy for local control. Chemotherapy is indicated in patients with nodal spread, or disseminated disease. Radiotherapy is restricted to therapy for localized disease only. (Sabiston, pp 1557–1559; Niederhuber, pp 764–765)

480–481. (480-D, 481-E) This patient has an inguinoscrotal mass from an incarcerated inguinal hernia. This has resulted in pain, irritability, and reflex vomiting. Prolonged

tion increases the risk of bowel is-
~~~he appropriate management is se-
th manual reduction, and surgical
repair within 24 hours. Delaying repair after
an initial episode of incarceration increases
the risk of further episodes of incarceration,
with potential bowel or testicular compromise. Failure to successfully reduce an incarcerated hernia mandates urgent surgical intervention. Testicular torsion is uncommon
in this age group and presents with a tender,
high-riding testicle. When suspected, urgent
surgical exploration is indicated. Inguinal
adenitis may be the result of an inflammatory
focus in the diaper area, with resultant
adenopathy, and secondary infection of the
inguinal nodes with a gram-positive organism. The infant is usually febrile, with a tender inguinal mass. Therapy includes systemic
antibiotics. An undescended testicle may present as an inguinal mass, with an empty
hemiscrotum. It is usually asymptomatic.
Management is elective orchiopexy at 2 years
of age. A noncommunicating hydrocele presents as an asymptomatic, fluctuant scrotal
mass that transilluminates. Surgical intervention is not required, as most will resolve
spontaneously by 1 year of age. *(Niederhuber,
pp 794–795)*

482–483. (482-A, 483-B) Patients with gross hematuria require aggressive diagnostic evaluation. A careful, planned approach will yield
the cause in the majority of patients. Painless
hematuria is often the first sign of a urinary
tract malignancy. After confirmation of hematuria, and exclusion of infection, all patients should have plain radiographs and
IVP. This is the optimal initial diagnostic approach to aid in distinguishing between upper tract (renal) pathology and lower tract
(lower ureteric and bladder) pathology. Further diagnostic evaluation will be guided by
these noninvasive studies. A voiding cystourethrogram is invasive. It is a limited
exam of bladder function and anatomy, and
although advanced invasive bladder tumors
may be demonstrated as a filling defect, it is
not sensitive for lower stages of bladder neoplasms. Cystourethroscopy is invasive and is
therefore not the initial exam in the evalua-

tion of hematuria. It is indicated in the evaluation of gross hematuria in patients with a
normal IVP. It is the optimal tool for evaluation of potential bladder pathology. An abdominal ultrasound or CT scan is indicated
in patients with a suspected renal mass, either by clinical examination or demonstrated
on IVP. Urine for cytology is useful for
screening of patients with suspected urinary
tract malignancy, but it is falsely negative in
approximately 20% of patients and should
not be used as the only diagnostic evaluation.
A transrectal ultrasound may be helpful in
evaluating the extent of invasion of a bladder
or prostatic neoplasm. Abdominal CT scan is
a superior imaging study for this purpose.
*(Sabiston, pp 1526–1529, 1548–1550; Niederhuber, pp
746–748, 760–761)*

484. (B) This child presents with progressive
cholestatic jaundice, as indicated by the elevated conjugated hyperbilirubinemia. Metabolic screening for inborn errors of metabolism and serologic evaluation for intrauterine
infections are important to exclude these
causes of intrahepatic cholestasis. Figure 4–15
depicts an acholic stool (absence of bile pig-
ments), which is usually indicative of complete biliary tract obstruction. In this clinical
setting, biliary atresia is the most probable
diagnosis. The most sensitive imaging study
is radioisotope scanning. Preimaging phenobarbital increases the diagnostic yield by
stimulating hepatic microsomal enzymes.
Abdominal ultrasound may show absence of
the gallbladder, but this study is operator dependent and does not evaluate hepatocyte
function and bile excretory pattern. CT or
MRI scans may demonstrate hepatic parenchymal changes (eg, extensive cirrhosis)
and the presence or absence of bile duct dilatation, but do not evaluate and differentiate
abnormalities of hepatocyte function or bile
excretory pattern. *(Niederhuber, pp 791–792)*

485–486. (485-C, 486-B) This patient has idiopathic
thrombocytopenic purpura (ITP), a disease
characterized by a low platelet count, normal
coagulation profile, increased megakaryocytes, and a normal-sized spleen. Patients
with ITP will often demonstrate excessive

bleeding in response to a minor injury. Circulating antiplatelet antibodies coat normal platelets, which are then sequestered by the spleen, with resultant platelet destruction. The majority of patients respond to initial therapy with systemic steroids. Splenectomy is indicated in patients who become steroid dependent with significant side effects, or in patients requiring increasing doses of steroids to maintain a satisfactory platelet count. The entire spleen must be excised, including any accessory spleens found at surgery. Residual splenic parenchyma would result in persistent platelet sequestration. Splenectomy is not indicated in the initial management of ITP. Platelet transfusion is rarely required. Spontaneous bleeding is unusual unless the platelet counts drop below 20,000/μL. When this occurs, if the patient is not responsive to steroids, platelet transfusion and urgent splenectomy is indicated. Antineoplastic chemotherapy is not used in the management of ITP. Expectant management is associated with significant risk, as the most life-threatening complication of ITP is spontaneous intracerebral hemorrhage. Bone marrow transplant is not indicated. ITP is a disease of peripheral platelet destruction, with normal or increased platelet production. (*Sabiston, pp 1193–1196; Niederhuber, pp 52, 370*)

487. **(E)** This patient has symptomatic anemia. The decreased oxygen-carrying capacity has resulted in decreased tissue perfusion. The heart attempts to compensate with increased contractility and heart rate, in an attempt to improve cardiac output and oxygen delivery. In this patient, however, this is inadequate, and has also placed excess metabolic demands on the myocardium with signs of ischemia. These changes can be ameliorated with a blood transfusion. Iron supplementation is indicated in the treatment of chronic iron-deficiency anemia. Restoration of iron stores and a normal red cell mass usually takes several months. It is therefore not appropriate in a patient with symptomatic anemia. Supplemental oxygen will not improve oxygen delivery in a patient with limited oxygen-carrying capacity and compensatory maximum oxygen extraction at the tissue

level. Intravenous fluid resuscitation will increase circulating blood volume, resulting in hemodilution and decreased red cell concentration. Calcium channel blockade is indicated for management of myocardial ischemia from primary coronary or myocardial pathology. (*Sabiston, pp 120–121; Niederhuber, p 52*)

488. **(A)** A febrile nonhemolytic transfusion reaction is usually caused by an interaction between recipient antibodies and leukocytes in the transfused blood. Treatment is discontinuation of the transfusion and antipyretics. If further transfusion is required, further reactions can be prevented by filtration of blood products for leukocyte reduction. Anaphylactic transfusion reactions are rare. Patients develop urticaria, flushing, hypotension, and bronchospasm. O blood type is characterized by the absence of ABO antigens on the red blood cell surface. Therefore, type O blood is universally accepted as the donor type for transfusion therapy, making an acute hemolytic transfusion reaction from ABO incompatability impossible. Delayed hemolytic reactions usually occur 1 to 3 weeks after a first transfusion and are manifested by an unexplained drop in hematocrit, associated with unconjugated hyperbilirubinemia. Acute bacterial infection transmitted through blood products is extremely rare, and has been reported only in association with platelet concentrates stored at room temperature. (*Sabiston, pp 124–125; Niederhuber, p 57*)

489. **(E)** Any patient with this history and point tenderness in the anatomic snuffbox must be assumed to have a scaphoid fracture. Undisplaced fractures may be difficult to visualize on initial radiographs, even when multiple views are obtained. The appropriate management is full immobilization of the scaphoid, which is achieved only with a cast that extends to include the thumb. X-rays should be repeated in 10 to 14 days, and if the fracture is confirmed, immobilization should be continued. Avascular necrosis is a common complication. Minor wrist injury with ligamentous sprain may be adequately treated with anti-inflammatory medication, application of

ice, an elastic wrist support, and restricted activity. However, these are not adequate therapy for a suspected scaphoid fracture. Furthermore, a wrist splint does not provide adequate immobilization of the scaphoid. *(Sabiston, pp 1415–1419)*

490.   **(B)** Symptoms of zinc deficiency include diarrhea, depression, alopecia, and perioral and periorbital dermatitis. Patients at greater risk for developing this syndrome include those with high gastrointestinal fluid losses, patients with multisystem trauma, and patients on prolonged parenteral nutrition. The symptoms resolve with zinc supplementation. Iodine deficiency results in hypothyroidism. Deficiency syndromes for selenium, silicon, and tin have not been described. *(Niederhuber, p 219)*

491–492.   **(491-B, 492-D)** In the initial postoperative period, the patient has a low pulmonary artery wedge pressure and poor urine output. Renal perfusion is compromised by hypovolemia, with subsequent inadequate preload and decreased cardiac output. The appropriate therapeutic intervention at this time is further IV fluid resuscitation. Diuretics are contraindicated in the patient with hypovolemia and are unlikely to improve urine output in the face of inadequate renal perfusion. A dopamine infusion or digoxin may improve cardiac contractility but will not result in improvement in cardiac output unless there is adequate preload. In a hypovolemic patient, nitroprusside will result in a significant drop in blood pressure. After receiving a fluid bolus, the patient develops distended neck veins and an elevated pulmonary wedge pressure, indicating biventricular dysfunction with increased left ventricular end-diastolic pressure, and increased left ventricular end-systolic volume. Cardiac output is low, and urine output has not improved. In a patient with a history of hypertension, this clinical picture is often due to increased afterload. Afterload reduction can be obtained with a nitroprusside infusion. *(Niederhuber, pp 154–159)*

493.   **(C)** This patient has an obstructed airway from maxillofacial trauma. The patient is stridorous, hypoxic, and cannot be ventilated with bag and mask. Immediate cricothyroidotomy is lifesaving. In the presence of severe facial trauma, orotracheal intubation is likely to be difficult because of distortion of landmarks and excessive oropharyngeal secretions. Nasotracheal intubation is contraindicated in this setting. A definitive tracheostomy is more time consuming than a cricothyroidotomy and requires specific surgical expertise. Stabilization of the airway is the first resuscitation priority, before placement of chest tubes to relieve potential pneumothoraces. *(Sabiston, pp 296–297; Niederhuber, pp 99–101)*

494.   **(E)** Frostbite is produced by formation of ice crystals in the tissue, with cessation of tissue perfusion. Appropriate initial treatment is rapid rewarming in warm water, to minimize further tissue damage. Dry heat can cause further tissue damage. With reperfusion, there is continued progression of tissue injury because of progressive microcirculatory thrombosis. Therefore, nonviable tissue should be allowed to demarcate over several weeks, with delayed debridement. A sympathectomy is not indicated acutely, since the vasculature in frozen tissue is already maximally dilated. *(Sabiston, pp 249–250; Niederhuber, pp 698–699)*

495–497.   **(495-B, 496-D, 497-A)** Ruptured cerebral aneurysms often occur in the setting of hypertension. The severe headache, nausea and vomiting, photophobia, and nuchal rigidity are the result of meningeal irritation from subarachnoid blood. Lumbar puncture is not necessary for diagnosis. Subarachnoid hemorrhage is visualized on CT scan, with definitive diagnosis of the aneurysm and its location by cerebral angiography. Early surgical clipping is the current neurosurgical approach, because of the significant risk of rebleeding in the first 24 hours after initial presentation. Hydrocephalus may occur as a late complication of subarachnoid hemorrhage and require serial lumbar puncture to drain CSF and control ICP. A hemorrhagic stroke can occur in association with malignant hypertension, and may have concurrent subarachnoid hemorrhage. Focal neurologic signs are usually present. Meningitis will produce similar signs of meningeal irritation, but usually with other systemic signs of infection and a clinical prodrome suggesting an infectious etiology. Lumbar puncture is diagnostic, and if a bacterial source is suspected, systemic antibiotics are initiated pending culture of CSF. Ischemic cerebrovascular accidents and transient ischemic attacks are not associated with subarachnoid hemorrhage and, hence, do not present with signs of meningeal irritation. Focal neurologic signs are usually present. Evaluation of a possible cause includes Doppler examination of the carotid arteries. Management includes anticoagulation and antiplatelet therapy. EEG measures brain electrical activity and is indicated in the diagnostic evaluation of seizures. *(Sabiston, pp 1349–1350; Niederhuber, pp 732–734)*

498. **(C)** This patient has developed a tension pneumothorax from dissection of carbon dioxide into the pleural space, either via an unrecognized defect in the diaphragm or via the retroperitoneal and retropleural spaces. Treatment is immediate decompression with a chest tube. Hypotension associated with a tension pneumothorax is secondary to decreased venous return from mediastinal shift. Intravenous fluids are indicated only if there is associated hypovolemia. Release of the pneumoperitoneum may prevent further carbon dioxide accumulation, but chest tube decompression is still required. A tension pneumothorax is a clinical diagnosis and does not require a chest x-ray for confirmation. Once the pneumothorax is adequately decompressed and the patient is stabilized, the laparoscopic procedure may continue. *(Sabiston, pp 793, 803–804)*

499–501. **(499-B, 500-A, 501-B)** This patient with diverticular disease has developed a colovesical fistula from diverticulitis, with localized sigmoid perforation into the adjacent bladder. Patients will present with signs and symptoms of a urinary tract infection, with air in the urinary stream and multiple fecal organisms

on urine culture. Cystoscopy is most useful in the diagnostic evaluation, with abnormalities found in 80 to 95% of patients, although it is unusual to precisely visualize the fistula. An air contrast barium enema may show evidence of diverticular disease and is useful to exclude other pathology. The diagnostic yield of cystography and colonoscopy are approximately 20%. Diagnostic laparoscopy is not indicated. This patient should be managed with broad-spectrum antibiotics and bladder drainage. When the acute inflammatory process has resolved, definitive surgical therapy can be performed electively. These patients will tolerate a gentle bowel prep and can then undergo a sigmoid colon resection and primary anastomosis. Outpatient management is not optimal, and oral antibiotics are not sufficient therapy. Clear fluids, magnesium citrate, and oral antibiotics are components of a surgical bowel prep. This should only be undertaken after treatment of the urinary tract sepsis and a period of bowel rest. A colovesical fistula is not a surgical emergency. Management of the complications of diverticular disease by proximal defunctioning colostomy is reserved for patients who are profoundly ill and require diversion of the fecal stream to control continued intra-abdominal and pelvic sepsis. This is not definitive therapy for a colovesical fistula, as it leaves a column of stool above the fistula, with continued fecal contamination of the urinary tract. A resection with Hartmann's procedure has the disadvantage of requiring a second major laparotomy to re-establish intestinal continuity. An abdominoperineal resection is not required for the management of diverticular disease. Diverticular disease does not involve the rectum. The sigmoid colon is the most common location for symptomatic diverticular disease resulting in a colovesical fistula. A total abdominal colectomy is therefore rarely indicated. *(Sabiston, p 991; Niederhuber, pp 309–311)*

502. **(D)** This patient presents with signs and symptoms of a sigmoid volvulus. Most commonly, this occurs in the elderly debilitated patient with a history of chronic constipation, resulting in the development of a long, re-

dundant, mobile sigmoid colon. Patients present with a clinical picture of an acute colonic obstruction. Abdominal radiographs will show a large dilated loop of colon originating in the left lower abdomen, and extending to the right upper abdomen. Management includes decompression with a rigid proctoscope, which will usually result in detorsion of the bowel. Placement of a sigmoid decompression tube is necessary to prevent recurrence. Urgent laparotomy is indicated in patients with fever, abdominal tenderness, and metabolic acidosis, suggesting colonic ischemia. Patients admitted to the hospital who do not undergo urgent decompression are at risk of developing colonic ischemia from the closed loop obstruction. A rectal decompression tube is insufficient for decompression, because the tip is located distal to the obstruction. Colonic enemas are ineffective in the face of a complete obstruction and may in fact further increase colonic distension. *(Sabiston, pp 1016–1017; Niederhuber, p 316)*

REFERENCES

Fauci AS, Braunwald E, Isselbacher KJ, et al., eds. *Harrison's Principles of Internal Medicine.* New York, McGraw-Hill; 1998.

Greenfield LJ, Mulholland M, Oldham KT, Zelenock GB, Lillemoe KD, eds. *Surgery: Scientific Principles and Practice.* Philadelphia: Lippincott-Raven; 1997.

Niederhuber JE. *Fundamentals of Surgery.* Stamford, CT: Appleton & Lange; 1998.

Sabiston DC, ed. *Textbook of Surgery,* 15th ed. Philadelphia: WB Saunders; 1997.

Schwartz SI, Shires GT, Spencer FC, eds. *Principles of Surgery.* New York: McGraw-Hill; 1994.

Zinner MJ. *Maingot's Abdominal Operations,* 10th ed., vols. I and II. Stamford, CT: Appleton & Lange; 1997.

Subspecialty List: Surgery

Question Number and Subspecialty

379. GI/Pediatric
380. GI/Pediatric
381. GI/Pediatric
382. GI/Pediatric
383. GU/Urology
384. GU/Urology
385. Critical care trauma
386. GI/Pediatric
387. GI/Pediatric
388. Trauma
389. GI/Pediatric
390. GI/Pediatric
391. GI/Pediatric
392. Neurologic surgery/Trauma & critical care
393. GI
394. GI
395. GU/Urology
396. Urology/Neoplasms
397. Critical care anesthesia
398. Trauma
399. Trauma
400. Endocrine critical care
401. Endocrine critical care
402. GI
403. GI
404. Head & neck/Pediatric
405. Infection
406. Head & neck/Pediatric
407. Head & neck
408. Head & neck/Neoplasm
409. Endocrine
410. Head & neck/Neoplasm
411. Biliary tract/Liver
412. Biliary tract/Neoplasm
413. Biliary tract
414. Neoplasm

415. Biliary tract
416. Breast/Neoplasm
417. Breast/Neoplasm
418. Breast/Neoplasm
419. Breast/Neoplasm
420. Breast/Neoplasm
421. Breast/Neoplasm
422. Breast/Neoplasm
423. Breast/Neoplasm
424. GI/Neoplasm
425. GI/Neoplasm
426. GI/Neoplasm
427. GI
428. GI
429. GI
430. GI
431. GI
432. GI/Neoplasm
433. GI/Neoplasm
434. GI/Neoplasm
435. GI/Neoplasm
436. GI/Neoplasm
437. Skin/Neoplasm
438. Skin/Neoplasm
439. GI
440. Pulmonary/Neoplasm
441. Pulmonary/Neoplasm
442. Vascular
443. Vascular/GI
444. Vascular/Cardiovascular
445. Cardiovascular/Vascular
446. Vascular/Cardiovascular
447. Vascular/Cardiovascular
448. Cardiovascular
449. Endocrine/Neoplasm
450. Endocrine/Neoplasm
451. GI/Neoplasm
452. GI/Neoplasm

453. GI
454. GI
455. GI
456. GI/Neoplasm
457. GI/Neoplasm
458. GI
459. GI
460. GI
461. GI
462. GI
463. GI/Neoplasm
464. GI/Neoplasm
465. GI/Neoplasm
466. Head & neck/Neoplasm
467. Head & neck/Neoplasm
468. GI/Pediatrics
469. GI/Pediatrics
470. Infection
471. Infection
472. Orthopedics
473. Critical care
474. Critical care
475. GI/Pediatrics
476. GI/Pediatrics
477. GI/Pediatrics

478. GU/Neoplasm
479. GU/Neoplasm
480. GI/Pediatrics
481. GI/Pediatrics
482. GU/Neoplasm
483. GU/Neoplasm
484. Biliary tract/Pediatrics
485. Hematology
486. Hematology
487. Critical care
488. Hematology
489. Orthopedics
490. Critical care/Nutrition
491. Critical care
492. Critical care
493. Trauma
494. Skin/Trauma
495. Cardiovascular/Neurosurgery
496. Cardiovascular/Neurosurgery
497. Neurosurgery
498. Anesthesia/Laparoscopy
499. GI
500. GI
501. GI
502. GI

CHAPTER 5

Psychiatry
Questions

Elizabeth A. Caspary, MD

DIRECTIONS (Questions 503 through 507): Each of the numbered items or incomplete statements in this section is followed by answers or by completions of the statement. Select the ONE lettered answer or completion that is BEST in each case.

Questions 503 and 504

503. A 20-year-old man is started on haloperidol (Haldol), 20 mg, each day for psychotic symptoms. Which of the following side effects would most likely be seen in the first 5 days of treatment?

   (A) restless shuffling and pacing
   (B) masked facies
   (C) muscle spasm in neck
   (D) writhing movement in fingers and hands
   (E) "rabbit" syndrome

504. Which of the following is least likely to cause the above signs?

   (A) thioridazine *mellanl*
   (B) thiothixene
   (C) chlorpromazine *thorazine*
   (D) haloperidol *haldol*
   (E) clozapine *clozaril*

   D₂ antagonist (H>L>atypical)
   haloperidol > thiothixene > chlorpromazine > thioridazine > clozapine

Questions 505 and 506

An 84-year-old man with no previous psychiatric history is referred by an internal medicine physician for psychiatric evaluation. For the past year, he has been successfully treated for prostatic cancer. About 2 months ago, his wife of 60 years died. He since has not been able to sleep at night, but naps during the day. He feels "lost" in the kitchen and is unable to make a meal for himself, although he claims to have been quite efficient at this in the past. He forgets where he puts things. He acknowledges being "scruffy-looking"—unshaven, crumpled clothes, mismatched socks. On the Mini-Mental Status Exam (MMSE), he scores 26; he was unable to successfully complete serial 7 subtractions and was unwilling to spell "world" backwards. He had little trouble with the language portion of the test. *↓ sleep ↓ ADL ↓ memory ↑ neglect ↓ concentration*

SIG E CAPS

505. Which of the following is the most likely diagnosis for this man?

   (A) acute psychotic reaction F *no psychotic sx*
   (B) grief reaction *possible but ↑ sxs than expected*
   (C) metastatic cancer to brain *sxs don't relate*
   (D) major depression
   (E) Alzheimer's disease

506. Of the following, which would be the most appropriate initial treatment?

   (A) psychotherapy ✗
   (B) electroconvulsive therapy (ECT) F *not life threaten*
   (C) diazepam F *no need for benzo*
   (D) thioridazine F *no psychotic sx*
   (E) venlafaxine •
   effexor

185

507. Which of the following sleep-related disorders is classified as a parasomnia associated with sleep–wake phenomena?

    (A) narcolepsy
    (B) hypersomnia
    (C) circadian rhythm sleep disorder
    (D) sleep paralysis
    (E) sleep bruxism

DIRECTIONS (Questions 508 through 512): For each item, select the ONE best lettered option that is most closely associated with it. Each lettered heading may be selected once, more than once, or not at all.

Identify the most likely diagnosis with the case descriptions below.

    (A) body dysmorphic disorder
    (B) conversion disorder
    (C) factitious disorder
    (D) hypochondriasis
    (E) malingering
    (F) pain disorder
    (G) panic disorder
    (H) somatization disorder

508. In spite of repeated efforts to reassure a 40-year-old woman that the stomach pain she is experiencing is not cancerous, she continues to worry and fear that she will die.

509. A 23-year-old violinist reports to his neurologist that he thinks he has had a stroke. He is unable to feel anything with his left fingers and is barely able to hold down the violin strings with this same hand because of "paralysis." The numbness he describes reaches to his wrist only, and he "even feels a band" around the wrist delineating the sensitive from the insensitive areas.

510. A 35-year-old woman complains that she has been to multiple doctors, none of whom have been able to effectively treat or even diagnose the cause of her chronic stomach pain and diarrhea, repeated problems swallowing, headache, and recurrent back pain. The symptoms have been present on and off for most of her adult life.

511. A 55-year-old man requests "some kind of pain medication that really works!" to relieve the "extreme" pain in his foot. He walks with a cane. He angrily claims that his previous employer does not care about what happened to him in an accident 1 year earlier in which his foot was struck by an iron rod. No fracture was found. He claims his doctor said he had a "severe contusion" and then states "the doctor didn't know anything."

512. A 40-year-old woman is brought to the emergency department after she had frantically called the paramedics because she thought she would die. She was experiencing sharp chest pain; shortness of breath; racing heartbeat; and cold, sweaty chills. Cardiac assessment proved negative for myocardial ischemia.

DIRECTIONS (Questions 513 through 581): Each of the numbered items or incomplete statements in this section is followed by answers or by completions of the statement. Select the ONE lettered answer or completion that is BEST in each case.

513. Of the following, which is considered an abnormal change in an elderly person?

    (A) decrease in brain weight
    (B) absence of sexual interest
    (C) decrease in acuity of all special senses (eg, vision, hearing)
    (D) decline in simple recall
    (E) none of the above

514. Which of the following changes in the sexual response cycle in the elderly is considered abnormal?

    (A) greater dependence on external stimulation during the period of sexual arousal
    (B) increased refractory period
    (C) decreased size and firmness of erection in men
    (D) decreased elasticity and lubrication of the vaginal barrel in women
    (E) none of the above

515. The treatment of choice for reversing anti-cholinergic delirium is

(A) dantrolene *fn NMS*
(B) bethanechol *specific for urinary retention*
(C) physostigmine *cholinergic*
(D) bromocriptine *dopamine agonist? for NMS*
(E) haloperidol *antipsychotic – vs anticholin*

✓ 516. Which of the following is inconsistent with the concept of dementia? *– ↓ intellectual, language, movements, perception*

(A) gradual decline in certain mental operations such as orientation, cognition, and memory *T* *In DSM – Aphasia, apraxia, Agnosia*
(B) presence of a specific language disorder such as aphasia, alexia, or agraphia *T not isolated neuro defect*
(C) onset of behavioral changes including apathy, eccentricity, and distractibility *T may be sudden or gradual*
(D) sudden loss of intellectual functioning, such as following an anoxic episode or a cerebrovascular accident *F*
(E) intellectual decline accompanied by neurologic abnormalities *T*

517. In the Diagnostic and Statistical Manual, 4th edition (DSM-IV), homosexuality is considered

(A) a disorder of sexual desire *F*
(B) a paraphilia *F*
(C) a sexual arousal disorder *F*
(D) a sexual aversion disorder *F*
(E) an alternative lifestyle *T*

518. In DSM-IV, an example of a sexual desire disorder is

(A) dyspareunia *F*] *(sexual pain)*
(B) vaginismus *F*
(C) pedophilia *F (paraphilic)*
(D) premature ejaculation *(orgasmic)*
(E) sexual aversion disorder *T @ hypoactive avoidance of genital sexual contact*

✓ 519. A patient reports that, on his way to the hospital, he saw a man feeding two squirrels in the park. He says that this means his future will be decided in 2 weeks. This man, he believes, is deliberately out to alarm him (the patient). One of the squirrels is scheming with the man; the other is innocent and trust-

ing. The term that best describes what this man is experiencing is

(A) illusions *T sensory misperceptions*
(B) hallucinations *F sensory input when not there*
(C) delusions *false ideas, not corrected by reasoning, not reality based*
(D) loosened associations *F*] *patterns of speech*
(E) neologisms *F*

Questions 520 and 521

A young mother seeks psychiatric help because she is unable to remember events surrounding her 3-year-old son's death after being struck by a car 2 months ago. She is worried that maybe she did something that put him at risk. Except for this brief time period, she is able to recall other events both before and after the tragedy.

520. Given the information above, what is the most likely diagnosis?

(A) depersonalization disorder *detached from body; observe*
(B) post-traumatic stress disorder *reexperience event, avoid stimuli similar, hyperarousal*
(C) dissociative amnesia *loss of recall*
(D) dissociative fugue *fugue identity @ travel*
(E) major depression *mood + affect disturbed*

521. Of the following treatments, which is the most appropriate to help this patient regain her memory?

(A) electroshock therapy
(B) individual psychotherapy *events, feelings, etc*
(C) chlordiazepoxide
(D) sertraline *antidepress*
(E) thioridazine *antipsychotic*

① No Amytal fn recall @ ② benzos for anxiety episode needs to be unconscious for healing

522. According to freudian theory, the term *primary process thinking* refers to

(A) the rational selection of one's personal goals
(B) a specific mode of thinking encouraged in psychotherapy
(C) the uncensored expression of primitive drives *– aggression, sexual energy, fantasy → DID can't be expressed: Uncons. freudian slips*
(D) the thought processes of psychotic individuals *F*
(E) the characteristic thought processes of an adult

2° process thinking = personal needs + desires expressed to outside world more socially accepted, rational

Questions 523 Through 525

A 44-year-old man presents with fears that his mathematical abilities have been slowly sucked out of his brain for the last 4 years. He believes an "alien force disguised as a human being" is responsible. To avoid contacting this being, he has isolated himself in a room in a boarding house. He has left his wife and children. After 10 years teaching math at a local high school, he resigned about 3 years ago. He supports himself by "collecting cans." His affect is blunted. His appearance is disheveled, unshaven, and unwashed.

523. Which of the following is LEAST suggestive of a schizophrenic disorder in this man?

   (A) delusional system F
   (B) 4-year history of symptoms
   (C) age of onset young adult M before F
   (D) decrease in level of functioning F
   (E) social isolation F

524. Of the following, the most likely diagnosis is

   (A) paranoid schizophrenia T
   (B) alcohol abuse and dependence F Ø hx
   (C) major depression with psychotic features F long course; mood has shorter cour
   (D) Alzheimer's disease ≈ Ø cog. impairment
   (E) Huntington's disease F Ø movement disorder

525. Considering the information thus far, which of the following would be the treatment of choice?

   (A) thiamine EtOH
   (B) haloperidol antipsych
   (C) clozapine 2nd line antipsych
   (D) amitriptyline TCA
   (E) lithium carbonate mood

526. Which of the following supports a diagnosis of anorexia nervosa? ♀, teens + YA

   (A) satisfaction with weight at least 20% below average weight recommended F
   (B) aversion to food-related activities (ie, menu planning, cooking) F take much cal
   (C) reasonably accurate perception of body image F

   (D) reduced fear of becoming fat once body weight is below 100 lb F
   (E) denial of the seriousness of the weight loss problem T

Questions 527 and 528

A 70-year-old man is brought to his primary care doctor by the man's son. According to his son, who had not seen his father for about a year, the father seemed to have some personality changes. He was no longer interested in his hobbies and seemed apathetic. He seemed to forget easily, and he repeatedly asked the same already answered questions. On at least two occasions, the father wandered out of the house and was found by neighbors, who thought he was confused.

527. Statistically speaking, which of the following dementias would this man most likely have?

   (A) Alzheimer's • 50-60%
   (B) Pick's
   (C) Parkinson's
   (D) vascular 15-30%
   (E) subcortical

528. If this man had Pick's disease, where would the preponderance of pathology be found?

   (A) cerebellum
   (B) caudate nucleus Huntingtons
   (C) hippocampus •
   (D) frontotemporal areas Pick's
   (E) parietotemporal areas Alzheimers or frontotemporal

529. The association between human immunodeficiency virus (HIV) infection and neuropsychiatric disturbance can be described by which of the following statements?

   (A) Dementia and delirium are the most common disorders in persons with acquired immune deficiency syndrome (AIDS).
   (B) Brain tissue typically remains free of HIV for the first 2 to 3 years after the initial infection. HIV in brain @ time of infectn
   (C) HIV-infected persons begin to show impaired performance on neuropsychiatric

refuse to maintain >85% body weight
preoccupy c feelings obese

tests ~~after~~ *before* neurologic symptoms of AIDS have appeared.

(D) ~~One quarter~~ *majority* of persons with AIDS perform inadequately on neuropsychiatric tests.

(E) ~~One third~~ *majority* of persons with AIDS have evidence of involvement of the central nervous system at autopsy. ·

Questions 530 and 531

A 40-year-old woman with a history of alcoholism and polysubstance abuse, a supervisor at a large legal firm, has had a marked increase in what she calls her usual "hyper feelings." The symptoms include a racing and pounding heart, sharp chest pain, flushed neck and face, lightheadedness, and shortness of breath. She is terrified she will collapse and die during one of these 10- to 15-minute episodes. She has been healthy all her life. A medical evaluation was done about 1 month prior for these same symptoms. The exam was unremarkable. She shares that her mother suffered a stroke approximately 3 months ago, and a sister was diagnosed with breast cancer around the same time.

530. At this point, the most likely diagnosis is

(A) autonomic changes secondary to menopause F *too young*
(B) early signs of myocardial infarction F *sts don't match, 1 mo ago*
(C) panic disorder T *sympathetic sxs + fear*
(D) hypochondriasis F *discrete episodes, not chronic*
(E) post-traumatic stress disorder F *Ø stressor, trauma*

531. Which of the following drugs would be the most appropriate long-term treatment for this woman's condition?

(A) alprazolam F *-hx of substance abuse*
(B) paroxetine *SSRI*
(C) risperidone F
(D) thioridazine F *] antipsychotic*
(E) propranolol F *-performance anxiety*

532. A 70-year-old woman was brought to the emergency department following her involvement in a minor car accident. She had sustained no injuries but was very upset and was therefore referred to a psychiatrist. After

speaking at length about her part in the accident and sharing her reactions, she still remained tremulous, anxious, and tearful. You decide to use an anxiolytic to help her. Of the following, which would be the best choice?

(A) diazepam L
(B) clorazepate L *] ↑SE (sedate, anti-cholinergic, resp↓, confusion, disorientation)   anxiety → elderly*
(C) lorazepam S
(D) buspirone *slow onset*
(E) temazepam *hypnotic*

533. Which of the following delusions would most likely be observed in a psychotically depressed person?

(A) "My mind's eye is perfused with a radiance of the gods."
(B) "I've been targeted by the FBI."
(C) "My body is rotting inside out." *mood congruent*
(D) "I have been hand-picked to be the world's leader; I am awaiting the signal to bring the masses together."
(E) "All I need to do is clutch the book to myself and all the knowledge pours into me."

534. The American court case *Wyatt* v. *Stickney* dealt with which of the following legal concepts?

(A) duty to warn F *Tarasoff*
(B) right to treatment
(C) informed consent
(D) confidentiality
(E) false imprisonment

535. Which of the following is a general characteristic of all personality disorders?

(A) rigid patterns of defense seen before age 18
(B) tendency to have short lapses of psychotic thinking F *(maybe borderline)*
(C) relatively well-developed sense of self F *poor sense of self*
(D) symptoms experienced as dystonic F *ego-syntonic*
(E) interpersonal relationships not necessarily impaired F *defense → impaired relations*

536. The drug of choice for the treatment of pathological separation anxiety in school-avoiding children is

(A) clonazepam benzo L
(B) haloperidol antipsychotic
(C) clonidine alpha agonist
(D) chlorpromazine antipsychotic
(E) alprazolam benzo I

537. The primary aim of methadone maintenance programs is

(A) gradual détoxification and eventual withdrawal from all opiates
(B) treatment of psychological factors underlying addiction so that detoxification can occur F
(C) satiation of "drug hunger" so addicts can focus on other aspects of their lives
(D) use of the opiate-antagonist agents to deter further opiate abuse F
(E) education of addicts about the dangers of narcotic abuse F

538. Infantile autism is a severe developmental disorder of early childhood that is characterized by

(A) symptoms and signs of schizophrenia occurring in an infant F
(B) head banging F
(C) gross impairment of communication before age 30 months
(D) preoccupation with morbid thoughts and bizarre use of objects after age 30 months but before 12 years F
(E) hallucinations and delusions F

539. Which of the following disorders could be prevented with proper perinatal care?

(A) Tay–Sachs disease F
(B) galactosemia
(C) phenylketonuria
(D) Down syndrome F
(E) cerebral palsy

540. Which of the following statements is true regarding treatment with clozapine?

(A) In certain severe psychotic disorders, it is used as the first drug of choice. F
(B) It has a low potency as a D_2 receptor antagonist. F atypical
(C) It has an unusually safe side effect profile, making it the drug of choice for the treatment of schizophrenia. F
(D) It has little impact on the improvement of negative signs of schizophrenia. F
(E) It has relatively low anticholinergic effects.

541. Delirium is distinguished from dementia by the presence of

(A) impaired judgment
(B) impaired memory
(C) clouding of consciousness
(D) thought disorder
(E) disorientation

Questions 542 and 543

A 56-year-old man with a dual diagnosis of schizophrenia and alcohol abuse and dependency was arrested for "driving under the influence." After 2 days in jail, he was noted to be acting agitated and "crazy," claiming that the guards were going to kill him that night. When questioned about his profuse sweating, he claimed that he had just come in from his job working in the heat and humidity. He was distracted by various noises, claiming that these were made by people watching him and waiting for him. He appeared to watch things that seemed to be moving on the walls. On further exam, it was noted that he was very tremulous, unable to follow an object with his eyes only, and quite ataxic.

542. The working diagnosis at this point is most likely

(A) acute exacerbation of schizophrenia F
(B) alcohol withdrawal delirium
(C) alcohol-induced persisting dementia F

(D) alcohol intoxication F

(E) malingering F

√543. Which of the following treatments should be avoided?

(A) thiamine, 100 mg IM need

(B) haloperidol, 2 to 5 mg IM Ⓗ for hallucin

Ⓒ chlorpromazine, 100 mg L orthostatic, anticholin

(D) chlordiazepoxide, 50 to 100 mg PO q4 to 6 hours } librium x-react

(E) lorazepam, 2 to 4 mg IM need

544. A 30-year-old ♂ accountant has not been able to leave his home since his wife of 3 years died. Before she died, he was dependent on her encouragement to leave the house, and in many cases she would drive him to his destination. He claimed that he became extremely anxious in traffic jams and elevators. In stores, he becomes so nervous and disorganized that he is unable to complete his shopping. One would expect this man's symptoms to best respond to which of the following? agoraphobia

(A) trihexyphenidyl antiparkinson

(B) propranolol β blocker

Ⓒ alprazolam benzo.

(D) risperidone antipsychotic

(E) pemoline stimulant

545. Among which of the following groups is the prevalence of alcohol-related disorders the lowest?

Ⓐ Asian-American T

(B) Native American and Eskimo F

(C) Hispanic F

(D) African-American F

(E) Caucasian F

50% lack EtOH dehydrogenase
→ ↑ unpleasant SE

white + AA ♂ highest

546. Characteristic features of dissociative identity disorder (multiple personality disorder) can be described by which of the following statements?

(A) Age of onset is in early adulthood. childhood, response to abuse

(B) It is an acute chronic reaction to profound, intolerable stress.

Ⓒ It is several times more common in women than in men. T

(D) Mild cases are seldom, if ever, encountered. F mild more likely

(E) Severity is calibrated by the number of distinct personalities that are revealed. F makeup of personalities

547. Which of the following is true regarding violence?

(A) Less than 70% 50% of homicides are committed with handguns.

(B) Rates of violent crime are about equal in urban and rural areas.

Ⓒ In the United States, homicide is the second leading cause of death among persons from 15 to 24 years of age. T

(D) In all areas, the predisposition to and frequency of violence is much higher in males. except: domestic violence

(E) Approximately 85% of homicides are alcohol related. F

548. Of the following, which is most characteristic of attention deficit disorder?

(A) ritualistic behavior OCD

(B) abnormalities in coordination

(C) pressured speech mania

(D) formal thought disorder psychosis

(E) fears about appearance and weight A/B

Ⓕ short attention span
low frustration tolerance
impulsive
perception/learning difficulties
Ⓓ

Questions 549 Through 551

A 65-year-old woman with a long history of schizophrenia is described as being in a "severe catatonic state." Approximately 1 week prior to the onset of this condition, her haloperidol dosage was increased from 5 mg/day to 20 mg/day to treat the presence of auditory hallucinations. These have begun to remit, but now the nursing staff caring for her say she is withdrawn; walks with a slow, shuffling gait; stares at the floor, shows little, if any, movement in her upper limbs; and has lost all expression in her face. The staff fear that her psychiatric relapse is deepening and that further increases in haloperidol are indicated. *parkinsonism*

549. In caring for this patient, which of the following would be the most appropriate next step?

(A) stat dose of haloperidol, 5 mg IM *F*

(B) stat dose of benztropine, 2 mg IM

(C) oral dose of benztropine, 2 mg *T*

(D) neurologic and vital signs evaluation by psychiatrist

(E) request for neurology consult

550. In evaluating this woman, her blood pressure is found to be 110/74, pulse 86 and regular, and temperature 97.4°F. Neurologic evaluation reveals "lead-pipe" stiffness in all extremities, a frozen facial expression, occasional pill-rolling in the right hand, small shuffling steps in walking, and a stiffly "bent-over" posture. Further medications include benztropine, 1.0 mg/day. The most likely diagnosis at this point is

(A) neuroleptic malignant syndrome *6 Sxs*

(B) tardive dyskinesia—severe *∅ sxs*

(C) pseudoparkinsonism ·

(D) exacerbation of schizophrenia—catatonic *bizarre posturing*

(E) major depression with psychosis *d/t affect w/l?*

551. Which of the following would be an appropriate choice for this woman?

(A) dantrolene *~NMS*

(B) benztropine ·

(C) fluphenazine/*prolixin (A)*

(D) amitriptyline *TCA*

(E) increase haloperidol *↓ antipsychotic*

552. Drug-induced extrapyramidal reactions may be correctly described by which of the following statements?

(A) These voluntary *involuntary* motor behaviors can be produced by a variety of psychoactive medications. *antipsychotic, stimulants, antidepress, Li, lead to early-dystonia, pseudoparkinism, akathisia*

(B) Late effects can appear several months after treatment is begun. *TD*

(C) They are irreversible despite reduction in or discontinuation of the causative medication.

(D) They are irreversible despite concomitant use of an anticholinergic agent.

(E) They occur as a consequence of postsynaptic dopamine receptor stimulation and decreased dopamine turnover in central nigrostriatal pathways.

553. A 37-year-old woman telephones to alert her psychiatrist that she has developed a severe pain in her right eye that has persisted for about 5 hours. She has no history of migraine headaches. The psychiatrist is treating her with 150 mg imipramine for major depression. She denies any recent injury or infection in this eye. She wears corrective lenses for nearsightedness. Of the following, which would be the most appropriate step? *names 2 glaucoma (anticholinergic)*

(A) Advise her to take an anti-inflammatory analgesic.

(B) Advise her to rest and call again in 8 hours if the pain has not subsided.

(C) Consult immediately with her ophthalmologist.

(D) Plan to evaluate her eye at her next psychiatric appointment in 2 weeks.

(E) Decrease imipramine to 125 mg/day.

554. For which of the following would a magnetic resonance imaging (MRI) scan provide the LEAST useful data?

(A) delirium or dementia of unknown cause

(B) substance abuse disorder with signs of cognitive deterioration

(C) marked personality change after age 50

(D) psychotic symptoms in a person with chronic schizophrenia

(E) anorexia nervosa with weight loss   ?

555. The mistreatment and abuse of children can be described by which of the following statements?

(A) As a result of more vigilant public health measures, the incidence of child abuse has declined.

[handwritten: many chld not reported]

(B) As a result of more vigilant public health measures, the death rate from child abuse has declined.

(C) As a result of aggressive public awareness campaigns, the reporting rate of child abuse is now about equal to the incidence rate.

(D) All states now require reporting of child fatalities that are due to maltreatment. *[handwritten: inconsistent]*

(E) Official estimates put the number of maltreated children at a million or more each year.

556. An otherwise healthy and unmedicated patient who meets DSM-IV criteria for major depression is administered the dexamethasone suppression test (DST). The patient receives 1.0 mg dexamethasone at 11:00 PM; blood is drawn at 8:00 AM, and at 11:00 PM the following day for serum cortisol determinations. Which of the following statements may be consistent with this clinical situation?

(A) Serum cortisol values of less than 5 mg/100 mL at 4:00 PM or 11:00 PM confirm the diagnosis of a depressive episode.

(B) Serum cortisol values of greater than 5 mg/100 mL at 4:00 PM and 11:00 PM eliminate the diagnosis of a depressive episode.

[handwritten: 40% of depressed pts show no suppression]
[handwritten: > 5mg/100mL — consider depression]
[handwritten: dexamethasone ⊖→ CRF release ⊖→ ↓ACTH → ↓cortisol (hypothal) (pit) (adrenal)]
[handwritten: seen c̄ depression + bipolar]

(C) Depressed patients who fail to suppress serum cortisol after dexamethasone tend to show a better response to somatic treatments such as tricyclics, monoamine oxidase (MAO) inhibitors, and ECT. *[handwritten: if abnl axes, more likely to respond to RX x ECT]*

(D) Normalization of response to dexamethasone during somatic treatment implies a predisposition for early relapse. *[handwritten: less risk]*

(E) The DST is nearly 95% accurate in identifying depressive states. *[handwritten: F]*

557. In which of the following conditions are the traditional antipsychotics contraindicated? *[handwritten: anticholinergic properties]*

(A) anticholinergic drug-induced toxic delirium

(B) agitation due to dementia

(C) acute manic states associated with bipolar disorder

(D) psychosis caused by being in unfamiliar and frightening surroundings, such as an intensive care unit

(E) psychotic depression

558. The endocrine abnormalities associated with anorexia nervosa can be described by which of the following statements?

(A) Primary pituitary gland dysfunction is the causative mechanism.

(B) Amenorrhea usually develops only after weight loss has become significant. *[handwritten: at begin weight lx]*

(C) Unlike affected women, affected men show little if any endocrine imbalances.

(D) Despite proper treatment for anorexia, affected endocrine systems rarely are restored to normal function. *[handwritten: F not starving]*

(E) none of the above

[handwritten: endocrine disturbances caused by starvation state ↓ GnRH/LH/FSH]

Question 559

A 27-year-old law school student is brought to the student health service by several of her housemates. They report that, during the past 2 weeks, the young woman has become increasingly agitated and intermittently euphoric, has neglected her studies and other usual activities, and has seemed to have difficulty paying attention to them when they interact with her. Her friends also reveal that the woman fears that neighbors are trying to bewitch her and believes that her friends want her "put away" because they are jealous of the job offer she expects to receive from a prestigious law firm. The on-call physician at the health service asks for a psychiatric consultation. The psychiatrist notes a mild left facial asymmetry, diminished response to pinprick and touch over the left leg, very brisk deep-tendon reflexes in both lower extremities, impaired coordination in the left hand, and difficulties in tandem walking. The young woman refuses voluntary hospitalization.

559. The legal aspects of hospitalizing this patient against her will are correctly described by which of the following statements?

(A) Either physician can legally hospitalize this patient. *Any physician can commit*

(B) Consultation with a psychiatrist is required before involuntary hospitalization for a mental illness.

(C) A close relative must concur with the decision.

(D) An emergency court hearing is required.

(E) There is little clinical justification for involuntary hospitalization in this case.

Questions 560 Through 562

A 45-year-old woman seen by her medical internist, has been experiencing fears that she may have a serious illness. She complains that after eating she experiences "a lot of gas" and abdominal pain, followed by diarrhea on occasion. Her heart at times seems to be beating rapidly, and she feels faint at times, has chest "discomfort," and wonders if she is having a heart attack. Multiple tests have identified only a mild irritable bowel syndrome. The woman's fears are not allayed by this. She makes repeated calls to be seen by her doctors as well as seeking consultation from other specialists. She insists that "there's something there" and believes the doctors are not taking her seriously.

560. Of the following, which is the most likely diagnosis?

(A) factitious disorder

(B) major depression

(C) reaction psychosis

(D) hypochondriasis *misperceptions + distortions of somatic s/s → preoccupy a illness*

(E) pain disorder

561. Which of the following is the most effective long-term way of managing this patient?

(A) transfer care to psychiatrist

(B) prescribe alprazolam

(C) establish regular follow-up visits with regularly scheduled physical exams *therapeutic alliance*

(D) refer for supportive group psychotherapy

(E) refer to a pain management clinic

562. Which of the following most appropriately describes this woman's disorder?

(A) more frequently seen in women than in men   *men = women*

(B) 20 to 25% prevalence rate in a general medical practice *4-9%*

(C) course of disorder usually of short duration (2 to 3 months) *chronic*

(D) associated with elevated erythrocyte sedimentation rate (ESR)

(E) absence of secondary gain a favorable prognostic indicator

563. During the course of psychotherapy with a woman who has a severe phobia of cars, it is discovered that her first sexual experience, which was a humiliating one for her, took place in an automobile. The defense mechanism illustrated by this phobia is called

(A) acting out F

(B) reaction formation

(C) displacement *emotion is severed from its original connections → attached to substitute*

(D) sublimation

(E) repression

564. Which of the following is true about somatization disorder?

(A) Having a biological parent with antisocial personality disorder has no correlation with risk of having a somatization disorder. *antisocial, substance abuse, somchzation*

(B) Symptoms typically begin before age 30. T

(C) Symptoms involve a single organ system. F *multi organ system*

(D) It generally remits within 6 months of onset. F *Sxs fluctuate, rarely remit*

(E) Prevalence rates for women range from 10 to 15%. F *0.2-2%.*

Question 565

A 65-year-old man is referred for a psychiatric evaluation by his primary care doctor. The doctor has noted that his patient seems less concerned about his personal hygiene; his clothes are mismatched, and he is no longer timely getting to his doctor's appointments. Additionally, the patient seems depressed, cries, and "no longer enjoys a good joke."

565. Which of the following would be the most therapeutic opening question in interviewing this man?

(A) "Tell me about your depression."

(B) "Why are you crying?"

(C) "Tell me what's been happening that brings you here." *open ended ?*

(D) "Your doctor tells me you don't match your clothes anymore—why not?"

(E) "Your doctor says you're depressed. How about an antidepressant to help you?"

✓**566.** Conversion disorder (also known as hysterical neurosis, conversion type) is distinguished by symptoms that

(A) suggest a physical disorder

(B) are expressive of a conscious psychological conflict *intrapsychic conflict*

(C) stem from the intrapsychic defense of sublimation

(D) are under voluntary control F

(E) are synonymous with symptoms of malingering F

✓**567.** The use of the thyrotropin-releasing hormone (TRH) test in the diagnosis of mood disorders can be described by which of the following statements?

(A) The test result is positive in almost three *¼* fourths of depressed persons.

(B) Reactive depression produces a positive test result. *major mood d/o.*

(C) Depression associated with bipolar disorder can produce a positive test result.

(D) The test is considered positive if it produces an abnormally brisk thyroid-stimulating hormone (TSH) response.

(E) Unlike the DST, the TRH test is unaffected by such exogenous factors as alcoholism or use of prescription drugs.

TRF → ↑TSH but ↓ ¼ depression

Questions 568 Through 570

A 25-year-old man presents in the emergency department for a 2-week problem of worsening urinary hesitancy. He has had problems getting his urine stream started and has noted a decrease in the force of the stream. Now it seems to just "dribble out." He denies any pain or burning, any medical problems, and any exposure to sexually transmitted diseases. For approximately 1 month, he has been taking thioridazine, 200 mg b.i.d., and benztropine, 2 mg q.i.d., and "sometimes (one or two benztropine)" PRN.

568. Given the above information, the most likely cause of this man's problem is

(A) anticholinergic side effects to the thioridazine and benztropine *(anti parkinson)*

(B) urethral stricture F *r/o*

(C) breakthrough of a psychotic delusion that he cannot urinate F *look for psychotics/s*

(D) injury from a perverse sexual practice he is not admitting to F *r/o*

(E) infection of the urethra F *r/o*

569. After further evaluation, it is determined that there is no significant distension of the bladder at this time; there are no signs of trauma, infection, or other lesion on external inspection of the genitals, and no enlargement of the prostate. At this point, you would

(A) give benztropine, 2 mg IM, for the side effect of thioridazine *anhchol*

(B) increase thioridazine to 200 mg t.i.d. *anhchol*

(C) administer bethanechol *stimulates parasyp*

(D) call in the urologist

(E) insert urinary catheter *if distended*

✓ 570. A safer choice of medication for this man would be   *↓ antichol SE : (A)*

(A) amitriptyline *TCA*

(B) haloperidol *H*

(C) chlorpromazine *N*

(D) loxapine *M*

(E) none of the above

571. Current data regarding suicide indicate that *♂ peak in teen + >45*

(A) the rate of completed suicide in men diminishes after the age of 45 years *F*

(B) men *commit* attempt suicide more often than women *F*

(C) women *attem* complete suicide more often than men *F*

(D) a past suicide attempt is a *good* poor indicator of current risk *F*

(E) discussing suicide with potential attempters may serve as a deterrent

572. A 78-year-old woman is seen by a psychiatrist for depression. She is fairly cooperative in responding to questions. She admits to feeling blue; she "catnaps" throughout the day and is up at night, and her appetite is very poor. She thinks of death frequently, but denies feeling suicidal. There is no past psychiatric history. On the MMSE, she obtains a score of 14. Her depressive symptoms have been present for "several days." Of the fol-

25-30 ∅ cognitive
20-25 mild cognitive
<20 @cognitive impair

lowing, which is highly suggested by the findings?

(A) impaired cognitive functioning

(B) psychosis not otherwise specified *F*

(C) bipolar disorder—manic *F*

(D) dysthymia *F*

(E) changes secondary to normal aging

573. Which of the following would LEAST benefit from treatment with ECT? *acute, life threatening sihd*

(A) severe depression in an elderly person *T*

(B) failure to respond to regular antidepressants *T*

(C) mania *F*

(D) chronic schizophrenia

(E) very severe, acute symptoms of depression *T*

✓ 574. Treatment with lithium has been associated with which of the following hormonal changes?

(A) ↑ decreased production of TSH

(B) ↓ increased release of thyroxine

(C) ↑ decreased TSH response to TRH

(D) ↑ decreased levels of parathyroid hormone

(E) increase in TSH production

Questions 575 and 576

A 40-year-old woman with no previous psychiatric history seeks help from her internist for a sleep problem. Initially, she is able to fall asleep but then sleeps fitfully, and finally around 4:00 AM decides to stay up. She averages approximately 3 to 4 hours of sleep per night, and this has been occurring for the last 3 weeks. She finds herself quite tired and "blue" during the day but is unable to nap. Mornings are "the worst" for her, but she feels better toward the end of the day. There has been a 15-pound weight loss because "I'm just not hungry." She denies any physical problems except for constipation. As a grade-school teacher, she feels extremely stressed but sees no way out and no way to improve the situation. At times, suicide seems like a possible option, and she admits to spending long hours brooding on how to do it. A physical exam is unremarkable.

575. At this point, the most likely diagnosis is

(A) borderline personality disorder F
(B) major depression *meets criteria*
(C) dysthymia F
(D) Alzheimer's disease F
(E) generalized anxiety disorder F

576. Of the following, the most appropriate treatment choice is

(A) olanzapine *atypical*
(B) paroxetine *SSRI   1st line agent*
(C) alprazolam *benzo*
(D) tranylcypromine *MAOI*
(E) ECT

577. Of the following, which is considered a negative symptom of schizophrenia?

(A) anhedonia
(B) loose associations F
(C) delusions of thought insertion F
(D) incoherence F
(E) stereotypic gestures F   *(+)ve sxs*

578. Which of the following medications is appropriate for treating children with attention deficit disorder?

(A) lithium F *mood*
(B) desipramine *TCA if not responsive to stimulant*
(C) alprazolam F *benzo*
(D) propranolol F *β block*
(E) perphenazine *antipsyc*

579. A middle-aged man with depression requests help for his symptoms of low self-esteem and feelings that "life is bad no matter what you do." He prefers to use no medication and expresses the desire to not be in therapy "for years." There is no previous psychiatric treatment. Of the following therapies, which would be the most helpful?

(A) psychoanalysis F   *↑ time*
(B) behavioral therapy
(C) cognitive psychotherapy *reds thus*
(D) supportive psychotherapy *↑ meds*
(E) group psychotherapy *after indiv. tx*

580. A 35-year-old woman is seen by her primary care physician for a physical exam. She tells him she has a twin brother who has bipolar disorder and has been worried that she will develop it. Of the following, which would be the most helpful for her to hear?

(A) "You're past the age when bipolar disorder develops, so don't worry about it."
(B) "There is no clear evidence that a bipolar disorder is genetically determined." F
(C) "The concordance rate for bipolar disorder for dizygotic twins is 19%."
(D) "The concordance rate for bipolar disorder for dizygotic twins is 79%." *monozygoti*
(E) "Prophylactic treatment with lithium is advisable." F

581. Of the following, which is considered a cortical dementia?

(A) Huntington's disease *-basal gang (motor)*
(B) Pick's disease *• aphasia apraxia, agnosia*
(C) Parkinson's disease
(D) occult hydrocephalus (normal pressure) *ventricle*
(E) none of the above

DIRECTIONS (Questions 582 through 615): Each set of matching questions in this section consists of a list of 4 to 26 lettered options followed by several numbered items. For each item, select the ONE best lettered option that is most closely associated with it. Each lettered heading may be selected once, more than once, or not at all.

Questions 582 Through 586

For each clinical description that follows, select the diagnosis with which it is most likely to be associated.

(A) childhood depression

(B) childhood schizophrenia

(C) conduct disorder

(D) attention deficit hyperactivity disorder

(E) infantile autism

582. A 9-year-old boy has had persisting difficulties in language and interpersonal relationships since the age of 2 years, and, although he can barely read, he is able to perform arithmetic calculations at the fifth-grade level.

583. An 11-year-old girl has become uncharacteristically and markedly withdrawn in the past 8 months, staying in her room so that she can "talk to the ghosts in the attic."

584. An 11-year-old girl has become markedly withdrawn in the past 8 months and has complained of persisting abdominal pain and constipation, for which no organic cause has been found.

585. A 5-year-old boy is reported by his kindergarten teacher to be distractible, impulsive, in need of continual supervision, but not hyperactive.

586. A 3-year-old boy spends hours rocking in a chair or spinning the blades of a toy windmill; his parents say he never cries when he falls.

Questions 587 Through 591

In the case studies below, identify the developmental stage that best describes the situation.

(A) anal

(B) autonomy

(C) basic trust

(D) formal operations

(E) generativity

(F) intimacy

(G) integrity

(H) latency

(I) oral

(J) preoperational

587. A 50-year-old professor makes attempts to be more conscious and mindful in her mentoring of students.

588. In looking back over his life, a 75-year-old man realizes that he made some mistakes but accepts these as part of what makes him who he is.

589. A 9-year-old boy imagines himself an Olympic skier, a fireman, and a doctor. He enjoys building huge space stations with building blocks.

590. A 24-year-old woman struggles with whether she should get married or go on with her doctorate degree.

591. A 16-year-old enjoys learning how to use deductive reasoning in a special science project.

Questions 592 Through 595

For each patient's psychiatric symptoms, select the most appropriate medication. Presume no medical problems other than those mentioned.

(A) amitriptyline

(B) clozapine

(C) divalproex

(D) fluoxetine

(E) hypericum perforatum

(F) olanzapine

(G) lorazepam

(H) propranolol

(I) temazepam

(J) thiothixene

592. A 23-year-old university student has lost interest in his master's degree program. His two friends who bring him to the psychiatrist say he has been isolating himself in his room and has covered all electrical appliances and outlets with duct tape claiming that "electromagnetic waves are disturbing the microchip in my brain." He acknowledges that he once took a medication for the same problem with the "microchip" but then he became unbearably restless, could not sit still, and felt that he was "crawling" inside. *psychosis→* **F**

F

593. A 36-year-old man complains that he cannot sleep at night. "I just can't settle down; my mind is constantly working." He describes being able to complete a lot of work, being highly energized, and having a lot of fun. He is afraid that without sleep he will "crash." Once before, he took a medication for depression. *mania → C*

C

594. A 65-year-old woman with a history of cardiac problems complains that she has lost her appetite, she cries frequently, and has lost interest in her grandchildren, her gardening, and her craft making. She thinks maybe it is time to die. **D**

D

595. A 50-year-old woman with a long history of taking trifluoperazine is noted to have repetitive chewing motions, and periodically protrudes her tongue. Her arms and shoulders seem to jerk fairly often, and there is a peculiar twisting movement in her right hand. She tried several of the "newer" medications that are not supposed to cause the movement problems, but then her auditory hallucinations started again. **B**

B

Questions 596 Through 600

Match the antidepressants below with the effect described.

(A) amitriptyline *TCA ↑sedat SHT, NE*

(B) nefazodone *inhibit 5HT + 5HT₂ blockade (0)trazod*

(C) paroxetine *SSRI inhibit*

(D) phenelzine *MAOi*

(E) venlafaxine *atypical ↓sedat 5HT, NE*

596. Primarily a selective serotonin reuptake inhibitor (SSRI) *c*

C

597. Both SSRI and serotonin type 2 (5-HT₂) receptor blockade *E*

B ✓

598. Strong sedation, strong serotonin effect, and norepinephrine effect *B*

A ✓

599. Little sedation, strong serotonin and norepinephrine effect *A*

E ✓

600. MAO inhibitory effect *D*

D

Questions 601 Through 605

For each clinical description, select the most appropriate pharmacotherapeutic agent.

(A) clozapine

(B) valproic acid

(C) haloperidol

(D) risperidone

(E) paroxetine

601. A 30-year-old man with a bipolar I disorder nonresponsive to lithium *B*

B

602. A 25-year-old woman with major depression *E*

E

603. A 20-year-old woman with a first psychotic episode *C*

C

604. A 26-year-old man with schizophrenia and tardive dyskinesia *A*

A

605. A 32-year-old woman with primarily negative symptoms of schizophrenia *D*

D

Questions 606 Through 610

Identify the following personality disorders with the symptoms listed below.

(A) antisocial
(B) avoidant
(C) borderline
(D) dependent
(E) histrionic
(F) narcissistic
(G) obsessive–compulsive
(H) paranoid
(I) schizoid
(J) schizotypal

606. Is quick to perceive a slight as an attack or assault on one's character F

607. Seems to not care what others think or feel; is aloof I

608. Preoccupied with feelings of superstitiousness; has a sixth sense; seems odd J

609. Chronic feelings of emptiness, fear of abandonment; unstable self-image C

610. Unwilling to take personal risks; perceives self as inept, unappealing, inferior B

Questions 611 Through 615

Identify the following defense mechanisms with the descriptions below.

(A) acting out
(B) altruism
(C) displacement
(D) intellectualization
(E) passive–aggressive behavior
(F) projection
(G) rationalization
(H) reaction formation
(I) sublimation
(J) suppression

611. Becoming angry with one's spouse at a party and deciding to wait until a more appropriate time to express it J

612. Becoming angry with one's spouse at a party and calling him or her a name in front of everybody A

613. A woman, wanting to have children but cannot, works as a nurse on a pediatric ward I

614. Afraid of her rage and anger, a woman presents as unusually meek and mild E

615. To accuse another of being angry and jealous when the feelings belong to oneself F

Answers and Explanations

503. **(C)** The various major extrapyramidal side effects (dystonia, akathisia, parkinsonism, and tardive dyskinesia) occur in a rather predictable time sequence if they are going to occur. To precisely and reliably predict their occurrence is not possible given the individual sensitivities to the antipsychotic medications as well as the potential of the antipsychotic to effect D_2 receptor blockade. Below are listed approximate order and time of appearance of these side effects:

Dystonias (muscle spasms)	Akathisia (restlessness) Parkinsonism (masked facies, "rabbit syndrome")	Tardive Dyskinesia (writhing movements)
Days	Weeks/Months	Years

(Kaplan and Sadock, pp 956–957)

504. **(E)** The question basically asks the question "which of the following drugs has the weakest potential to produce D_2 receptor blockage?" In order of decreasing strength, these line up as follows: haloperidol > thiothixene > chlorpromazine > thioridazine > clozapine. *(Kaplan and Sadock, p 1029)*

505. **(B)** Although one would be careful to rule out other causes of this man's symptoms, the most likely precipitant is the recent death of his wife. He has moved beyond the first stage of grief, that of shock and denial, to a period of time when there is intense preoccupation with the deceased. During this pe-

riod, there are not only the thoughts and dreams of the dead but also fatigue, sadness, some withdrawal, and loss of interest in previously enjoyed activities. There are variable degrees of disorganization. This is what is seen in this man as evidenced by his disheveled appearance. The score of 26 on the MMSE suggests no cognitive impairment as one would expect if there were Alzheimer's disease. It is possible that at some point if the grief reaction becomes pathological, he could develop a psychotic reaction or major depression. With adequate support, a psychologically healthy person would be expected to achieve resolution of the grief process. *(Stoudemire, Clinical Psychiatry, pp 595–596)*

506. **(A)** The most appropriate initial therapy for this person would be psychotherapy in which he is allowed time to share his feelings and reactions to what has happened. Care should be given to avoid anxiolytics since these may actually delay resolution of the grief process. At times, they are helpful to contain extreme, paralyzing distress. Thioridazine (an antipsychotic), venlafaxine (an antidepressant), and ECT should be avoided, unless of course the severity of the grief response deepens and indications for use of the medications is apparent. *(Stoudemire, Clinical Psychiatry, pp 596–598)*

507. **(D)** As a group, the parasomnias are behavioral or physiological events that occur during sleep, and do not involve falling asleep or staying asleep as seen in the dyssomnias. Specific parasomnias occur during specific sleep stages and involve the activation of physiological systems (autonomic nervous

system, motor system, etc) during inappropriate times. In sleep paralysis, a person seems to be "caught" between being seemingly awake mentally and yet "asleep" physically, unable to move. Other examples of parasomnias include sleep bruxism (a stage 2 phenomenon), sleep terror, and sleepwalking. Narcolepsy, hypersomnia, and circadian rhythm sleeping disorder are associated with falling or staying asleep. (*APA, pp 579–592*)

508–512. (508-D, 509-B, 510-H, 511-E, 512-G) Complaints involving both psychological and medical conditions are difficult to diagnose and treat. At times, medically identifiable causes are present, but the psychological factors contributing to the discomfort complicate the diagnosis and treatment, and lead to frustration in both physician and patient. At other times, no identifiable cause for pain or other physical symptoms can be found; nevertheless, the patient still has the symptoms. Questions arise: Is the patient lying? Is there some deep psychological problem? Could there be a medical disorder in the early stages of development that gives rise to physical symptoms but no clear physical signs to make the diagnosis? One group of psychiatric disorders addresses some of these issues—the somatoform disorders. The table below aids in identifying these:

Panic disorder is a kind of anxiety disorder. Discreet periods of extreme sympathetic nervous system symptoms occur, including tachycardia, sweating, shortness of breath, and others, during which time a person experiences extreme fear. Malingering is the deliberate manufacture of false or exaggerated symptoms to avoid an unpleasant situation such as jail time or military duty. In a factitious disorder, there is the deliberate production of signs and symptoms of illness in order to assume the sick role. (*APA, pp 445–474, 683*)

513. (B) For those older persons who were interested and active in sex in their younger years, there will be continued interest and activity in their older years. Availability of a partner and good health are important factors. (*Kaplan and Sadock, pp 63–64; Wedding, p 82*)

514. (E) As they age, both men and women experience changes in the various phases of the sexual response cycle. Some of these changes are results of decreases in sex hormones. In spite of these changes, persons who have been sexually active and who have an available partner will generally remain sexually active into old age. (*Stoudemire, Human Behavior, pp 118–119; Wedding, pp 89, 117; Kaplan and Sadock, pp 63–64*)

515. (C) Severe anticholinergic reactions, such as delirium, should be treated with intramuscular or intravenous injection of physostigmine, 1 to 2 mg IV (1 mg every 2 minutes) or IM every 30 to 60 minutes. The first dose should be repeated in 15 to 20 minutes if no improvement is seen. Such peripheral anticholinergic side effects as urinary retention can be treated with bethanechol. Dantrolene and bromocriptine, not effective in the treat-

SOMATOFORM DISORDERS

Disorder	Symptoms	Psychological Factors	Duration
Somatization	Multiple physical complaints involving multiple organ systems	Yes	Begins before age 30; occur over a period of years
Conversion	Motor or sensory functions involved	Yes	Usually begins after age 10, before age 35; short duration (weeks)
Pain	Pain in one or more anatomic sites, severe enough to warrant clinical attention	Yes	Appears at any age; variable duration
Hypochondriasis	Misinterpretation of a bodily sign or symptom leading to fear of dying	Yes	Most usually appear in early adulthood; cause is usually chronic

ment of anticholinergic reactions, are two drugs that have been tried in the treatment of neuroleptic malignant syndrome, a rare but extremely dangerous neuroleptic-induced disorder. Haldol, having anticholinergic effects, is contraindicated. (*Kaplan and Sadock, pp 878, 946, 981*)

516. **(B)** Dementia is a loss of intellectual functioning. Other neurologic operations are also affected in dementia, such as language, skilled movements, and perception. However, isolated neurologic defects like aphasia are not classified as dementias. Likewise, sensory defects or hemiplegia of body parts would not be included. Nonetheless, many of these neurologic abnormalities may precede or follow the onset of intellectual dysfunction, thereby taxing the diagnostic acumen of the clinician. Dementia does not necessarily mean a gradual loss of these functions, for it may be of sudden onset (eg, following a stroke). It is a syndrome resulting from a variety of diseases affecting the brain and, in many cases, is remediable with proper diagnosis and treatment. Irrespective of the cause of the disorder, the symptoms are a function of the locus and not the type of disease. Therefore, atrophy affecting the frontal lobes or a tumor involving the same areas may present in a similar fashion. Additionally, there are typical and often prominent behavioral changes that may become evident much earlier in the evolution of the disorder than do problems with orientation, cognition, or memory. (*Stoudemire,* Clinical Psychiatry, *pp 114–118; Kaplan and Sadock, pp 332–338*)

517. **(E)** Homosexuality is considered an "alternative lifestyle" rather than a disorder. In 1973, the American Psychiatric Association eliminated homosexuality as a diagnostic category and removed it from the DSM-IV. (*Kaplan and Sadock, p 682*)

518. **(E)** DSM-IV describes two disorders of sexual desire: hypoactive sexual desire and sexual aversion. The sexual aversion disorder is characterized by the aversion to and active avoidance of genital sexual contact with a sexual partner, which causes marked distress

or interpersonal difficulty, and the dysfunction is not later accounted for by some other axis I disorder. Both dyspareunia and vaginismus are classified as sexual pain disorders. Pedophilia is classified with the paraphilias. Premature ejaculation is considered an orgasmic disorder. (*APA, pp 496–532, 838*)

519. **(C)** Delusions are false ideas that cannot be corrected by reasoning and that are not based on reality. Psychotic patients often experience ideas or delusions of reference and misinterpret incidents or events in the outside world as having direct personal reference to themselves. Delusions may occur in a variety of psychiatric disorders, including schizophrenia, paranoia, mania, depression, and organic brain syndromes. The bizarre nature of the delusion described in the question is more characteristic of schizophrenia than of other types of psychiatric ailments. Illusions are sensory misperceptions that occasionally may be experienced even by normal individuals. Psychotic persons may report hallucinations, which are sensory experiences that cannot be substantiated by normal observers. Loosened associations and neologisms are patterns of speech often noted in psychotic individuals. (*Kaplan and Sadock, pp 282–283*)

520. **(C)** Dissociative amnesia is loss of ability to recall information occurring within a certain time period, usually related to a severely stressful event as occurred with this woman. In depersonalization disorder, a person feels detached from his or her own body or mental processes and feels as if he or she is standing apart and acting as observer. In post-traumatic stress disorder, there is a persistent re-experiencing of the traumatic event in a variety of ways, persistent avoidance of stimuli associated with that event, and persistent symptoms of arousal. It is possible for the arousal to be a part of this larger symptom complex. In dissociative fugue, the person forgets his identity, travels, and may even establish a new identity. Symptoms of major depression involve mood, inability to experience pleasure, appetite and sleep disturbance, fatigue, and other disturbances of affect and mood. (*Kaplan and Sadock, pp*

622–664; Stoudemire, Clinical Psychiatry, *pp 202, 372–375, 382)*

521. (B) Individual therapy, which would include exploring the events recalled surrounding the incident, reactions to the child's death, feelings about motherhood, as well as other issues, is considered the most effective treatment for dissociative amnesia. If other symptoms indicate another disorder (eg, major depression, psychosis), then treatment would include appropriate drugs or ECT. In some cases, there is a role for hypnosis on sodium amobarbital interview to help recall. Benzodiazepines may be helpful to reduce anxiety. Integration through psychotherapy of the events of the traumatic episode into one's conscious state is important for recovery. *(Kaplan and Sadock pp 662–664; Stoudemire,* Clinical Psychiatry, *pp 202, 372–375, 382)*

522. (C) Freud understood the phenomenon of thought as a synthesis of two processes. Primary process thought is the expression of primitive drives, including aggression, sexual energy, and fantasy. These and other drives (or instincts) collectively constitute the id. Their direct expression is unacceptable in the outside world, which demands a large degree of conformity, restraint, and rationality. Hence, productions of the id are relegated to the unconscious, although they may become conscious in disguised ways, such as in dreams or as "freudian slips" of the tongue. Secondary process thinking is the process by which our personal needs and desires are communicated to the outside world (and to ourselves) in a more socially acceptable form. Their organization is based on more or less rational processes and on an acceptance of the demands of reality. *(Wedding, p 257)*

523. (C) Schizophrenia usually develops in young adulthood. The mean age of the first psychotic break is in the early twenties for men. Of men with schizophrenia, 9 to 10% have developed the disorder by age 30. Women tend to develop the disorder at an older age. Developing the disorder at age 40 is unusual. *(Andreason and Black, pp 187–190, 205–215, 249–254; Tomb, pp 214–216)*

524. (A) The preoccupation with a rather well-developed delusional system and later age at onset suggest paranoid schizophrenia. A case can be made for undifferentiated schizophrenia because of the apparent disorganization in personal habits and the flattening of affect. There is no history of alcohol abuse and dependence to support the diagnosis. The long period of symptoms, bizarreness of paranoid delusion, and decline in functioning are more characteristic of schizophrenia. The time course of a major depression is much shorter. Usually, there is not the profound decline in functioning. No symptoms of memory impairment or loss of cognitive functioning has occurred that would suggest Alzheimer's or Huntington's dementias. Additionally, in Huntington's dementia, one would expect a prominent movement disorder seen in subcortical dementia. *(Andreason and Black, pp 187–190, 205–215, 249–254; Tomb, pp 214–216)*

525. (B) The treatment of choice for persons with a schizophrenic disorder is an antipsychotic drug. The choice of which of the many antipsychotics to use is based in such factors as past history of response, side effect profile of a particular drug, and the patient's response to a drug. Listed here are two antipsychotics, haloperidol and clozapine. At this time, clozapine is generally reserved for persons who have not responded to more traditional antipsychotics, those who have extreme extrapyramidal reactions, and particularly those who have developed tardive dyskinesia. Its cost and the cost of monitoring for agranulocytosis, a potentially deadly side effect, limit the use of clozapine. Haldol, a relatively low-cost neuroleptic, is considered a first-line drug in the treatment of schizophrenia. *(Andreason and Black, pp 187–190, 205–215, 249–254; Tomb, pp 214–216)*

526. (E) Anorexia nervosa is an eating disorder that predominantly affects women in their teens and in early adulthood. It is defined as refusal to maintain a minimal normal weight, at least 85% of that weight considered normal for that person's age and height, and a morbid preoccupation with feeling obese. Common strategies to lose weight include avoidance of all fats and carbohydrates, self-induced vomiting, obsessive physical activity, and abuse of laxatives or diuretics or both. Despite apparent aversion to gaining weight, anorectics frequently take very special care in preparation and consumption of food and may delight in preparing gourmet feasts for others. Menstrual irregularity and amenorrhea are also commonly reported but are not essential factors in making the diagnosis. It is not yet clear whether such menstrual problems are simply secondary to starvation or whether they reflect a more pervasive endocrine dysfunction. Perhaps the most striking clinical feature of this bizarre disorder is the misperception of body image. Regardless of the method of confrontation, including use of mirrors or photographs, sufferers see themselves as overweight. The patient often refuses to agree that there is any problem whatsoever. Numerous factors, including developmental, family, endocrine, and gastrointestinal disturbances have been implicated in anorexia nervosa, but the etiology has yet to be clearly established. Most commonly, the course consists of a single episode followed by remission. Some patients may suffer a series of relapses and remissions. Mortality rates have been estimated to be as high as 20%. *(Kaplan and Sadock, pp 721–725)*

527. **(A)** Alzheimer's is the most common form of dementia. Of persons with dementia, 50 to 60% will have Alzheimer's. Vascular dementia is the second most common, accounting for about 15 to 30% of dementias. *(Kaplan and Sadock, pp 328–329)*

528. **(D)** Pathological changes will be seen in the frontotemporal cortex in patients with Pick's disease. Alzheimer's, also a cortical dementia like Pick's, has pathological changes in the parietotemporal areas. *(Kaplan and Sadock, p 331)*

529. **(A)** HIV can enter the central nervous system (CNS) soon after initial infection and can lead to impaired cognitive functioning discernible on neuropsychiatric tests well before obvious symptoms are present. By the

time AIDS has developed, most affected persons will demonstrate neuropsychiatric disturbance on testing and CNS involvement on autopsy. The most common organic mental disorders associated with AIDS are dementia and delirium. *(Andreason and Black, pp 533–535; Kaplan and Sadock, pp 379–381)*

530. **(C)** This woman describes discrete, recurrent panic attacks in which there is fear and discomfort. Several symptoms are named: racing, pounding heart; chest pain; flushing; lightheadedness; shortness of breath; and fear of dying. Medical evaluation indicates no underlying physical causes to these symptoms. The possibility of autonomic changes secondary to menopause is relatively remote considering that she is 40 years of age. Menopause most commonly occurs after age 48. Myocardial infarction also seems remote— the pain is not characteristic angina pain; being premenopausal, there is low risk for an MI, and the recent medical evaluation revealed no cardiac abnormalities. Hypochondriasis is a consideration here but is unlikely because of the discrete periods of panic symptoms, suggesting more the diagnosis of panic disorder. Another consideration, post-traumatic stress disorder, requires as the first criteria the occurrence of a trauma outside the limits of what is normal human experience. Though sad and painful, the two stresses listed here (stroke and breast cancer) are not outside the realm of what is normal. *(APA, pp 394–395, 427, 462)*

531. **(B)** Paroxetine would most likely be the best choice. It is an SSRI antidepressant, which is not only effective in treating depression, but also effective in the management of panic disorder. Alprazolam, a benzodiazepine, is especially effective for the treatment of panic disorder. A very serious consideration here is the implication of this woman's history of substance abuse. The risk of exposing this woman to alprazolam, and the problems of abuse and dependence that very likely will occur, may eliminate this as a drug of choice in this case. Propranolol may be of some help in treating this woman. Risperidone and thioridazine are both antipsychotics and not in-

dicated for panic disorders. *(Kaplan and Sadock, p 1301)*

532. **(C)** Lorazepam, because of its relatively short half-life, intermediate rate of onset and absence of active metabolites, would be an appropriate medication for this elderly woman. Diazepam and clorazepate both have long half-lives as well as active metabolites. These properties easily lead to more severe side effects in older patients, such as prolonged sedation, respiratory depression, confusional states, and disorientation. Temazepam, though it has no active metabolites and a relatively short half-life, is very sedating and is used to promote sleep. Buspirone, a nonbenzodiazepine, is an effective antianxiety agent, but it may take up to a week to exert its effect. The woman in this case needs medication that will help her quickly. *(Andreason and Black, p 685; Kaplan and Sadock, p 1301)*

533. **(C)** Patients with severe psychotic depression will often have delusions that are mood congruent and reflect the depth of their despair and self-abhorrence. Patients with mania are more likely to have delusions that are mood congruent that would reflect their grandiosity, paranoid feelings, inflated self-esteem, and feelings of having special powers. *(Andreason and Black, pp 256–257)*

534. **(B)** The legal concept of "right to treatment" has been developed in order to clarify societal responsibility to provide care and active intervention for hospitalized individuals (particularly from involuntary commitment) rather than simply provide custodial services or removal from the community at large for those persons thought to be dangerous. The 1971 Alabama case of *Wyatt* v *Stickney* was a class-action suit against several state psychiatric hospitals on behalf of a group of patients who had been civilly committed to those institutions. The court ruled that such persons have the constitutional right to receive individual treatment sufficient to give each a reasonable opportunity for cure or improvement of the mental condition necessitating the involuntary confinement. *(Kaplan and Sadock, p 1310)*

535. **(E)** Maladaptive, immature, and rigid patterns of defense begin early in the lives of persons with personality disorders. Before age 18 is considered the period of development for these patterns. In general, persons with these disorders have a poor sense of identity and poor sense of self. Immature defenses, including acting out, splitting, passive–aggressive behavior, projection, and so forth, lead to serious interpersonal problems. Such persons experience their symptoms as egosyntonic for the most part except under some circumstances (eg, rejection from others, incarceration, hospitalization during which ego-dystonic feelings may result). Generally, these people do not lapse into psychotic behaviors, with the exception of the borderline disorder in which brief periods occasionally occur. *(Kaplan and Sadock, pp 220, 775–776)*

536. **(A)** School phobia accounts for 8% of the referrals to child guidance clinics. Children entering kindergarten, first grade, and high school are most prone to experience phobic symptoms. The phobia may coexist with a separation anxiety disorder or a depressive disorder, as well as other phobic disorders. Clonazepam, a benzodiazepine, has been useful in the treatment of both phobias and depression and has been successfully used in school phobia. *(Kaplan and Sadock, p 1234)*

537. **(C)** Since the initiation of such programs in the mid-1960s, methadone maintenance therapy has become the most widely used modality in the treatment of heroin abuse. The philosophy of the program is based on the view that heroin abuse leads to physiologic changes that cause addicted persons to require opiates or face an overwhelming "heroin hunger." This biochemical deficiency of opiates persists even after detoxification and social rehabilitation. Thus, abstinent individuals who were previously addicted remain at high risk for relapse and an eventual downward physical and social spiral. One solution is long-term maintenance with methadone, a synthetic opiate. Methadone maintenance is likened to the use of insulin in diabetes or digitalis in congestive heart failure.

A controlled addiction with methadone has several advantages over heroin addiction: There is no need for multiple injections as methadone is given PO, no need for illegal drug trafficking or stealing to pay for drugs, and no persistent drug craving to divert addicts from other important areas of their lives. U.S. federal law requires that a methadone maintenance program provide a variety of services in addition to simply dispensing medication. These services include group therapy, individual and family counseling, and vocational training. Addicted persons are thus encouraged to rejoin the mainstream of society even as they continue potentially permanent methadone maintenance. *(Kaplan and Sadock, pp 1055–1056; Tomb, p 156)*

538. **(C)** Infantile autism usually presents before the age of 30 months. It is characterized by lack of responsiveness to other human beings, gross and global communication impairment, peculiar repetitive habits, and, very often, low intelligence quotient (IQ). It is this early pervasive lack of responsiveness that differentiates infantile autism from childhood schizophrenia, mental retardation, childhood-onset pervasive developmental disorder, and developmental disorders of language—all of which either present at a later age or without such global dysfunction in communication and affective life. *(DSM-IV, pp 66–71; Kaplan and Sadock, pp 1179–1186)*

539. **(E)** Cerebral palsy is more typically a consequence of perinatal trauma. Careful management of the infant during and after delivery can help prevent this disorder. Genetic counseling, which includes measurements of enzyme levels (Tay-Sachs disease and galactosemia), karyotype analysis (Down syndrome), and tolerance tests (phenylketonuria), helps in the primary prevention of mental retardation through early diagnosis and subsequent intervention in the genetically caused disorders. *(Kaplan and Sadock, pp 1144–1145)*

540. **(B)** Clozapine, as compared to most traditional neuroleptics, has a low potency as a D_2 receptor antagonist. Clinically, this means the less frequent appearance of extrapyramidal syndromes. It is not without its side effects, however. Clozapine has considerable anticholinergic potential, there are dose-related seizures, and there is the problem of agranulocytosis, which until recently required a weekly white blood cell count (WBC). This rule has recently been relaxed to allow WBCs every 2 weeks for those patients taking clozapine who have gone 6 months without a significant reduction in their WBC. Because of these side effects, clozapine has been limited to use by persons whose schizophrenia is refractory to other antipsychotics or who have suffered severe extrapyramidal side effects. Clozapine has been particularly helpful in alleviating some of the negative signs of schizophrenia. *(Kaplan and Sadock, pp 1069–1073)*

541. **(C)** The hallmark of delirium is fluctuation in level of consciousness. Periods of lucency may be interspersed with periods of clouding and unresponsiveness. Impaired judgment, impaired memory, and disorientation are seen in both delirium and dementia. Disordered thought is seen in both and tends to be disorganized in delirium and impoverished in dementia. Another distinguishing feature is that the onset of delirium usually occurs within hours or days, whereas the onset of dementia may be insidious throughout a period of weeks to months. *(Kaplan and Sadock, pp 326–327; Stoudemire, Clinical Psychiatry, pp 101–107)*

542. **(B)** According to the case study, this man can be presumed to have been without alcohol for at least the 2 days he has been in jail, and therefore the emerging symptoms would be most attributable to withdrawal and delirium. Withdrawal symptoms included autonomic hyperactivity, hand tremor, hallucinations, illusions, and agitation. Added to these were the signs of delirium, disorientation, irritability, agitation, disorganized thought, inability to focus and concentrate, and development of symptoms over a short time. A diagnosis of exacerbation of schizophrenia does not adequately explain these symptoms and their development shortly after the withdrawal of alcohol. The signs and symptoms are not consistent with dementia, in which one would expect a longer period for symptom development and a clouding of consciousness. Though malingering might be considered, especially for an incarcerated individual, the history of recent alcohol intoxication with abrupt withdrawal makes alcohol withdrawal delirium a more consistent diagnosis. *(Andreason and Black, pp 385–389; APA, pp 124–132, 683; Tomb, pp 149–151)*

543. **(C)** Because of chlorpromazine's potential to cause orthostatic hypotension, as well as its anticholinergic properties, it would not be the most appropriate choice in this man whose autonomic system is already compromised. Haloperidol, with its low anticholinergic/hypotension profile, is a better choice to manage hallucinations. Care must be taken because of its potential to lower the seizure threshold. Chlordiazepoxide and lorazepam, both benzodiazepines, are used to control the signs of alcohol withdrawal. These are cross-tolerant with alcohol, have relatively long half-lives, and are relatively inexpensive. Thiamine replacement, along with folic acid and multivitamins, is essential to prevent the development of permanent neurologic damage. *(Kaplan and Sadock, pp 399–400, 1029)*

544. **(C)** The symptoms described here suggest an anxiety disorder, specifically agoraphobia, in which there is a fear of being in places from which one may not easily escape. As in other anxiety disorders, benzodiazepines are especially effective. Alprazolam, a short-acting form, is particularly helpful. Propranolol, a beta blocker, has had limited success in the treatment of agoraphobia. Trihexyphenidyl, an anticholinergic, antimuscarinic drug is used to treat neuroleptic-induced side effects. Neither risperidone, an antipsychotic, nor pemoline, a stimulant used in attention deficit disorder, are indicated here. *(Kaplan and Sadock, pp 978–979; Stoudemire, Clinical Psychiatry, pp 234–242)*

545. **(A)** It is believed that about 50% of Japanese, Chinese, and Korean persons lack a form of aldehyde dehydrogenase that eliminates acetaldehyde, the first breakdown product of

alcohol. Consequently, these persons experience unpleasant side effects to drinking, such as flushed face and palpitations, and therefore are less likely to drink. In the United States, both white and African-American males have high rates of alcohol-related disorders. Native American and Eskimo persons also have a high prevalence rate of alcohol-related disorders. Across all cultures, men outnumber women in these disorders. *(Kaplan and Sadock, pp 392–394, 396; APA, pp 200–202)*

546. **(C)** Dissociative identity disorder usually develops in children in response to extremely traumatic conditions, such as abuse. A chronic disorder that typically stays undetected until adulthood, dissociative identity disorder affects women quite a bit more often than men. The number of distinct personalities is less of a determinant of severity than is the makeup of the personalities themselves. Mild cases of dissociative identity disorder do occur. *(APA, p 271)*

547. **(C)** More than 70% of homicides in the United States are committed with handguns. A particularly vulnerable group are those 15 to 24 years of age, in whom homicide is the second leading cause of death. Alcohol consumption plays a role in approximately 50% of homicides. The predisposition to and frequency of violence is much higher in males, except in domestic violence where the frequency between men and women is about equal. Violent crime rates are highest in urban metropolitan areas compared to rural areas. *(Kaplan and Sadock, pp 154–155, 392)*

548. **(B)** Characteristic features of childhood attention deficit disorder include short attention span, abnormalities in coordination, emotional lability, low frustration tolerance, impulsiveness, and perceptual and learning problems. Hyperactivity may or may not be associated with the disorder. Ritualistic behaviors are seen in childhood autism and in obsessive–compulsive disorders. Pressured speech is seen in a variety of disorders, especially and characteristically in mania. Formal thought disorder refers to a disturbed form or process of thought (versus content of thought) and is seen in schizophrenia. Fears about appearance and weight are seen in their most severe form in anorexia nervosa. *(Kaplan and Sadock, pp 281, 1194–1196; Stoudemire,* Clinical Psychiatry, *pp 29, 431–440)*

549. **(A)** Because of the possibility of other clinical conditions (specifically pseudoparkinsonism) being present in this woman, which would contraindicate further neuroleptics, it is essential to further investigate the etiology of this woman's problems without assuming that her mental illness is the causative factor. The first steps in caring for this patient need to be taken by the psychiatrist before requesting consultation. Specifically, one would want to determine the precise nature of physical signs already present, as well as determine this person's autonomic stability ascertained by vital signs. Until evaluation is completed, medications should be given. *(Stoudemire,* Clinical Psychiatry, *pp 164–165; Tomb, pp 212–213)*

550. **(C)** The signs of bradykinesia (apparent apathy, slowed movements, difficulty initiating movement, masked facies) suggest a parkinsonian syndrome secondary to neuroleptic use. The temporal relationship of the increased neuroleptic and increased susceptibility as an older woman, along with the Parkinson signs, help support this as the most likely diagnosis. The bradykinesia and apathy do suggest a severe depression, and at times it is difficult to separate this out as well as separating out an exacerbation of catatonic schizophrenia. In the latter, one might expect more bizarre posturing. The signs of normal autonomic activity—blood pressure, pulse, and temperature—do not support a diagnosis of neuroleptic malignant syndrome. A diagnosis of tardive dyskinesia is also not supported. In tardive dyskinesia, one would see an increase in movements, characteristically choreiform or tic-like movements. In this woman, there is a significant decrease in all movements. *(Stoudemire,* Clinical Psychiatry, *pp 164–165; Tomb, pp 212–213)*

551. **(B)** The treatment of choice for this drug-induced parkinsonism is the use of anticholinergic agents, of which benztropine is a most common example. This woman is already on a small dosage at 1 mg/day, which is, in this situation, not enough to control the emergence of the syndrome. It would also be advisable to decrease the haloperidol or switch to another neuroleptic with fewer extrapyramidal side effects. Increasing haloperidol or changing to fluphenazine would most likely increase the problem. Dantrolene is used in the treatment of neuroleptic malignant syndrome. Amitriptyline is useful as an antidepressant agent. *(Stoudemire,* Clinical Psychiatry, *pp 164–165; Tomb, pp 212–213)*

552. **(B)** A wide variety of agents (eg, antipsychotics, stimulants, antidepressants, lithium, levodopa) used therapeutically in clinical psychiatry can produce, as side effects, characteristic extrapyramidal syndromes. These abnormal involuntary motor behaviors can be divided into the following two main groups: (1) early effects, occurring within several days of initiation of drug therapy; and (2) late effects, which appear after several months of drug treatment. Early abnormal movements include acute dystonia (intermittent or sustained muscle spasms), a pseudoparkinsonian syndrome (bradykinesia, akinesia, rigidity, resting tremor), and akathisia (a state of motor restlessness subjectively experienced by the patient, along with tension, restless sensations in the legs, and inability to tolerate inactivity). These syndromes are often reversible with either reduction or discontinuation of the causative medication or the use of concomitant anticholinergic medication (benztropine, diphenhydramine). Involuntary movements called tardive dyskinesia (TD) may appear later in the course of treatment (usually after 3 months). These abnormal movements consist of a variable mixture of facial grimaces and orofacial dyskinesia, as well as truncal and extremity athetosis, dystonia, chorea, and hemiballismus—all of which may worsen with stress, decrease with drowsiness or sedation, and disappear in sleep. The syndrome may be reversible, especially by medication tapering, or may become permanent and irreversible. It is thought that the underlying pathophysiologic mechanism in-

volves initial postsynaptic dopamine receptor blockade by the psychoactive medication as well as increased presynaptic dopamine turnover. These events lead to increased sensitivity of the postsynaptic dopamine receptors and, thus, dopamine system (nigrostriatal) overactivity. The behavioral manifestation becomes observable as abnormal involuntary movements. *(Tomb, pp 212–213; Kaplan and Sadock, pp 955–960)*

553.   **(C)** The onset of severe, persistent eye pain is always a cause for concern. In a patient medicated with a drug with anticholinergic side effects, such as imipramine, there is a potential for the development of narrow-angle glaucoma. A delay in the diagnosis and treatment of this will lead to irreparable harm to the eye. In this case, the psychiatrist would act immediately to facilitate appropriate evaluation and treatment, which would best be provided by her ophthalmologist. *(Andreason and Black, p 668)*

554.   **(D)** When deciding to order an MRI of a patient, the physician needs to determine of what clinical value it will be, keeping in mind that the clinical value will be different than the research value. In persons with long-standing schizophrenia, research has shown various changes that occur in the brain structures. Seeing these changes in the brain of one's own patient may satisfy one's curiosity but, practically speaking, may have no clinical implications. On the other hand, if a person has developed behavioral changes, the MRI may help identify the etiology, which then points to treatment. The MRI may also be used to monitor further deteriorating or restorative changes in the brain as the person is treated. *(Andreason and Black, pp 106–115)*

555.   **(E)** A million or more children are maltreated each year, according to U.S. government estimates. So few cases are reported compared with the actual incidence that accurate data are impossible to compile; however, child maltreatment and abuse do not seem to be diminishing. Estimates of the number of deaths caused by child abuse are hampered by the inconsistent reporting requirements of the various states; recent estimates put the toll at as many as 2000 to 4000 or more deaths each year. *(Kaplan and Sadock, p 847)*

556.   **(C)** The DST is a neuroendocrine test widely used in psychiatry. At least 40% of patients who meet the current diagnostic criteria for major depression fail to show suppressed serum cortisol values after receiving an oral dose (usually 1.0 mg) of dexamethasone, a potent synthetic glucocorticoid. Normally, such a dose acts to shut off hypothalamic production of corticotropin releasing factor (CRF), leading to decreased secretion of adrenocorticotropic hormone (ACTH) by the pituitary and diminished cortisol secretion by the adrenal gland. Patients with unipolar depression (repeated major depressive episodes) as well as those with bipolar depression (episodes of mania and depression) can manifest an abnormal response to dexamethasone. Therefore, the DST does not appear useful in distinguishing between these two categories of depressed patients. A negative result (ie, normal suppression of serum cortisol after dexamethasone) does not rule out the diagnosis of major depression—it is simply noncontributory. More recent clinical reports indicate that those depressed patients who manifest a disorder in their hypothalamic–pituitary–adrenal axis (abnormal DST) are more likely to respond to pharmacotherapy or ECT. Nonsuppressors who convert to normal suppressors (DST repeated) during the course of somatic treatment also appear less likely to suffer relapse when the somatic treatment is stopped. *(Andreason and Black, pp 118–119; Kaplan and Sadock, pp 256–258)*

557.   **(A)** Because most antipsychotic drugs have some anticholinergic properties, they are contraindicated in atropinic psychoses. Although lithium is the drug of choice for treating an acute manic state, concurrent use of an antipsychotic agent is often required. This is because of lithium's slow (7 to 10 days) onset of action. Similarly, antipsychotic drugs can be helpful in the early treatment of psychotic depression, especially until antidepressant

therapy takes hold. Psychosis associated with unfamiliar surroundings such as the intensive care unit often responds to a low-dose regimen of a potent antipsychotic agent (eg, haloperidol); so, too, does the agitation associated with dementia. Acute hallucinogenic drug-induced states are usually self-limited and respond as well or better to antianxiety drugs. (*Kaplan and Sadock, p 981*)

558. **(E)** The endocrine disturbances that exist in association with anorexia nervosa arise as a consequence of starvation and thus do not represent primary dysfunction in the hypothalamus or its target organs, such as the pituitary and adrenal glands. Release of gonadotropins is impaired, and secretion activity shows pubertal or even prepubertal diurnal changes. Other hormone systems, such as the thyroid, operate abnormally, although they revert to normal when affected persons gain back weight. Half of affected women developed amenorrhea at the beginning of their weight loss. Men with anorexia nervosa are by no means immune from hypothalamic dysfunction. (*Hales and Frances, pp 193–194*)

559. **(A)** In most states, any licensed physician, on evaluation of an individual, has the legal authority to mandate involuntary hospitalization of those persons who are either gravely disabled or a danger to themselves or others. In the case described in the question, the patient presents with the rather acute onset of heretofore never experienced psychiatric (paranoia, delusion, euphoria, grandiosity, agitation) and neurologic (facial weakness, sensory deficit, incoordination, abnormal reflexes) symptoms of significant concern. Her capacity to function has declined (by history) over the past 2 weeks, and there is an indication (locking herself in her room) that her judgment is sorely impaired. Additionally, the nature of the presenting symptoms is such that further decline is expected. Thus, the patient could meet criteria for grave disability and can be hospitalized against her will. The duration of such forced hospitalization for observation, evaluation, or treatment varies by law from state to state. Al-

though any physician may order involuntary hospitalization for grave disability or dangerousness, many physicians in general or emergency practice are unfamiliar with psychiatric illnesses and therefore consult a psychiatrist colleague as part of the decision-making process. It is always advisable to inform a patient's nearest relative of impending hospitalization. However, in cases of grave disability or dangerousness, the physician is empowered to hospitalize based exclusively on his or her clinical judgment. (*Tancredi, pp 799–806*)

560–562. **(560-D, 561-C, 562-E)** Hypochondriasis is a somatoform disorder in which misperceptions or distortions of somatic signs and symptoms lead to preoccupation with fears of having a serious illness. In factitious disorders, one deliberately manufactures signs and symptoms to enter the sick role. The preoccupation with fear of serious illness is not part of the factitious disorder. Major depression is characterized by symptoms of depression, sleep disturbance, appetite disturbance, and so forth. It may be complicated by hypochondriasis. In the case study, no supporting evidence for major depression (for which she would have been evaluated) is provided. This woman's symptoms as described are not of a psychotic level; thus, reactive psychosis would be inappropriate. In pain disorder, pain in a specific body site is the predominant focus, unlike the predominance of fear seen in hypochondriasis. Care of these patients is best managed supportively by developing a therapeutic alliance with them. Anticipating their needs by establishing regular office visits and physical exams with them will help allay fears as well as reassure them of one's concern that if an occult condition becomes evident it will be diagnosed early. Certainly, regular consultation with other specialists is in order to manage these patients. Though the course of hypochondriasis tends to be chronic, there are indications that factor in for a good outcome. One of these is the absence of secondary gain. This disorder is seen equally in both men and women. The prevalence in a general medical practice is approximately 4 to 9%. There is no relationship between hypochondriasis and increased ESR. *(Stoudemire, Clinical Psychiatry, pp 288–291)*

563. **(C)** In the defense mechanism of displacement, an emotion is severed from its original connection with a person or event and attached to a substitute person or object. With its origin thus disguised, the emotion may be more safely expressed. In the example described in the question, anxiety associated with sexual feelings is displaced onto the setting in which they occurred, with resulting phobic anxiety. *(Kaplan and Sadock, p 221)*

564. **(B)** Typically, somatization symptoms begin before age 30 and occur over several years. The symptoms tend to fluctuate but rarely completely remit. Studies show that both genetic and environmental factors contribute to the risk of developing this disorder. Additionally, family studies show a correlation among antisocial personality disorders, substance-related disorders, and somatization disorders. The prevalence rate for women ranges from 0.2 to 2%. *(APA, pp 446–449)*

565. **(C)** In starting an interview, generally an open-ended question will allow the patient the freedom to tell his story. Choice A assumes the person is depressed; the patient may object if he feels already diagnosed "and hasn't had the opportunity to talk." Choices B and D may be seen as critical and do not directly address the issue of what brings this patient to the psychiatrist. The patient may experience these as unempathetic. Choice E is premature. As the consulting psychiatrist, you must perform a thorough evaluation to determine the nature and treatment of this patient's problem. *(Stoudemire, Clinical Psychiatry, pp 63–75)*

566. **(A)** Conversion disorder (hysterical neurosis) is defined as the presentation of physical symptoms suggestive of a medical illness that are actually rooted in and expressive of an underlying intrapsychic conflict. A classic example is that of a patient who suddenly finds that his hand is paralyzed. According to psychoanalytic theory, the symptom of paralysis expresses a conflict over the expression of anger. Through the process of repression, the conflicted impulse to strike out is relegated to the unconscious. The symptom then is a compromise expression of the conflict and is symbolic of the conflict. The unacceptable impulse itself remains unconscious. Conversion disorder is distinguished from malingering, in which there is conscious, voluntary production of physical symptoms. *(APA, pp 452–457)*

567. **(C)** In addition to the use of dexamethasone as a hormonal indicator of the presence of biologic depression, the hormone thyrotropin-releasing factor also has been employed. Injection of this hypothalamic peptide normally would result in a brisk elevation in thyrotropin (TSH), but in one fourth of persons with a major mood disorder (ie, not with a reactive depressive syndrome), the TSH response is slowed. As is true with the DST, the accuracy of the TRH test is affected by various factors, including the presence of thyroid disease, alcoholism, and such drugs as lithium, estrogens, and thyroid extract. *(Kaplan and Sadock, pp 256–258)*

568–570. **(568-A, 569-C, 570-B)** Given the temporal relationship in the start of two anticholinergic drugs and the onset of the urinary hesitancy in an otherwise healthy young male, it would be reasonable to conclude that the drugs are causing the problem. Certainly, a rapid assessment regarding the possibility of other causes (eg, infection, trauma, stricture) is important. Careful, attentive listening for any hint of psychotic delusion involving urination is important to screen for. The manner in which the patient describes his symptoms is invaluable in facilitating diagnosis. Also remember that a real medical condition can be described in bizarre, distorted terms, making assessment more difficult and complicated.

Drug-induced urinary hesitancy may be treated by discontinuing the causative medications. Additionally, bethanechol, 10 to 30 mg three to four times each day, may be administered. Bethanechol acts by stimulating the parasympathetic nervous system. The tone of the detrusor urinae muscle increases, producing a contraction strong enough to initiate micturition and emptying of the bladder. Giving benztropine, an anticholinergic, would only heighten the problem. Unfortunately, some patients understand that benztropine is "for the side effect" of their antipsychotic medication but do not understand the difference between the extrapyramidal effect and the anticholinergic effects. Increased thioridazine would also increase the urinary problem. Calling in a urologist would be indicated if the initial treatment failed to work or if the emergency department physician were not able to "get beyond" an extremely distorted, disorganized presentation by the patient. If the bladder were extremely distended and the patient very uncomfortable, insertion of a urinary catheter would be a reasonable course of action. In the patient described, the bladder is not distended.

Of the medications listed, haloperidol would be the safest choice since its anticholinergic effects are low compared to these as well as other antipsychotics. For loxapine, these effects are in the mid-range. Both chlorpromazine and amitriptyline have high anticholinergic potential. Additionally, amitriptyline is an antidepressant, not an antipsychotic drug. *(Kaplan and Sadock, p 946; Tomb, pp 210–211)*

571. **(E)** Although clinical experience is invaluable in the assessment of suicide potential, there is no checklist of clinical manifestations that allows reliable prediction of whether or not a patient will proceed to attempt suicide. However, it is helpful to be armed with some basic information on the demographics of suicide. The rate of completed suicide in men peaks in adolescence and again after the age of 45. The rate of completed suicide in women peaks after the age of 55 years. Women attempt suicide four times as often as men, but men complete suicide three times as often as women. In both sexes, the rate of completed suicide increases in later life. History of a past suicide attempt is a strong indicator of current risk. Forty percent of depressed people who complete suicide have a history of earlier unsuccessful attempts. Inex-

perienced clinicians may cling to the myth that asking about suicidal thoughts may put a dangerous new idea in the patient's mind. This assumption may stem from the anxiety clinicians experience in acknowledging the extreme nature of the patient's situation. Such well-intentioned failure to address the topic of suicide may only reinforce the patient's sense of hopelessness and isolation, thus increasing suicide risk. A nonjudgmental, understanding invitation to frankly discuss suicide may demonstrate that others do care and that perhaps it is possible that the patient's problem can be accepted. This is not to be confused with another pervasive myth about suicide—that people who talk do not act. Eight out of ten individuals who commit suicide give some clear warning of their plans before the act. Broaching the subject of suicide is only the first step in a comprehensive approach to suicide evaluation and intervention. *(Kaplan and Sadock, pp 864–868)*

572. **(A)** One of the most significant findings here is, the woman, cooperative with the exam, has the score of 14 on the MMSE. A score of 25 to 30 indicates no cognitive impairment, 20 to 25 suggests possible mild impairment, and less than 20 is very strongly suggestive of cognitive impairment. This degree of change on the MMSE is not a normal sign of aging. Additionally, there are no signs of psychosis or mania. Even if there were, in this woman with no previous psychiatric history, one would not likely consider psychosis not otherwise specified or mania. The time frame for dysthymia is not met by the "several days" length described here. *(Stoudemire, Clinical Psychiatry, pp 111–117)*

573. **(D)** ECT has been useful in treating catatonic schizophrenia and some schizophrenias that are fairly new in onset. It has not been useful in chronic schizophrenia. ECT has been most useful in the treatment of affective disorders, namely severe depressions that are debilitating, have severe vegetative symptoms, have failed to respond to the usual antidepressants, or when there may be severe suicidal symptoms. *(Andreason and Black, p 692; Stou-*

demire, Clinical Psychiatry, *pp 541, 542; Kaplan and Sadock, pp 1116–1118)*

574. (E) Thyroid function studies should be obtained to establish baseline values in a person about to begin lithium therapy. Lithium can cause a number of thyroid-related abnormalities, including reduction in thyroxine release, increase in TSH production, and heightened response of TSH to TRH. Lithium can also raise parathyroid hormone levels, although not to clinically significant levels. *(Stoudemire,* Clinical Psychiatry, *pp 535–536)*

575. (B) This woman's symptoms meet the criteria for a major depressive episode. She has had a depressed ("blue") mood for at least a 2-week period, a significant weight loss, insomnia, fatigue and loss of energy, and thoughts of suicide. Because her symptoms seem to be limited to 3 weeks, dysthymic disorder would most likely not be considered. There are no indications for an organic mental disorder that would suggest Alzheimer's disease. Generalized anxiety disorder is characterized by excessive anxiety and worry for about 6 months. For a diagnosis of borderline personality disorder, patterns of instability in relationships, self-image, affect, and impulsivity would have been present in early adulthood. None of that is described here. *(APA, pp 327, 432; Stoudemire,* Clinical Psychiatry, *pp 199–204)*

576. (B) For a first, relatively acute episode of major depression, a tricyclic or SSRI is usually considered a first-choice drug. The SSRIs, considered as effective as the tricyclics, are often favored by clinicians because of their greater safety profiles and faster onset of action. Olanzapine is an example of an antipsychotic drug. Alprazolam is a benzodiazepine that, at higher doses, does have some antidepressant value. Its addictive potential does not make it a drug of choice for depression. Tranylcypromine is an effective MAO inhibitor antidepressant selected for use after a depression has failed to respond to the tricyclics and SSRIs. ECT is also used after other treatments have failed. In very severe, debilitating depressions, however, a clinician

may choose ECT as a first treatment. *(Andreason and Black, pp 283–287; Kaplan and Sadock, pp 567–572)*

577. (A) Negative symptoms of schizophrenia reflect the absence or deficiency of a mental function that is normally present. Anhedonia, or the inability to experience pleasure, is an example of such. Positive symptoms of schizophrenia reflect aberrance or distortion of these mental functions. Loose associations, delusions of thought, insertion, incoherence, and stereotypic gestures are all examples of these distortions. *(Andreason and Black, pp 205–207)*

578. (B) The antidepressant desipramine has been found effective for treating some cases of attention deficit disorder and offers help to those children not responsive to the usual treatment with stimulants (methylphenidate, pemoline). The remaining choices have not been found useful in treating this condition. They are lithium, a mood stabilizer; alprazolam, a benzodiazepine anxiolytic; propranolol, a beta blocker; and perphenazine, an antipsychotic. *(Stoudemire,* Clinical Psychiatry, *pp 437–439)*

579. (C) Cognitive psychotherapy would be helpful to this man to see and understand how cognitive distortions about himself, others, and the future bring about his depressive feelings. Psychoanalysis, a process lasting several years with a weekly commitment of 3 to 4 sessions, would require this person to be willing to explore and work through issues and conflicts that have their source in childhood. Behavioral therapy has as its goal the disruption of inappropriate behaviors with the substitute of more appropriate behaviors. It is intended for the treatment of phobias and various psychosomatic disorders (eg, migraine, hypertension). Supportive psychotherapy could also be of some value. This is used frequently in conjunction with medication. Group therapy may be of some value after this patient has had the opportunity to work in a one-to-one situation in which understandings about himself have developed. Proper preparation is essential before entering group therapy. *(Stoudemire,* Clinical Psychiatry, *pp 481–499)*

580. **(C)** There is strong evidence for a genetic predisposition to bipolar disorder. Some of the evidence comes from twin studies. The concordance rate for monozygotic twin is 79%, but for dizygotic twin it is 19%. Advising the patient that she is past the age when bipolar disorders develop, using lithium to prevent the disorder, or saying that no genetic link has been determined is very misleading and clinically incorrect. *(Stoudemire,* Clinical Psychiatry, *pp 213–214)*

581. **(B)** Pick's disease is considered a cortical dementia, with the preponderance of pathological findings found in the frontotemporal area. Aphasia, apraxia, and agnosia are signs sometimes seen in these patients. Huntington's disease and Parkinson's disease are caused by pathological changes in the basal ganglia. Pathological changes are seen in the ventricles in occult hydrocephalus. Signs seen in subcortical dementia more characteristically involve motor disorders: rigidity, tics, gait difficulties, and incoordination. *(Kaplan and Sadock, pp 1294–1295; Stoudemire,* Clinical Psychiatry, *pp 121–122)*

582–586. **(582-E, 583-B, 584-A, 585-D, 586-E)** Infantile autism, called a pervasive developmental disorder in DSM-IV, typically is diagnosed when children do not demonstrate the acquisition of communication skills. Ability to form interpersonal relationships also is grossly impaired. Other behavioral manifestations of infantile autism include unusual repetitive mannerisms (eg, spinning), marked anxiety during environmental changes, and high pain threshold. As to be expected, school performance is poor, though autistic children may display isolated areas ("islands") of normal or superior intellectual functioning. Behavioral manipulation is useful in trying to contain the behavior of autistic children. Unlike infantile autism, childhood schizophrenia usually develops later in childhood and follows an intermittent course. Deterioration in social or school functioning is a characteristic presenting feature, along

with hallucinations, delusions, and other manifestations of psychosis. Phenothiazine drugs offer effective treatment. Symptoms and signs of depression in children are similar to those in adults. However, children may not be able to recognize depressed feelings. Persistence of puzzling physical problems in association with apathetic, withdrawn behavior is a common presentation. The use of antidepressants is controversial; family and individual counseling often can be quite helpful. Attention deficit hyperactivity disorder once was called *hyperactivity* and *minimal brain dysfunction.* Characteristic signs include impulsivity, distractibility, inattention in school, and (usually but not universally) hyperactivity. A variety of pharmacologic agents, including imipramine, dextroamphetamine, and methylphenidate (Ritalin), have been recommended for treatment of attention deficit hyperactivity disorder. *(APA, pp 66–71, 77–91; Kaplan and Sadock, pp 1193–1199)*

587–591. **(587-E, 588-G, 589-H, 590-F, 591-D)** The various stages listed are found in the theories of development of Freud, Piaget, or Erickson. The anal, oral, and latency periods are from Freud's stages of psychosexual development. The latency period occurs between the ages of about 5 and 11 years. It is a period of industry, mastery, experimentation by the child. Basic trust, autonomy, generativity, intimacy, and integrity are stages in Erik Erikson's stage of life cycle. The period of generativity (ages 40 to 65) involves a "giving" to the next generation (eg, altruistic work, guidance, social concern). Integrity, a stage occurring sometime after age 65, is the acceptance of one's life. Intimacy (ages 21 to 40) is that period of life in which there is the development of lifelong attachments to others and the productive living of one's life. Formal operations is a stage in Piaget's cognitive development stages in which the adolescent develops the ability to think in a logical and symbolic way. *(Kaplan and Sadock, pp 142, 216, 235)*

592. **(I)** This man's symptoms are psychotic in nature and somewhat bizarre. Additionally, the information strongly suggests that he is very

sensitive to the extrapyramidal effects of the traditional antipsychotics. Olanzapine, a new antipsychotic with very few extrapyramidal effects, would be a good choice here. *(Kaplan and Sadock, pp 1076–1078)*

593. **(C)** A hypomanic state is described here. This is seen in bipolar I and bipolar II disorder. A treatment of choice is the mood stabilizer divalproex. If psychotic symptoms were present, the addition of an antipsychotic would be indicated. *(Kaplan and Sadock, p 262)*

594. **(D)** This woman is exhibiting signs of severe depression. Because of her cardiac condition, avoiding an antidepressant with negative cardiac effect is important; therefore, amitriptyline would be eliminated. Fluoxetine, an SSRI, would be an appropriate choice. *(Kaplan and Sadock, p 945)*

595. **(B)** Signs of tardive dyskinesia are evident in this woman. She also was tried on several "newer" medications, one of which may have been olanzapine. This would have to be determined. Assuming this is so, a possible good choice is clozapine, which does not contribute to the development of tardive dyskinesia. *(Kaplan and Sadock, pp 1070–1071)*

596–600. **(596-C, 597-B, 598-A, 599-E, 600-D)** The drugs listed in this question are examples of the various classes of antidepressants. These classes include the tricyclics, the SSRIs, the MAOIs (monoamine oxidase inhibitors), the triazolopyridines, and the phenylethylamines. Understanding the site of action, neurotransmitter(s) involved, and side effects characteristic of these classes is helpful in selecting an antidepressant for a particular patient. SSRIs which are comparable in their antidepressant effects to the older tricyclics but significantly safer when taken in larger doses, as in suicidal overdose, are frequently used as the first choice in the treatment of depression. An example here is paroxetine. Drugs that both inhibit serotonin reuptake and block 5-HT$_2$ receptors are characteristic of the triazolopyridines. The overall effect of these actions is believed to decrease both de-

pression and anxiety in patients. There are two drugs in this class: trazodone and nefazodone.

Strong sedation caused by histaminergic and cholinergic activity is seen in the older antidepressants—the tricyclics. These also have both serotonin and norepinephrine effects that are important in decreasing depression. Amitriptyline is the drug example listed here. Drugs demonstrating little sedation and significant serotonin, norepinephrine, and dopamine effects are more characteristic of the phenylethylamines. They are effective in managing depression because there is no histaminergic activity and little sedation is seen. Venlafaxine is an example. MAOIs increase the concentrations of serotonin, norepinephrine, and dopamine by inhibiting their degradation. The MAOIs, although effective as antidepressants, are used relatively infrequently because of the potential development of a hypertensive crisis induced by consuming tyramine-containing foods while on the MAOI. An example here is phenelzine. *(Kaplan and Sadock, pp 971–981; 988–992, 1003–1004)*

601–605. **(601-B, 602-E, 603-C, 604-A, 605-D)** Valproic acid is an anticonvulsant used as a mood stabilizer. It is found useful in the treatment of mania in a bipolar disorder. It has also been valuable in the treatment of rapid cycling bipolar patients. Paroxetine is an example of an SSRI, which is a newer form of antidepressant. The SSRIs are being found to be as effective as the tricyclic antidepressants. Haloperidol is an example of a neuroleptic or antipsychotic medication useful in the management of acute psychosis, as well as long-term care. Clozapine is a newer atypical antipsychotic medication. It is not associated with tardive dyskinesia as are the older neuroleptics. This makes it a drug of choice for individuals who have developed signs of tardive dyskinesia after using other neuroleptics. Problems with agranulocytosis prevent clozapine's being used as a "first-line" neuroleptic. Risperidone, also a newer atypical antipsychotic, is helpful for those persons suffering from primarily negative symptoms of schizophrenia. *(Andreason and Black, pp 656–664; Stoudemire, Clinical Psychiatry, pp 163, 165, 221, 537)*

606–610. (606-H, 607-I, 608-J, 609-C, 610-B) Persons with personality disorders are rigidly bound to the use of patterns of defense and various traits that distinguish the disorders. All have problems with interpersonal relationships. *(Kaplan and Sadock, p 731, 734–737, 739–740, 743)*

611–615. (611-J, 612-A, 613-I, 614-H, 615-F) Defense mechanisms provide a means for dealing with anxiety and affect. The mechanisms chosen range from the very narcissistic and immature to mature. In suppression, a person makes a conscious decision to put the conflict aside until it can be dealt with more appropriately. On the other hand, in acting out, there is little or no attempt to contain the affect, and it is directly expressed as in name calling. Sublimation provides a channel for the indirect expression of a need or affect. Its use is positive and socially acceptable. In reaction formation, the person acts as if the strong need or affect did not exist and acts out the opposing feeling. In projection, unacceptable feelings and thoughts are denied as part of the self and instead are "put on" the other person. *(Kaplan and Sadock, pp 220–221)*

REFERENCES

American Psychiatric Association (APA). *Diagnostic and Statistical Manual of Mental Disorders*, 4th ed., revised. Washington, DC: American Psychiatric Association; 1994.

Andreason NC, Black DW. *Introductory Textbook of Psychiatry*, 2nd ed. Washington, DC: American Psychiatric Association; 1995.

Hales RE, Frances AJ, eds. *Psychiatry Update: American Psychiatric Association Annual Review*, vol. 6. Washington, DC: American Psychiatry Press; 1987.

Kaplan HI, Sadock BJ. *Synopsis of Psychiatry: Behavioral Sciences Clinical Psychiatry*, 8th ed. Baltimore: Williams & Wilkins; 1998.

Stoudemire A, ed. *Clinical Psychiatry for Medical Students*, 2nd ed. Philadelphia: JB Lippincott; 1994.

Stoudemire A, ed. *Human Behavior: An Introduction for Medical Students*. Philadelphia: JB Lippincott; 1990.

Tancredi LR. Emergency psychiatry and crisis intervention: some legal and ethical issues. *Psychiatry Ann* 1982;12:799–806.

Tomb DA. *Psychiatry*, 5th ed. Baltimore: Williams & Wilkins; 1995.

Wedding D. *Behavior and Medicine*, 2nd ed. St. Louis: Mosby; 1995.

Subspecialty List: Psychiatry

Question Number and Subspecialty

503. Assessment
504. Assessment
505. Psychopathology/Assessment grief
506. Intervention tx fn grief
507. Psychopathology parasomnia
508. Psychopathology
509. Psychopathology
510. Psychopathology
511. Psychopathology
512. Psychopathology
513. Development/Assessment
514. Assessment/Development
515. Intervention
516. Psychopathology/Assessment dementia
517. Psychopathology
518. Psychopathology
519. Assessment define delusion
520. Assessment
521. Intervention
522. Psychodynamics
523. Assessment/Psychopathology
524. Assessment/Psychopathology
525. Intervention
526. Psychopathology
527. Assessment
528. Psychopathology
529. Psychopathology HIV
530. Assessment/Psychopathology
531. Intervention
532. Intervention
533. Assessment/Psychopathology
534. Legal, ethical
535. Psychopathology
536. Child psychiatry/Intervention
537. Intervention
538. Child psychiatry/Psychopathology

539. Child psychiatry/Psychopathology
540. Psychopharmacology
541. Assessment
542. Psychopathology/Assessment
543. Intervention tx fn EtOH withdrawl
544. Psychopathology
545. Epidemiology
546. Psychopathology
547. Epidemiology
548. Assessment
549. Intervention pt evaluation
550. Assessment
551. Intervention
552. Assessment EPS
553. Assessment
554. Assessment MRI
555. Child psychiatry/Epidemiology
556. Assessment
557. Intervention
558. Psychopathology anorexia
559. Legal, ethical commit
560. Legal, ethical
561. Legal, ethical
562. Legal, ethical hypochondriasis
563. Psychodynamics
564. Epidemiology
565. Assessment
566. Psychopathology conversion
567. Assessment TRF testing
568. Assessment
569. Intervention
570. Intervention antipsychotics
571. Epidemiology
572. Intervention
573. Intervention
574. Psychopathology Li SE
575. Psychopathology/Assessment
576. Intervention depression tf

577. Psychopathology/Epidemiology
578. Child psychiatry/Intervention *ADHD tx*
579. Intervention
580. Intervention/Psychopathology
581. Psychopathology
582. Child psychiatry/Assessment
583. Child psychiatry/Assessment
584. Child psychiatry/Assessment
585. Child psychiatry/Assessment
586. Child psychiatry/Assessment
587. Assessment *dev. str*
588. Assessment
589. Assessment "
590. Assessment "
591. Assessment
592. Intervention
593. Intervention
594. Intervention
595. Intervention
596. Psychopharmacology

597. Psychopharmacology *antidepress*
598. Psychopharmacology "
599. Psychopharmacology "
600. Psychopharmacology
601. Intervention
602. Intervention
603. Intervention
604. Intervention
605. Intervention
606. Assessment *PD*
607. Assessment
608. Assessment
609. Assessment
610. Assessment
611. Psychodynamics
612. Psychodynamics
613. Psychodynamics
614. Psychodynamics *defens mecha*
615. Psychodynamics

Rx / Tx = 9
assess = 8
psychopar 8
dynamics = 1
epd = 2

CHAPTER 6

Preventive Medicine
Questions

*Tilahun Adera, PhD, C.M.G. Buttery, MD, MPH,
and W.R. Nelson, MD, MPH*

DIRECTIONS (Questions 616 through 689): Each of the numbered items or incomplete statements in this section is followed by answers or by completions of the statement. Select the ONE lettered answer or completion that is BEST in each case.

616. Rheumatic fever and rheumatic heart disease are late complications of untreated or inadequately treated group A beta-hemolytic streptococcal infections. Which factor among the following has been demonstrated to increase the incidence of the disease?

    (A) genetic profile of patient
    (B) the strain or serologic type of the *Streptococcus*
    (C) low socioeconomic conditions
    (D) endemic rather than epidemic streptococcal infections
    (E) northern hemisphere versus southern hemisphere

617. Glomerulonephritis, like rheumatic fever, is a complication of beta-hemolytic streptococcal infections but differs from rheumatic fever because

    (A) it most frequently occurs in children between 10 and 14 years old
    (B) recurrent attacks are rare
    (C) all strains of streptococci are equally associated
    (D) the latent period is 20 to 30 days
    (E) the prevalence is similar in most population groups

618. Ingestion of toxic substances are unlikely to demonstrate renal impairment at an early stage of exposure because

    (A) few substances are toxic to the kidneys
    (B) concentration of substances in the kidneys is poor
    (C) the kidneys are able to compensate for toxic damage
    (D) the latent period is insufficient to allow detection
    (E) individuals are hesitant to report renal disease symptoms

619. While blindness is common in elderly people, much can be prevented by ensuring access to

    (A) residence in a nursing home
    (B) corneal surgery for near vision
    (C) cataract surgery
    (D) treatment of glaucoma
    (E) refractive correction

620. While poliomyelitis outbreaks have been controlled by use of vaccines, the occurrence of outbreaks is most likely from transmission from

    (A) green monkeys in Africa
    (B) mosquitoes of the species *Aedes aegypti*
    (C) contaminated vaccine
    (D) polluted water sources
    (E) poorly cooked food

621. Because of the widespread use of diphtheria toxin immunization, the number of cases of diphtheria occurring in the United States each year has declined while remaining much more common in undeveloped countries. It is important that immunization be ensured by

(A) giving two doses of vaccine by 6 months of age

(B) enhancing herd immunity by ensuring that all children play outdoors

(C) providing only acellular vaccines

(D) using tetatus–diphtheria (Td) vaccine for persons over 7 years of age

(E) focusing on early use of antibiotics in an injured adult

622. Leprosy (Hansen's disease) is a chronic infection with a long incubation period (1 to 20 years). The prevention of leprosy is effective only if

(A) the entire community is skin-tested when a case is found

(B) patients with leprosy are isolated in a sanitarium

(C) all contacts with the index case are identified and examined

(D) there is widespread notification of the community

(E) family members are immunized

623. Immunization against typhoid fever has been available for many years. Vaccine should be administered when

(A) natural disasters destroy water and sewage systems

(B) taking a rural vacation

(C) traveling in countries with endemic typhoid

(D) antibiotics are not readily available

(E) carriers are found in the community

624. Brucellosis is commonly seen among workers in meat processing plants. The organism results in

(A) each Brucella species producing its own distinct human illness

(B) frequent recurrence of Brucella infections

(C) person-to-person transmission commonly

(D) a chronic relapsing infection

(E) particulate airborne infection

625. Greater attention has been given to cardiovascular disease, specifically heart disease, in women recently. We now know that

(A) men have fewer heart attacks than women

(B) the underlying cause of heart disease in women in now well understood

(C) older women have greater low-density lipoprotein (LDL) levels than high-density lipoprotein (HDL)

(D) estrogen has not been found to be protective to women's cardiovascular systems

(E) women show their earliest symptoms of cardiovascular disease as angina

626. Primary preventive measures are preferred to secondary prevention. Which of the following best exemplifies primary prevention?

(A) annual sigmoidoscopy

(B) routine immunization

(C) mammography

(D) prostate-specific antigen (PSA) testing

(E) isolation of disease contacts

627. Among other agents, the food industry uses which of the following chemicals most commonly?

(A) sugar

(B) vinegar

(C) sulfites

(D) carbon dioxide

(E) benzoic acid

628. While there have been a number of well-documented food poisoning outbreaks in recent years, the one action that overwhelmingly causes such an outcome is

(A) unhygienic food-handling methods
(B) improper storage of rodenticides
(C) inadequate cooking
(D) the use of unlabeled products
(E) use of old untensils

629. Concern with training in geriatrics has increased over that for pediatrics. The population change driving this concern is due to the great increase in rate of population growth among

(A) 45 through 54 year olds
(B) 55 through 64 year olds
(C) 65 through 74 year olds
(D) 75 through 84 year olds
(E) over 85 years of age

630. Prior to sending treated water into the community distribution system, the final treatment provided by a water treatment plant is

(A) coagulation
(B) sedimentation
(C) disinfection
(D) alkalinization
(E) adsorption

631. The elderly are subject to frequent falls, often from medication use. The underlying cause of the excess fracture rate is

(A) Alzheimer's disease
(B) Parkinson's disease
(C) obesity
(D) deteriorating eyesight
(E) osteoporosis

632. The health hazards related to tobacco smoking have received considerable attention in recent years. The public has concentrated on cancer of the lung as the most important association. However, studies from Framingham have indicated other organs or systems are affected. Which of the following is also identified in the Framingham studies?

(A) bone
(B) spleen
(C) cerebrovascular system
(D) thyroid
(E) auditory system

633. High blood leads are seen among children living in older houses in which the interiors are coated with lead paints. Which is the optimal age to examine blood for high lead content?

(A) birth
(B) while still in the crib
(C) 6 months to 1 year of age
(D) on entry to school
(E) yearly intervals

634. Following a patient's visit, the occupational health physician confirms a potential cancer. He refers the patient for surgical treatment. A similar case occurred in this factory during the past year. The occupational medicine physician should

(A) inform the patient's supervisor as a reason for scheduling a work change
(B) tell management that this was the second case to occur at this location in the last year
(C) tell both management and union representatives that this problem occurred twice in the last year
(D) begin a search for possible carcinogens, but inform neither workers nor management
(E) report the occurrence to the state's occupational health agency

635. A young woman who works full time is making her first prenatal visit to her obstetrician. Because her work involves climbing ladders, with the risk of falling, the physician should

    (A) advise the patient not to work
    (B) recommend that the patient seek alternative work
    (C) recommend no change in employment but suggest avoiding risk
    (D) suggest that the patient perform all her normal duties except climbing ladders
    (E) write to the employer, requesting reassignment of the patient

636. Figure 6–1 represents a bimodal increase in numbers of deaths in London, during the winter of 1952 to 1953, compared with the previous year. This phenomenon is most likely caused by

    (A) failure to apply a standard case identification
    (B) a progressive epidemic
    (C) two separate disease etiologies
    (D) failure of a public health intervention
    (E) herd immunity

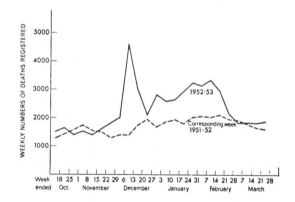

Figure 6–1. Numbers of deaths in London during the winter of 1952 to 1953.

637. The only organization that cannot develop statutes is

    (A) United States Congress
    (B) state legislatures
    (C) state institutions
    (D) county boards
    (E) city councils

638. Documentary evidence in a court of law may be

    (A) inadmissible
    (B) a copy of a medical record
    (C) a piece of an ancient manuscript
    (D) a medical record
    (E) circumstantial evidence

639. Which of the following agents is recommended to control limited outbreaks of meningococcal meningitis in the home, nursery schools, and public schools?

    (A) rifampin or ceftriaxone
    (B) gamma globulin
    (C) group A meningococcal vaccine
    (D) group C meningococcal vaccine
    (E) quadrivalent meningococcal vaccine

640. It may be legitimate to detain individuals in a mental health facility involuntarily. This situation may arise when

    (A) a person has bizarre fantasies and actions
    (B) persons are mentally incompetent and unable to manage their own affairs
    (C) a close relative submits a petition that an individual is actually and presently insane
    (D) the individual's continued liberty poses a danger to himself or others
    (E) a person has visual and aural hallucinations

641. Schedules for the routine immunization of young children are developed jointly by the Advisory Commission on Immunization Practices (a federal commission) and the American Academy of Pediatrics. Which of the following vaccines is recommended for routine vaccination for all children in the United States?

    (A) anthrax vaccine
    (B) rabies vaccine

(C) *Hemophilus influenzae* b (Hib) vaccine

(D) hepatitis A vaccine

(E) typhoid vaccine

642. The cost of health services continues to increase. The highest proportion of health services use is associated with

(A) age

(B) sex

(C) race

(D) education

(E) income

643. When disaster has struck, anywhere in the world, which of the following factors has been the greatest problem in coping with its effects?

(A) lack of government resources

(B) triage of casualties

(C) failure of management

(D) lack of telecommunications

(E) lack of volunteer helpers

644. Market forces leading to development of managed care systems have been accompanied by a slowdown in the rate of increase in health care costs. The majority of third-party coverage is arranged through employer-based programs and

(A) Americans have become less demanding for expensive treatments

(B) physicians have increased their participation in single-specialty group practices

(C) hospitals have reduced their specialized services

(D) patients are more likely to be admitted to the hospital with chronic diseases

(E) utilization studies have been replaced by quality management and control in hospitals

645. Physicians in private practice are more likely to group together, either in partnerships or in formal group practices that may be incorporated, than they did in the past. Which of the following statements is true regarding physicians who associate with each other in these ways?

(A) Physician productivity is higher in small groups than in large groups.

(B) Because of the complexity of large groups, physicians find it difficult to take vacations or educational leave.

(C) Physicians in large groups have larger patient loads.

(D) More work is delegated to allied health employees in large groups.

(E) Large prepaid group practices realize substantial economies in the cost of ambulatory care.

646. Although individual physicians and small health care facilities wish to provide health care for all those who request it, the charges for the services provided must be reimbursed. If some individuals are allowed to ignore their bills, either practice income decreases or patient charges increase. The final step in handling accounts receivable is to

(A) refer accounts older than 30 days to a collection agency

(B) write off accounts not paid within 6 months

(C) avoid legal proceedings even if long overdue

(D) take them to a small-claims court

(E) obtain a court judgment and subsequent enforcement

647. Concerning confounding variables, it may correctly be stated that the confounder

(A) must relate to the sample population containing the disease

(B) must relate to only the total population from which the sample was drawn

(C) must be related to the disease under investigation and to the risk factor

(D) must relate to the disease but not to the risk factor

(E) must relate to the risk factor but not necessarily the disease

648. Bacterial contamination of cooked foods prepared for use on site is by far most likely to occur when food is

(A) pasteurized

(B) canned

(C) flash frozen

(D) dried

(E) bulk stored in refrigerators

Questions 649 and 650

Use Table 6–1 to answer the following two questions.

Table 6–1. SUMMARY OF DATA COLLECTED IN A COHORT OR CASE-CONTROL STUDY

	Risk Present	Risk Absent
Disease Present	A	B
Disease Absent	C	D
Total	A + C	B + D

649. What is the relative risk in those with the risk factor compared to those without the risk factor?

(A) $\dfrac{a/(a+c)}{b/(b+d)}$

(B) $\dfrac{a/c}{b/d}$

(C) $\dfrac{ad}{bc}$

(D) $\dfrac{a+c}{a+b+c+d}$

(E) $\dfrac{b+d}{a+b+c+d}$

650. What is the odds ratio?

(A) $\dfrac{a/(a+b)}{c/(c+d)}$

(B) $\dfrac{ab}{cd}$

(C) $\dfrac{ad}{bc}$

(D) $\dfrac{a+c}{a+b+c+d}$

(E) $\dfrac{ac}{bd}$

651. *Hemophilus influenzae* meningitis infections have responded dramatically to the introduction of an appropriate vaccine. Prior to the introduction of the vaccine, *H influenzae* infection

(A) had a peak incidence among children 6 to 7 months old

(B) 90% of infections occurred in children 4 to 8 years old

(C) was rarely associated with epiglottitis

(D) was more common in white than in black children

(E) epidemics were frequently observed

652. Jehovah's Witnesses usually refuse to consider a recommended blood transfusion. A 5-year-old child with hemophilia and dangerously low hemoglobin levels needs such a transfusion, but the Jehovah's Witness parents refuse to accept the recommendation. How are principles of autonomy best resolved?

(A) The hospital's representatives respect the parents' right to consent and support their refusal.

(B) The physician explains the need, in simple words, to the child who refuses the transfusion.

(C) The hospital requests a local court to exercise the rights of the child through the appointment of a surrogate guardian.

(D) The local court gives the physician the right to decide if the transfusion is warranted.

(E) The hospital Chaplain is usually given the final authority in these matters.

653. Epidemiology, the study of the distribution of disease (events) in time and space, can be said to be

(A) related to environmental influences on populations

(B) related to infections transmitted within populations

(C) due to psychological causes

(D) the result of ingestion of chemical toxins

(E) not fully understood, but it does not occur randomly

654. Stratified random sampling is correctly described as

(A) based on selecting every "ith" individual

(B) random sampling of separate segments of a population

(C) randomly grouping the population

(D) sampling a cluster

(E) none of the above

Questions 655 Through 662

In a study on the association between hypertension and myocardial infarction (MI), the findings of a questionnaire sent to *the whole population (1000 persons),* all of whom responded, are presented in Table 6–2. A randomly chosen *sample of 100 members* of the same total population is examined. The results obtained are shown in Table 6–3.

Table 6–2. WHOLE POPULATION

History of Hypertension	History of MI	
	Present	*Absent*
Present	15	185
Absent	5	795

Table 6–3. SAMPLE OF 100 MEMBERS

History of Hypertension	History of MI	
	Present	*Absent*
Present	4	36
Absent	1	59

655. The reported prevalence of hypertension in the population per 1000 is

(A) 150

(B) 185

(C) 200

(D) 220

(E) 250

656. The prevalence of MI per 1000 hypertensive persons in this community is

(A) 10

(B) 15

(C) 19

(D) 75

(E) 81

657. The prevalence of MI per 1000 persons in the community is

(A) 5

(B) 10

(C) 15

(D) 20

(E) 25

658. The statistical test that could best be used to determine whether there is a significant increase in the history of MI among those persons who have hypertension in comparison with those without hypertension is

(A) *t*-test, single-tailed

(B) *t*-test, two-tailed

(C) test of variance

(D) *P* value

(E) chi-square test

659. If we compare the population sample examined with the whole population that responded to the questionnaire, which of the following statements accurately describes the available information?

(A) The sample group confirms the findings of the questionnaire.

(B) As expected, there is a higher "real" incidence of hypertension than reported.

(C) As expected, there is a higher "real" incidence of MI than reported.

(D) There is a statistical test that could be applied to assess the significance of the differences.

(E) The data as presented are not really adequate for further statistical examination.

660. The approximate odds ratio of having MI if one is hypertensive as opposed to normotensive, as computed from the questionnaire, is

(A) 3

(B) 4

(C) 9

(D) 13

(E) 21

661. Using the data for the examination of the *sample cases*, the approximate odds ratio for having an MI in relation to hypertension is

(A) 2.1

(B) 4.7

(C) 6.6

(D) 8.0

(E) 9.2

662. The chi-square test is used to compare

(A) proportions of different experimental results

(B) data that can be examined with a Student's *t*-test

(C) data from observations and expectations

(D) only data that cannot be expressed as percentages

(E) means of two groups

663. A series of biologic measurements are made in a population, and is shown below. The percentage of readings likely to fall below 1 standard deviation (SD) less than the mean is

(A) 2%

(B) 10%

(C) 16%

(D) 25%

(E) 30%

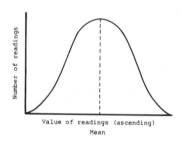

Figure 6–2. Biologic measurements of a population.

664. The standard error of the mean (SEM)

(A) corresponds to the SD

(B) quantifies the variability of the population

(C) summarizes data about the population

(D) quantifies variability in the estimate of the mean

(E) is usually greater than the SD

665. A study assessing mean fasting triglyceride levels is performed on 200 women of childbearing age. *Ninety* of the women used oral contraceptives, while *the remainder* did not. Among the oral contraceptive users, the mean triglyceride level was 95 mg/dL, with an SD of 42.4. For the nonusers, the mean was 73 mg/dL, with an SD of 53.9. When performing a *t*-test on this population, one must calculate the "degrees of freedom." What are the degrees of freedom for this population?

(A) 11.5

(B) 22

(C) 156.5

(D) 198

(E) 200

666. Epidemiologic data are frequently collected in groups, such as blood pressure readings: 120 to 129, 130 to 139, and so on. To analyze each group mathematically, the group value used is

(A) a modal group value

(B) a lowest group value

(C) a mean group value

(D) a highest group value

(E) an assigned group value

667. The causative organism of cholera, *Vibrio cholerae*, was first isolated by Koch in 1883. There have been seven pandemics of cholera, with the most recent subsiding only in the 1980s. With humans as the usual reservoir, the organism spreads as man travels. The most likely mode of spread is by

(A) contaminated fomites

(B) specific strains of mosquitoes

(C) food cleaned in contaminated water

(D) person-to-person transmission in crowded airplanes

(E) contaminated droplets from air conditioning systems

668. A dermatitis often called "swimmers' itch" manifests as a rash that is caused by

(A) contact with stingrays

(B) infection with blood flukes

(C) contact with jellyfish

(D) scrapes against rocks while swimming

(E) contact with irritant seaweed

669. While the etiology of multiple sclerosis (MS) has not been identified, epidemiologists have shown that

(A) blacks and Asians have a higher incidence of MS than whites

(B) males and females have a similar incidence of MS

(C) prevalence increases as latitude increases

(D) more cases are noted in urban than in rural areas

(E) migration to warmer climates decreases the likelihood of developing the disease

670. Of 125 persons who drowned, 11 wore life jackets but 114 did not. Which of the following statements is justified?

(A) The use of life jackets diminishes the risk of drowning.

(B) The population that uses life jackets may be small.

(C) No explanations of the phenomenon may be deduced.

(D) The investigation does not report the weather conditions.

(E) Most drownings occur due to falls from bridges.

671. Cytomegalovirus (CMV) infections have attracted increasing attention since recent outbreaks caused by poor management of some major potable water systems in the United States. The presence of CMV in humans and the environment results in

(A) its not being one of the diseases causing secondary infection among acquired immune deficiency syndrome (AIDS) patients

(B) infants acquiring CMV infection only during passage through the cervix

(C) children infected with CMV being a hazard to staff and other children in day care centers

(D) transfusion's not being one of the avenues for transmission of CMV

(E) its being detected best by antibody testing

672. Passive immunization by use of immune globulin will

(A) prevent the development of congenital rubella in children of infected pregnant women

(B) modify or prevent the development of measles in the first 6 months of life

(C) fail to modify or prevent the development of mumps in exposed individuals

(D) modify or prevent the development of chickenpox in exposed individuals

(E) prevent the development of hepatitis A in food industry workers

673. Administration of chelating agents, such as ethylenediaminetetra-acetic acid (EDTA) and penicillamine, for the treatment of heavy-metal poisoning (such as lead)

(A) requires prophylaxis for persons exposed to metal dust and fumes

(B) is rarely necessary because the toxic effects of the metal poisoning are quickly reduced

(C) should be performed only on patients (adults or children) with symptomatic disease

(D) minimizes absorption of the metal from the gastrointestinal tract

(E) can be performed without removing the patient from exposure to the metal

674. The treatment of choice for basal cell carcinomas of possible occupational origin is

(A) application of 5-fluorouracil (5-FU)

(B) liquid nitrogen cryosurgery

(C) electrosurgery

(D) curettage

(E) scalpel excision

675. Job-related noise is a hazard that occurs in many industries and should require hearing protection. The danger is cumulative, being related to the number of hours of exposure each day over a number of years. Of the following occupations, the one that is most likely to result in hearing damage without proper protection is

(A) scraper-loader operator

(B) aircraft ramp attendant

(C) engineer in diesel engine room

(D) oxygen torch operator

(E) riveting machine operator

676. To assess workers exposed to inhaled materials, pulmonary function tests are

(A) of little value without simultaneous gas exchange analysis

(B) expensive in relation to the results yielded

(C) unable to yield positive results before the onset of symptoms

(D) discriminatory in determining cause

(E) appropriate for medical surveillance of occupational disease

Questions 677 and 678

A hypothetical screening test is proposed for detecting a certain disease, which can be verified by more elaborate clinical examination. The *test* is applied to 600 persons in an apparently normal population. The *test results* are positive in 200 cases. Of these, 100 persons are discovered on clinical examination to have the disease, but 50 individuals who have negative test results are also proved to have the disease on clinical grounds.

677. The sensitivity of the test is

(A) 16.7%

(B) 22.2%

(C) 66.7%

(D) 77.8%

(E) 87.5%

	D(+)	D(−)
T(+)	100	100
T(−)	50	350

678. The specificity of the test is

(A) 16.7%

(B) 22.2%

(C) 66.7%

(D) 77.8%

(E) 87.5%

679. Epidemics of hepatitis A virus (HAV) are found worldwide. Additionally,

(A) the distribution of disease has little relation to socioeconomic conditions

(B) in more advanced developing countries, community hygiene has little relation to outbreaks

(C) this virus has not been a cause of day care infant epidemics

(D) the greatest increase in infection has occurred among young adults

(E) only raw meat has been associated with hepatitis A epidemics

Questions 680 Through 684

680. A group of male workers between the ages of 20 and 39 years are being screened for lung disease by spirometry. Nine subjects are examined. Their forced expiratory volume in 1 second (FEV_1) divided by forced vital capacity (FEV~/FVC%) results are 80, 76, 73, 61, 64, 79, 64, 64, and 78. The *mean* is

(A) 61

(B) 64

(C) 71

(D) 73

(E) 76

681. Using the same values as in the previous question, the *modal* reading is

(A) 61

(B) 64

(C) 71

(D) 73

(E) 76

682. Using the same values as in question 680, the *median* value is

(A) 61

(B) 64

(C) 71

(D) 73

(E) 76

683. Using the same readings as in question 680, the *range* is

(A) 17

(B) 18

(C) 19

(D) 20

(E) 21

684. The variance of the set of values listed in question 680 is 58.75. The SD is

(A) 5.8

(B) 6.5

(C) 7.7

(D) 8.5

(E) 9.0

685. The crude mortality rate in Sweden was 0.010 per year, while in Costa Rica it was 0.008 per year. All age-specific mortality rates, except those for the oldest-age category, were higher in Costa Rica than in Sweden. From this data, one can infer that

(A) the difference is too small for any deductions to be made

(B) it is healthier to live in Sweden than in Costa Rica

(C) it is healthier to live in Costa Rica than in Sweden

(D) a greater proportion of the Swedish population is in the older-age categories

(E) a greater proportion of the Costa Rican population is in the older-age categories

Questions 686 Through 689

Table 6–4 relates to a hypothetical case control study of cigarette smoking and lung cancer.

Table 6–4. CIGARETTE SMOKING AND LUNG CANCER

Cigarette Smoking	Lung Cancer		
	Cases	Controls	Totals
Yes	75	25	100
No	25	75	100
Totals	100	100	200

686. What is the odds ratio in this example?

   (A) 3
   (B) 6
   (C) 9
   (D) 12
   (E) 20

687. Using the same table, what is the risk ratio?

   (A) 3
   (B) 6
   (C) 9
   (D) 12
   (E) cannot be calculated

688. Normally odds ratios and relative risk calculations would result in approximately similar answers if:

   (A) The overall size of the series is too large to estimate relative risk.
   (B) If the number of controls were increased, the two ratios would be similar.
   (C) The number of controls is twice as many as the cases.
   (D) The odds ratio is not appropriate for this series.
   (E) The disease is rare.

689. An investigator in a community hospital decides to examine all patients for a problem with alcoholism. In addition to recall bias, which is the most obvious error *in selecting all patients admitted* to a community hospital?

   (A) observer bias
   (B) selection bias
   (C) detection bias
   (D) interpretive bias

DIRECTIONS (Questions 690 through 720): Each set of matching questions in this section consists of a list of 4 to 26 lettered options followed by several numbered items. For each item, select the ONE best lettered option that is most closely associated with it. Each lettered heading may be selected once, more than once, or not at all.

Questions 690 Through 693

Workers in certain occupations are exposed to diseases for which animals are the reservoir. These workers may then become the source of infection to others. For each of the occupations listed, choose the infectious disease the workers are most likely to acquire and transmit.

   (A) anthrax
   (B) brucellosis
   (C) Lyme disease
   (D) murine (endemic) typhus
   (E) salmonellosis

690. Butcher

691. Granary and warehouse worker

692. Livestock worker

693. Rancher

Questions 694 Through 696

For each of the organizations listed, select the type of health care planning used by that organization.

   (A) population-based planning
   (B) institution-based planning
   (C) financial planning
   (D) program planning
   (E) morbidity planning

694. Local health departments

695. Prepaid health plan or health maintenance organization (HMO)

696. Maternal and child health care system

Questions 697 Through 701

For each of the diseases listed, select the arthropod vector responsible for its transmission.

    (A) *Aedes aegypti*
    (B) *Anopheles* species
    (C) *Pediculus humanus corporis*
    (D) *Xenopsylla cheopis*
    (E) *Sarcoptes scabiei*

697. Epidemic typhus

698. Malaria

699. Dengue fever

700. Colorado tick fever

701. Yellow fever

Questions 702 Through 706

For each of the regulatory agencies, choose the function for which the organization has responsibility.

    (A) Food and Drug Administration (FDA)
    (B) United States Department of Agriculture (USDA)
    (C) Environmental Protection Agency (EPA)
    (D) United Nations Food and Agriculture Organization (FAO)
    (E) World Health Organization (WHO)

702. Controls the use of pesticides in the United States

703. Retains authority to remove from the market any food with excess pesticides or other toxic substances

704. Defines action levels for polychlorinated biphenyls (PCBs) in fish

705. Enforces standards in the sale of meat

706. Mounts international control programs for the eradication of communicable disease

Questions 707 Through 710

For each disease-causing organism, choose the corresponding incubation period.

    (A) up to 3 hours
    (B) 12 hours (6 to 24 hr)
    (C) 12 to 16 days
    (D) 24 hours
    (E) 12 to 48 hours (1 to 6 days)

707. *Clostridium perfringens*

708. *Clostridium botulinum*

709. *Staphylococcus aureus*

710. *Salmonella*

Questions 711 Through 715

Several groups of organic compounds are associated with serious toxic effects when used as described. Select the choice that matches the description in the question.

    (A) nitrosamines
    (B) epoxy compounds
    (C) PCBs
    (D) formaldehydes
    (E) organophosphorus compounds

711. Used in transformers because they withstand high temperatures

712. Used as insecticides and responsible for more deaths on a worldwide basis than any other group of substances

713. Highly toxic and dangerous as a solvent; used in the manufacture of rubber, dyes, and lubricating oils

714. Used in the production of resins, plasticizers, and solvents

715. Used in the manufacture of textiles and materials; often found in manufactured homes

Questions 716 Through 720

Various gases and fumes are widely recognized for their toxic effects. For the gases described, select the choice that fits the description.

(A) carbon monoxide
(B) methane
(C) hydrogen sulfide
(D) ozone
(E) sulphur dioxide

716. A colorless, pungent gas occurring naturally in the stratosphere, which can be produced by electric arcs

717. A colorless gas that rapidly paralyzes the nasal receptors; found in sewers

718. A colorless, odorless, flammable gas sometimes encountered in mines and wells

719. An odorless, colorless, tasteless gas produced by partial combustion of tobacco and fuels

720. A colorless, pungent gas encountered in drilling petroleum

Questions 721 Through 725

For the secondary prevention techniques identified, choose the appropriate frequency of use.

(A) no recommendation
(B) yearly for women over age 50
(C) first trimester of pregnancy
(D) every 1 to 2 years for women aged 50 to 69
(E) every year after two negative tests
(F) every 3 years following an initial examination
(G) yearly for all over age 50

721. Mammography

722. Cervical cytology (Pap smear)

723. Occult blood testing and flexible sigmoidoscopy

724. Screening for hepatitis B

725. Prostate cancer screening

Questions 726 Through 730

For each of the clinical indications, choose an option for use of immune globulin.

(A) indicated
(B) not proven effective
(C) not routinely indicated
(D) contraindicated

726. Hepatitis A prophylaxis

727. Hepatitis B prophylaxis

728. Hepatitis C prophylaxis

729. Measles prophylaxis

730. Rubella prophylaxis

Questions 731 Through 737

For each of the infectious diseases of childhood, select the appropriate incubation period.

(A) 1 to 7 days
(B) 6 to 8 days
(C) 7 to 10 days
(D) 10 to 21 days
(E) 30 to 50 days

731. Diphtheria

732. Chickenpox

733. Infectious mononucleosis

734. Mumps

735. Pertussis

736. Tetanus

737. Rubella

Questions 738 Through 748

For each of the conditions listed, select the organism associated with it.

   (A) coagulase-positive *Staphylococcus aureus*
   (B) beta-hemolytic *Streptococcus*
   (C) *Hemophilus influenzae*
   (D) *Mycoplasma pneumoniae*
   (E) *Hemophilus pertussis*
   (F) *Helicobacter pylori*
   (G) *Escherichia coli*
   (H) *Rickettsia prowazekii*
   (I) *Giardia lamblia*
   (J) *Clostridium perfringens*

738. Chronic diarrhea in a homosexual male

739. Impetigo

740. Chronic cough and low-grade fever in children and adolescents

741. Spasmodic cough with inspiratory stridor in a child

742. Nursery epidemics of watery diarrhea

743. Furunculosis

744. Gastric ulcer

745. Acute otitis media

746. Food poisoning at a banquet

747. Epidemic typhus

748. Toxic shock syndrome

Questions 749 Through 753

For each of the following body sites, select the carcinogen most likely to produce carcinoma upon industrial exposure.

   (A) skin
   (B) lung
   (C) bladder
   (D) scrotum
   (E) liver
   (F) bone
   (G) blood (leukemia)
   (H) pleura

749. Asbestos

750. Benzidine

751. Radon

752. Ultraviolet (UV) radiation

753. Radium

Questions 754 and 755

When making recommendations to a state general assembly against routine premarital screening, the State Health Commissioner used the following data to arrive at his conclusions. An average state population of 1000 young adults had a prevalence of 1 in 1000 with human immunodeficiency virus (HIV) positivity. The best screening test available had a sensitivity of 98% and a specificity of 95%. From this data:

754. How many people in this population would have screened false positive?

   (A) 98
   (B) 9
   (C) 150
   (D) 60
   (E) 120

755. How many people would have screen as false positive?

   (A) 2,000
   (B) 3,250
   (C) 4,995
   (D) 6,851
   (E) 7,999

Questions 756 Through 760

Interventions at different stages of disease have different aims. Match the following levels of prevention with the aims.

    (A) secondary prevention
    (B) primary prevention
    (C) tertiary prevention
    (D) casual prevention
    (E) indefinite prevention

756. Aims to diagnose symptomatic clinical disease as early as possible

757. Aims at decreasing susceptibility of the individual who is still free of disease

758. Aims at modifying the course of clinical disease

759. Aims at preventing the onset of disease

760. Environmental control of the causes of disease

Questions 761 Through 764

Match the most appropriate study design with the statements.

    (A) cross-sectional study
    (B) randomized, controlled trial
    (C) cohort study
    (D) case-control study

761. This study design avoids self-selection of study subjects to different exposure groups.

762. It is generally difficult to ascertain the antecedent-consequent aspects of the hypothesized relationship.

763. Multiple disease outcomes associated with smoking can be assessed.

764. Multiple exposures associated with lung cancer can be assessed.

DIRECTIONS (Questions 765 through 794): Each of the numbered items or incomplete statements in this section is followed by answers or by completions of the statement. Select the ONE lettered answer or completion that is BEST in each case.

765. In a cohort (follow-up) study, the population at risk at the beginning of the follow-up period should consist of

    (A) persons with and without the disease
    (B) persons with diverse exposure levels and disease
    (C) persons of comparable age, gender, and race
    (D) persons with homogeneous disease probability
    (E) persons who are susceptible but free of prevalent disease

766. Among the observational study designs, a major advantage of the prospective cohort design is that

    (A) it provides a relatively quick answer
    (B) it allows one to take advantage of existing outcome data
    (C) it is easy to assemble a comparison group
    (D) it allows one to measure incidence
    (E) it is relatively cheap

Questions 767 and 768

The distribution of cases and controls by coffee-drinking habits are shown below for an unmatched case-control study of pancreatic cancer and coffee drinking (fictitious data).

Coffee Drinking (cups/day)	Cases (no.)	Controls (no.)
0	9	32
1–2	94	200
3–4	53	80
5+	60	65
	216	377

767. What is the odds ratio of pancreatic cancer in those who drink five or more cups of coffee compared to those who drink no coffee?

(A) 1.0

(B) 3.3

(C) 2.4

(D) 1.7

(E) 5.9

768. Based on the above table, which of the following statements is correct? (Hint: calculate the odds ratio for each "coffee drinking category" using 0 cups per day as reference, and look at pattern.)

(A) The data suggest that the risk of pancreatic cancer increases with rising levels of coffee consumption.

(B) The data do not suggest that the risk of pancreatic cancer increases with rising levels of coffee consumption.

(C) There is no suggestion of a dose–response.

(D) The dose-response calculation is invalid because it uses the 0 cups per day category as a reference.

(E) There is neither dose nor response in this question.

769. On January 15, 1996, a health survey was performed in an elementary school of a developing country. All the schoolchildren were examined for conjunctivitis, and 2% of the children were diagnosed with the disease. From these data, one can determine

(A) the incidence of conjunctivitis

(B) the prevalence of conjunctivitis

(C) both incidence and prevalence of conjunctivitis

(D) neither the incidence nor prevalence of conjunctivitis

(E) the attributable risk

770. The probability of testing positive if the disease is truly present is called

(A) specificity

(B) sensitivity

(C) positive predictive value

(D) negative predictive value

(E) none of the above

771. The proportion of true positives among those who have positive test results is called

(A) specificity

(B) sensitivity

(C) positive predictive value

(D) negative predictive value

(E) none of the above

772. A certain test has a sensitivity of 95% and a specificity of 95%. When given to a population of 1000 persons, the positive predictive value of the test is

(A) 95%

(B) 90%

(C) 10%

(D) 2.5%

(E) unable to be derived from this information

773. Which of the following is the best study design to test the efficacy of a new drug?

(A) ecological study

(B) randomized, controlled trial

(C) cohort study

(D) case-control study

(E) case series study

Questions 774 Through 778

In a cohort study of cigarette smoking and coronary heart disease (CHD), 1000 cigarette smokers and 1000 nonsmokers were followed over a 10-year period. During the study, 160 of the cigarette smokers developed CHD, while 60 of the nonsmokers experienced such an event. Assuming no losses to follow-up and no deaths from other causes, answer the following questions.

774. The incidence rate of CHD (per 1000 person-years) among smokers is closest to

(A) 6

(B) 11

(C) 12

(D) 16

(E) 23

775. The incidence rate of CHD (per 1000 person-years) among nonsmokers is closest to

(A) 6

(B) 11

(C) 12

(D) 16

(E) 23

776. The rate ratio for CHD is closest to

(A) 0.4

(B) 2.3

(C) 2.7

(D) 4.2

(E) 3.8

777. The 10-year risk difference is closest to

(A) 40%

(B) 10%

(C) 15%

(D) 25%

(E) 30%

778. The attributable risk percent is

(A) 32.5%

(B) 45.5%

(C) 50.0%

(D) 53.0%

(E) 62.5%

Questions 779 Through 782

In an unmatched case-control study of induced abortion and breast cancer, 15 of 100 cases reported a history of induced abortion while 10 of 200 controls reported such an event.

779. The odds of exposure among cases is

(A) 2.208

(B) 0.453

(C) 0.176

(D) 0.112

(E) 3.354

780. The odds of exposure among controls is

(A) 2.201

(B) 0.452

(C) 0.184

(D) 0.053

(E) 3.353

781. The odds ratio for exposure is

(A) 2.20

(B) 0.45

(C) 0.18

(D) 0.11

(E) 3.35

Questions 782 and 783

The mean systolic blood pressure in normal, healthy individuals was found to be 120 mm Hg, with an SD of 10 mm Hg. Assuming that the blood pressures were normally distributed, provide estimates for the following questions.

782. The proportion of subjects who have a systolic blood pressure above 130 mm Hg is

(A) 12%

(B) 16%

(C) 34%

(D) 95%

(E) 99%

783. The proportion of subjects who have systolic blood pressure between 100 and 140 mm Hg is

(A) 95%

(B) 68%

(C) 99%

(D) 34%

(E) 12%

784. A 3-year-old child recovers from a severe episode of bloody diarrhea, hemolysis, and uremia. The child's case is linked to other cases across the country by statistical association with consumption of hamburgers obtained from a nationwide supplier of ground beef. The best method for preventing this illness in the general population is

(A) cooking ground beef to be well done and washing of fruit and vegetables

(B) regulations enforcing worker hygiene in the workplace

(C) a testing program for enteric disease in livestock

(D) regulations enforcing sanitary conditions in slaughterhouses

(E) a ban on imported meats and produce

785. Death certificates list causes of death using diagnostic names familiar to physicians. Deaths can then be aggregated into categories of disease such as atherosclerotic coronary artery disease, for example. Another approach would be to use what is known about the etiology of the disease and calculate what the underlying causes of death are. This was done in 1993 for the calendar year 1990. In that year, the most common underlying cause of death was

(A) unintentional injury

(B) use of tobacco products

(C) use of alcohol products

(D) communicable diseases

(E) sedentary lifestyle/poor diet

786. Since 1990, the growth of managed care programs has been explosive. What has been the predominant force behind this?

(A) patient advocacy groups requesting comprehensive care

(B) the efforts of elected officials to reform the health care system

(C) the overwhelming desire of Americans to have a seamless, one-payor health care system

(D) the desire of employers and other purchasers of care to reduce their costs

(E) the increasing number of health care providers

787. An insurance company insures several groups of people. The first group consists of young, healthy employees of a large software development company. The second are schoolteachers who are generally older and a little less healthy. The third is a group of construction workers who are older and not very healthy. The company bases its premiums for each group on how they utilize health services and what they cost. The first group pays $150/month in premiums, the second $225/month, and the third $400/month. A common expression for this approach is called

(A) community rating

(B) customer-driven rating

(C) experience rating

(D) market rating

(E) employee-driven rating

788. A 28-year-old nursing home aide has skin tests for tuberculosis (purified protein derivative [PPD] testing). Her tests have always been read as negative, but this year, she developed 20 × 25-mm induration. She feels well and has no cough; a baseline white count and liver function test is normal, and a recent HIV antibody test is negative. Her physician orders a chest x-ray, which is negative. The next step in management is to

(A) begin three-drug antituberculosis therapy

(B) educate the patient on the symptoms of tuberculosis and repeat the chest x-ray in 1 month

(C) isolate her from her family and other close contacts

(D) immunize the patient with bacillus Calmette–Guérin (BCG) vaccine

(E) begin isoniazid, 300 mg daily

Question 789

Twenty-four hours after a large church supper, guests begin to complain of nausea, abdominal cramps, and watery diarrhea. The health department surveys all the guests and develops the following data, based on presence of illness and food ingested:

	Attack Rate of Persons Eating Food	Attack Rate of Persons Not Eating Food
Pickles	23%	40%
Potato salad	45%	58%
Tuna salad	90%	10%
Baked beans	56%	35%
Ham biscuits	71%	35%
Barbecue chicken	15%	60%
Ice cream	32%	49%
Iced tea	47%	1%

789. The implicated food item is

(A) ham biscuits

(B) baked beans

(C) iced tea

(D) potato salad

(E) tuna salad

790. A young mother has an income below the federal poverty level. She applies to her local social services agency for health insurance for her child and is enrolled in a statewide program funded with state and federal tax dollars, which provides complete medical care for her child. The likely name for this program is

(A) Medicaid

(B) Medicare

(C) Blue Cross/Blue Shield

(D) The Robert Woods Johnson Foundation

(E) Women, Infants, and Children program (WIC)

791. A young child finds a bat lying on the floor of his room. The child picks it up to show it to his mother, and it bites him on the hand. The bat then escapes, flying out an open window. What disease poses the most serious threat to the child's health?

(A) rabies

(B) Lacrosse encephalitis

(C) distemper

(D) tularemia

(E) tetanus

792. An outbreak of influenza occurs across the United States in the early winter. Of individuals contracting influenza, a large proportion had received vaccinations earlier in the fall. The most likely explanation is

(A) the vaccine was manufactured improperly

(B) the vaccine used did not contain antigen specific to the outbreak strain

(C) a systemic storage problem with a major shipper damaged the vaccine

(D) due to unusually cold weather, people were more susceptible

(E) the virus was especially virulent

793. A family is scheduled to move into a home that is 15 years old. Its water supply is a well, and sewage is discharged to an on-site septic system. In preparation for the move, they obtain a series of water tests from the well. All of the results show the presence of coliform bacteria. This means

(A) they are at risk of acquiring a coliform bacterial infection

(B) the well water has been mixed with untreated surface or groundwater

(C) nothing—this is a common finding in the country

(D) the groundwater is extensively contaminated and the house is unlivable

(E) they can live in the house but must seek medical care at the first sign of illness

794. Municipal water systems serving large numbers of citizens must adhere to standards of quality. These standards are mandated by

(A) local governments

(B) state legislatures

(C) regional councils

(D) executive mandate

(E) the Safe Drinking Water Act

795. The mortality rates from two countries are being compared. Despite vast differences in their economy, level of public services, birth rates, and education, the difference in crude mortality rate is the opposite of what is expected: The more developed country has the higher crude mortality rate. To determine whether this is a real difference, the proper step is to

(A) verify a difference in health status of residents by doing a health survey

(B) examine the causes of death to determine the reason for the difference

(C) recalculate the rates using 5-year aggregate data

(D) calculate an age-standardized death rate for each country

(E) compare the mortality rates for cities of equal size in each country

796. An HMO has its annual medical directors meeting, at which time new treatments are discussed. A recent study has just clearly demonstrated that a new drug can lower blood pressure significantly, although monitoring tests for renal function are required. They consider adding the treatment to their list of approved treatments but are handicapped by one of the real disadvantages of making treatment decisions based on clinical outcomes alone. This disadvantage is that

(A) clinical tests cannot reliably tell which treatment works best

(B) clinical trials ignore the difference in costs between treatments

(C) results of clinical trials cannot possibly be applied to real-world situations

(D) effects noted in the study population will not show up in the general population

(E) the advantages of improvement in clinical outcomes are always too significant to ignore

797. The U.S. Preventive Services Task Force made the following recommendations for breast cancer screening: for women aged 50 to 70 years, screening mammography and clinical breast exam every 1 to 2 years. They did not recommend routine screening mammography for women in the general population less than 50 years of age. The best explanation for this is that

(A) screening mammography in women less than 50 is not as sensitive as in those over 50

(B) screening mammography in women less than 50 is more difficult due to tissue density

(C) women under the age of 50 are still likely to have high estrogen levels

(D) breast self-examination in the younger group is more sensitive in detecting cancers than mammography

(E) the benefit of detecting cancers in the younger age group was outweighed by the risks screening caused in that age group

798. The infant mortality rate for a population is expressed as the number of deaths in the first year of life divided by the number of live births in the same period. In the United States, the infant mortality rate for 1997 was approximately

(A) less than 5 infant deaths/1000 live births

(B) between 5 and 10 infant deaths/1000 live births

(C) between 10 and 15 infant deaths/1000 live births

(D) between 15 and 20 infant deaths/1000 live births

(E) over 20 infant deaths/1000 live births

799. Infant mortality rates are often used to compare the health status of populations. In 1997, what was the approximate comparison between the infant mortality rate for white infants and black infants?

(A) The infant mortality rate for black infants was one fourth the rate for white infants.

(B) The infant mortality rate for black infants was one half the rate for white infants.

(C) The black infant mortality rate was approximately the same as the white infant mortality rate.

(D) The black infant mortality rate was approximately twice the white infant mortality rate.

(E) The black infant mortality rate was approximately three times the white infant mortality rate.

DIRECTIONS (Questions 800 through 807): Each set of matching questions in this section consists of a list of 4 to 26 lettered options followed by several numbered items. For each item, select the ONE best lettered option that is most closely associated with it. Each lettered option may be selected once, more than once, or not at all.

Questions 800 Through 804

For each scenario below, select the public health method it represents.

(A) evaluation of vital records
(B) investigation
(C) active surveillance
(D) health survey
(E) case-control study
(F) policy development
(G) consultation
(H) passive surveillance

800. Local health departments systematically collect information on the appearance of measles (rubeola) in their locality and send it, by way of state health department offices, to the Centers for Disease Control and Prevention (CDC). At each step, the data are analyzed and interpreted.

801. In the wake of public alarm over the possible food-borne transmission of Creutzfeldt–Jakob disease, epidemiologists at the CDC systematically call pathologists and neurologists from selected large urban areas in an attempt to identify cases.

802. The National Center for Health Statistics routinely selects a sample population and asks individuals questions about their health problems and health care.

803. Having determined that an outbreak of fever, shock, and pulmonary edema without a known etiology is occurring in the Southwestern United States, a team of experts is dispatched to the area for the purpose of finding the cause and stopping the outbreak.

804. In the face of ongoing prevalence of meningitis caused by type B *Hemophilus influenza,* state officials advocate and then obtain state laws requiring immunization for school entry in order to increase immunization levels.

Questions 805 Through 807

For each situation below, select the category of prevention it represents

(A) primary prevention
(B) secondary prevention
(C) tertiary prevention
(D) selective prevention
(E) community prevention
(F) preventive therapy

805. A community hospital conducts a screening for hypercholesterolemia by setting up stations and testing blood samples. Persons with elevated cholesterol are referred for dietary counseling, exercise programs, and possible treatment.

806. State officials conduct a program providing public service messages outlining the dangers of smoking and urging adolescents not to start. The program is a success, in that surveys indicate fewer adolescents begin smoking.

807. A patient has severe respiratory disease as a result of years of smoking. He successfully quits smoking and improves his respiratory function.

Answers and Explanations

616. (C) In the past, age, race, sex, latitude, altitude, and dampness have all been thought to affect the incidence of rheumatic fever. Although the earliest reports and studies came from temperate zones, tropical zones are now reporting a higher incidence. All types and strains of group A beta-hemolytic streptococci have been associated with the condition. Available data suggest that the environment facilitates transmission through crowding, seen typically in lower socioeconomic communities.

617. (B) The peak incidence of poststreptococcal glomerulonephritis occurs between the ages of 3 and 7 years. Not all strains of streptococci are equally associated with glomerulonephritis. Because these strains are not evenly spread throughout the communities, the prevalence of poststreptococcal glomerulonephritis can vary widely between different population groups. There is little tendency for the condition to recur, and therefore there is little indication for secondary preventive measures.

618. (C) Renal function tests are relatively insensitive in detecting early renal damage, mainly because the kidneys demonstrate tremendous reserve and therefore an ability to compensate for loss of function. In fact, the presence of toxic substances in the body is unlikely to affect the kidney because of the rich blood supply to this organ. Because of the kidney's resistance to injury, the length of the latent period before the onset of disease makes association with a particular toxin difficult to determine. It is therefore likely that there are many more substances that eventually will prove toxic to the kidneys but that have not at present been identified.

619. (C) There is a markedly higher frequency of impaired vision of the elderly in nursing homes than in the community. While it is not frequently recorded as a reason for nursing home admission, people with impaired vision experience many other limitations. Cataract is the leading cause of blindness in both communities. Maximizing visual ability by appropriate refraction obviously improves mobility and ability to function but does not prevent blindness.

620. (D) The virus is excreted in stools and pharyngeal secretions. Transmission occurs mainly by the fecal–oral route, particularly where sanitation and personal hygiene are poor, as in developing countries. The WHO, with the assistance of Rotary International, has called for global eradication by the year 2000. There is no known reservoir for poliovirus except humans.

621. (D) Children in developing countries often injure themselves. The resulting frequent contact with soil enhances their herd immunity. The pediatric schedule is three initial doses and a booster of diptheria–pertussis–tetanus (DPT). All persons over 7 years of age must receive the Td vaccine to avoid severe local reactions. Injuries contaminated with soil require debridement and booster doses of vaccine.

622. **(C)** The long incubation period has led to difficulties in studying the epidemiology of Hansen's disease. Numerous studies have indicated that close personal contact is the most significant factor in the risk of infection. Leprosy is a disease of prolonged close contact. Testing of entire communities is not an effective method of disease control. Testing and examination is performed on all close continued contacts of the index case. While immunization is a goal, an effective vaccine is not yet available.

623. **(C)** Vaccination against typhoid fever is less effective than antibiotic treatment. It has only a 60 to 70% effectiveness. While past vaccines had unpleasant side effects, the newer ones still under population testing have few side effects and appear to be more efficacious. Most cases (62%) are contracted as a result of overseas travel. In certain areas of the world, the incidence remains high. It is in such endemic areas that vaccine is still advised. There has been no indication that immunization after earthquakes or other cataclysmic disasters is either necessary or effective.

624. **(D)** Human illnesses caused by the various species of *Brucella* organisms tend to be quite similar. All have a tendency to be a chronic infection as well as relapsing and recurring. Infection is rarely airborne but can be encountered in laboratory and abattoir workers. Person-to-person spread is rare. The mode of infection is principally from direct contact with infected animals or by the ingestion of infected milk.

625. **(E)** Researchers have reported significant disparities between men and women in heart disease. An excess risk is documented in Western society through studies such as the Framingham study and studies in Finland. There appears to be relative protection from estrogens among younger women. Cardiac disease is more likely to present as angina in women. Older women carry more cholesterol as HDL than LDL compared to younger women. In Eastern Europe, cardiovascular disease is increasing rapidly in women, while in the United States, the age-specific decline in cardiovascular disease is greater among women than men.

626. **(B)** Routine immunization of individuals at risk, whether children or adults, is primary prevention because it occurs before signs, symptoms, or deviation from health occur. No disease is present, even in a presymptomatic phase. Risk factor identification, such as identification of a high-risk community, is also primary prevention. The early or presymptomatic recognition of disease, using sigmoidoscopy, PSA testing, or mammography, is secondary prevention. The isolation of disease contacts, or of individuals with disease, is tertiary prevention.

627. **(A)** Sugar and salt are the most commonly used chemical preservatives in the food industry. At concentrations of 65% or greater, sugar prevents the growth of bacteria, yeasts, and molds. Bacteria rarely survive in concentrations greater than 25%. Salt is also an effective preservative but, because of its taste is not as readily acceptable as sugar. From a health standpoint, both substances have disadvantages. Benzoic acid, prohibited in some countries, is permitted in concentrations of as much as 0.1% for certain foods in the United States. Carbon dioxide is rarely used, except in carbonated beverages. Sulfites act as enzyme and microbial inhibitors.

628. **(A)** Although all of the phases of the food preparation process may present opportunities for contamination, the major problem is related to food handling rather than to the quality of the food itself. The principles of correct food handling are generally known, but in practice, hygiene has to be maintained by the individual food handlers. The methods and equipment may be sufficient to allow for the preparation of hygienic food, *but* if the technique falls below acceptable standards, problems are likely to arise.

629. **(E)** About 80% of persons over the age of 65 maintain functional independence, but the proportion diminishes with increasing age, so that only 54% of men and 38% of women live at home independently after age 85. Data from the National Center for Health Statistics show that those over 85 are the faster-growing segment of the population. Quality-of-life issues become very important at this age.

630. **(C)** Disinfection with chlorine is the process used to ensure that potable water continues to contain minimal active, infectious organisms as its passes through the distribution system. It is the final step in the process prior to entering the distribution system. The main purpose is to protect the water from infectious organisms that may enter the system by infiltration. Coagulation is used to purify drinking water by removing suspended material, colloidal material, microorganisms, and, to some extent, dissolved substances. After coagulation or flocculation, the water is allowed to sediment in tanks. Synthetic organic chemicals are removed by adsorption, generally in activated carbon filters. Alkalinization of water may be necessary to counteract the corrosive effects that may result from the lowered pH, caused by the other purifying processes. Acidic water is particularly damaging to plumbing and heating systems.

631. **(E)** There are many intrinsic factors that lead to falls in the elderly. Iatrogenic causes from medication prescribed commonly impair stability of gait. However, it is osteoporosis, particularly in the elderly female, that results in the excess fractures, usually of the femur. Although the elderly are more likely to have Alzheimer's and Parkinson's diseases, poorer eyesight, and diabetes, these are not as important as osteoporosis in fractures among the elderly.

632. **(C)** No association has been found between smoking and disease of the bones, spleen, thyroid, and auditory system. A number of studies have shown the increased rate of diseases of the cerebrovascular system due to smoking.

633. **(C)** The age at which children most frequently ingest the largest amounts of lead is during the crawling and walking stage, which is also the oral–anal stage of development that occurs between the ages of 6 months and 2 years. Until children are mobile, they are unlikely to come into contact with objects that might have been coated with lead-based paint. After 2 years, children normally have less tendency to put unusual objects in the mouth.

634. **(D)** The code of ethical conduct for physicians providing occupational medicine services recommends that such physicians should treat as confidential whatever is learned about individuals served, releasing information only when required by law or because of overriding public health considerations. The occurrence of two similar cases of an illness in a year could be attributed to chance and should not at this stage indicate such a possible risk as to introduce the concept of an overriding public health problem. The occurrence of two similar illnesses in a single year does not indicate a timely need for specific concern. Employers are entitled to advice regarding their workers' physical ability to perform their duties but are not entitled to diagnoses or details of a specific nature. Physicians employed in industry need to communicate to employers and employees, in an accurate yet wise and discrete manner, any information about health hazards.

635. **(B)** The situation described in the question calls for clinical judgment by you as the personal physician. Advice should be given to patients and not to their employers. Unless there is extreme urgency, it is proper to advise the patient to cease work. Telling a patient to avoid risk is impractical, difficult to interpret, and cannot be applied effectively. For her to perform all her normal duties without climbing ladders requires a modification of her job description that may be inappropriate. The patient would have to discuss this with her employer. The appropriate recommendation is for the patient to seek alternative work within her company. The patient should discuss her needs with her employer and refer to your advice. Only if requested by the patient should the physician communicate directly with the employer.

636. **(C)** The shape of the accompanying graph exhibits different characteristics of peaks from two separate epidemics. The first peak coincided exactly with the great fog in London of December 1952 and its effect on chronic obstructive pulmonary disease (COPD). The second peak, in January through February, coincided with an outbreak of influenza. If herd immunity had developed, a steady decline in the number of cases recorded would have occurred after the initial peak. A progressive epidemic would normally produce a steadily increasing number of cases. Application of specific control measures is most likely to produce a steadily diminishing number of cases reported. Ineffective case identification normally leads to low levels of reporting, particularly at the outset of an epidemic.

637. **(C)** A statute is any enactment, resolution, ordinance, or public law decided and ratified by any legal body to which authority has been given or delegated. Thus, the United States Congress has jurisdiction in federal affairs; state legislatures have authority in their own states but may not enact statutes that conflict with federal authority (overriding). Similarly, state legislatures may delegate authority in defined areas to county boards or city councils. Physicians therefore have to be familiar not only with federal law, but also with their own state laws and local laws enacted by county boards or city councils. State institutions (eg, universities or mental health hospitals) may have their own internal regulations, which apply to their population (eg, students). However, internal regulations are not applicable to the general population and are not statutes.

638. **(D)** Documentary evidence in a court of law is, in general, the complete actual document that may prove a point relevant to the case. Part of a document is not acceptable, because there may be relevant information in the part not provided. Although copies of medical documents may be used in preparing and examining evidence, the actual record is required for presentation in court. Relevant documentary evidence is always admissible in court.

639. **(A)** Both rifampin and ceftriaxone have been recommended for the chemoprophylaxis of close contacts of cases of meningococcal meningitis. Gamma globulin has not been shown effective for prevention of meningococcal disease. Most outbreaks are caused by strains of groups A, B, C, and W-135. A vaccine for groups A, C, Y, and W-135 is available but is used only when the source has been isolated and typed, which is rarely the case when prophylaxis must be started immediately. Meningococcal vaccine has been shown to be effective in Finland. The immunogenicity of vaccines for groups A and C is poor, especially in children. The search continues for a widely acceptable vaccine.

640. **(D)** Before a person can be involuntarily confined to an institution, a competent professional must decide that the person is dangerous to himself or others. A person who is mentally incompetent is more appropriately protected by the legal appointment of a guardian to make the necessary decisions and manage property. A person who merely has strange fantasies may be neither mentally incompetent nor a danger to himself or others. Persons with auditory and visual hallucinations do not necessarily pose a threat of danger or injury to themselves or others and therefore are not candidates for confinement.

641. **(C)** Hib vaccine is recommended for routine immunization of children. Anthrax is used to vaccinate military troops in selected overseas deployment. Rabies vaccine is used for postexposure prophylaxis when children are bitten by potentially rabid mammals. Hepatitis A vaccine is used for children at special risk of such infection. Typhoid vaccine is not routinely recommended for use in the United States.

642. **(A)** Persons aged 65 and over constitute 11% of the population but consume 29% of the expenditure for health care. By contrast, those under age 19 represent 31% of the population but account for only 12% of health care expenditures. While women use health services more frequently than men (primarily because of problems associated with the reproductive cycle), their use is less than the use by older age groups. The effects of race are closely related to income. When adjusted for health status, the poor make fewer visits to physicians than the nonpoor. Higher levels of education relate to appropriate health care use.

643. **(C)** Since the 1950s, the single most important failure in coping with disasters has been poor management by those in charge. There has been no significant problem with resources needed or with triage of casualties. Neither has there been evidence of poor response to the need for volunteer helpers. Telecommunications have improved continuously, especially with satellite communications available.

644. **(E)** In spite of the high cost of health care services, Americans utilize and demand more health care than any other nation. Single-specialty group practices are being replaced by multispecialty groups that use generalists to monitor the use of services provided by specialists. Specialized services availability is unchanged. Patients with chronic diseases are more likely to be provided ambulatory care than were such patients in the past. Economies are being produced by hospitals' and managed care organizations' accounting for specialists as cost centers, rather than revenue producers, largely through quality management and control.

645. **(A)** Most studies have demonstrated that economies of scale are achieved when physicians practice together rather than alone. These economies peak at a relatively low scale: between two and five practitioners. There is no real support for the notion that large-scale group practices produce substantial economies. Physicians in large groups find it necessary to press for such benefits as longer vacations, more educational leave, and lighter patient loads.

646. **(E)** A bill is legal evidence of a contract to pay for services rendered. The reputation of a small health care facility or a small practice may be worth more than collecting 100% of accounts receivable. Some patients must be reminded of their obligation to pay medical bills just as they pay other bills. A small-claims court is a partial solution to collecting unpaid debts. When initial collection efforts fail, a legal judgment must be obtained and enforced as a good business practice.

647. **(C)** Variables whose effects are entangled with other variables are known as confounders. To adjust for these confounding variables, some data adjustment may be needed. For a variable to be a confounder, it must be related both to the disease (or condition) of interest and to the risk factor being investigated.

648. **(B)** Food prepared for use on site, but not for immediate consumption, must be stored. While canning, flash freezing, pasteurization, and drying are all appropriate methods of storage, all are subject to mishandling. The one storage method most likely to lead to contamination is bulk storage rather than storing in individual portions. Bulk storage results in slow cooling of the central portions of the food mass, leading to bacterial growth.

649. **(A)** The relative *risk* estimates the magnitude of an association between exposure and disease. It indicates the likelihood of developing a disease from exposure to a risk compared to a group not exposed to the risk. It is the ratio of the incidence of the disease in the exposed group, $a/(a + c)$, divided by the incidence in the nonexposed group, $b/(b + d)$.

650. **(C)** C is correct. In a case-control study, participants are selected based on disease status. It is not usually possible to calculate the incidence rate of the disease because the denominator population from which the sample was drawn is not known. Therefore, the formula for relative risk, which works well for a cohort study (in which the denominator data are known), cannot be applied to data from a case-control study. The risk can be estimated

by calculating the ratio of the odds of exposure among cases to that among the controls.

651. **(A)** The peak incidence (150/100,000 per year) is in children 6 to 7 months old. Ninety-five percent of cases of *H influenzae* meningitis occur in children less than 5 years of age. The incidence in black persons is three times as high as for white persons. Epiglottitis occurs most commonly among children 2 to 4 years of age. True epidemics have not been observed, but clusters of cases may be seen in households, day care centers, and so forth.

652. **(C)** The law has generally recognized that the parents do not necessarily exercise autonomy appropriately on behalf of their child. It also recognizes that children cannot exercise autonomy for themselves, and that children should not be required to make complicated decisions about their own care. For children, and for adults who are unable to make medical decisions, a surrogate decision maker is normally named by a court of appropriate jurisdiction.

653. **(E)** A fundamental assumption of epidemiology is that disease does not occur randomly. Epidemiology studies the distribution and determinants of disease and the frequency of their occurrence. Each of the factors listed may play a part; none is truly predominant.

654. **(B)** Sometimes it is possible to identify subgroups or strata of a population. Randomly sampling these segments, called strata, may reduce sampling error. Systematic sampling, selecting every "ith" individual, is not necessarily random, depending on how lists are constructed. Random groups would presumably be based on random selection of individuals, and little benefit would derive from studying such groups. Random groups produce more hazards statistically than randomized strata. Clusters are somewhat different; they may be small groups of the population occurring in specific areas, such as families, villages, or wards. The characteristics of clusters are not necessarily those of the population, but more those of location. Cluster sampling may be useful but does not have the same outcome as a stratified sample. *(Hill, p 16)*

655. **(C)** Prevalence is the number of existing cases of a disease occurring in the total population at a given period of time. In this study, the prevalence rate is calculated based on reported figures (15 + 185). The actual figure, as demonstrated by the investigation of the sample, is likely to be higher.

656. **(D)** In the tables that accompany the question, the number of hypertensive persons in the community is 200. The number of patients with hypertension who also report a history of myocardial infarction (MI) is 15. The prevalence is therefore 15 in a population of 200, which may be translated as a rate of 75 per 1000.

657. **(D)** In the study described in the question, the prevalence rate is the total number of cases occurring in the community, divided by the number of members in the community, multiplied by 1000. This is a point prevalence rate: the number of individuals who have had an MI at the time the questionnaire is administered. Thus, the prevalence is $(20 \div 1000)\,1000 = 20/1000$.

658. **(E)** The chi-square test is the most appropriate statistical test in the situation described in the question. It is designed to describe with a single number how much the frequencies in each cell of a box of paired readings differ from the frequency we would expect if there were no relationship between the observed readings. If the observed readings are similar to expected readings, the chi-square will be a small number. If there is a greater difference, the chi-square will be larger. The mathematical equation is:

$$\chi^2 = \Sigma \frac{(O - E)^2}{E}$$

659. **(E)** In a questionnaire relating to history, patients' knowledge as to whether or not they

have hypertension or have had an MI might be sufficiently accurate to allow further statistical analysis. The data provided in this questionnaire are not adequate for more detailed statistical analysis. The questionnaire (Table 6–2) relies on memory recall, which at best is questionable, for comparison with an actual examination (Table 6–3). Criteria for establishing a diagnosis of MI and, if possible, actual blood pressure readings, as well as a definition of hypertension, are required. The crux of epidemiologic analysis is a detailed criterion for establishing a diagnosis. With this additional information, relevant statistical tests could be applied. In the absence of this information, any further statistical analysis is likely to lead to misleading results.

660. **(D)** The odds ratio (OR) is determined as the odds of hypertension in those with MI relative to the odds of hypertension in those without MI:

$$OR = \frac{15/5}{185/795} = \frac{15 \times 795}{5 \times 185} \approx 13$$

661. **(C)**.

$$OR = \frac{4/1}{36/59} = \frac{4 \times 95}{1 \times 36} = 6.6$$

Thus, the sample data underestimates the effect of hypertension on MI.

662. **(C)** The general formula of chi-square is

$$X^2(df) = \Sigma \frac{(O-E)^2}{E}$$

where O = observed count in category and E = expected count in category if the null hypothesis is true. It is designed to make comparisons of proportions, but the data must be presented in raw numerical form. The test is designed for the comparison of paired or independent samples, for example, the proportion of persons exposed to a certain level of radiation developing leukemia compared to the number of those who also develop the disease but who have not been exposed.

663. **(C)** For a normal distribution, the proportion of the population falling below 1 SD from the mean is 16%.

664. **(D)** The SEM and the SD measure two very different things. The SEM is always smaller than the SD. Some medical investigators are persuaded erroneously to use the SEM in reporting data. The SD quantifies the variability in the population, but the SEM quantifies variability in the estimate of the mean from different samples in the same population. The mean of a sample population may not reflect the mean of the whole population. However, the mean value of the collection of all possible sample means will equal the mean of the original population.

665. **(D)** One group contains 90 women, among whom there are 89 degrees of freedom, and the other contains 110, with 109 degrees of freedom. Thus, for the whole series, there are 198 degrees of freedom. Degrees of freedom are not based on the measures or deviations, but on the number of individuals being *studied (less the first individual for whom there is no variation)*.

666. **(E)** An assigned value is generally used for each group class. This is frequently indicated by Xi, where Xi is the value assigned to each member of the *i*th class, usually taken as *i*th class interval. This value may be either the mean or the mode of the sample readings within the class. This method is generally considered to be more accurate than either the lowest or highest reading.

667. **(C)** Humans are the usual reservoir of *Vibrio cholerae*. It tolerates exposure and drying poorly. It survives longest in water, especially if the water is at temperatures of 18 to 23°C (60 to 70°F). It does not spread on infected clothing (fomites). Direct person-to-person transmission probably does not occur. Contaminated water is the main source of infection (eg, frequent exposure to polluted surface water through bathing, food preparation, and utensil washing). Although flies may transport small numbers of vibrios from

excreta to food, lack of multiplication makes it unlikely that flies play an important part in transmission. Mosquitoes are not vectors.

668. **(B)** "Swimmers' itch" is caused by penetration of the skin by cercariae, the fluke stage of schistosome organisms. The normal hosts are usually aquatic birds, with mollusks serving as intermediate hosts. The cercariae die in the skin and cause a pruritic papular rash. The cercariae of three forms of schistosomiasis are pathogenic for humans: *Schistosoma mansoni, Schistosoma haematobium,* and *Schistosoma japonicum.* These give rise to blood fluke disease, which affects 75% or more of the population in endemic areas. Swimmers' itch, unlike schistosomiasis, may be contracted in the United States.

669. **(C)** The geographic pattern of MS has been established in many countries. The greater the latitude (the further north or south from the equator), the greater the prevalence. Consideration of viruses such as measles are thought to be a contributory cause, but no definitive conclusion can be drawn. Blacks and Asians have a lower incidence of MS than whites. There is no difference in prevalence between rural and urban areas. Females have an incidence 50% higher than males. Persons born in warmer climates retain the same susceptibility to the disease even when they move to an area where MS is more prevalent.

670. **(C)** No denominator data are provided, only numerators. Measures of disease or event occurrence are dependent on the size of the population in which the disease occurs or event takes place. In this example, the sizes (denominators) of the two populations among which the events took place (those who did and did not wear life jackets) have not been provided. It is possible that the size of the population of life jacket users may be small in comparison with the size of the population of nonusers. Confounding variables, such as drowning when falling from a bridge or drowning in stormy weather, are not mentioned but might be relevant. Based on the data provided, no explanations of the differences between life jacket use and nonuse are appropriate.

671. **(C)** Close contact with body secretions such as urine and saliva are a hazard to staff, visitors, and other children in day care centers. CMV is the greatest secondary infection of AIDS patients, affecting 40% of patients. The risk of transfusion-acquired CMV is greatest when patients receive blood from multiple donors. Infants can be infected not only during passage through the cervix, but also from breast milk and the mother's saliva. Culturing urine remains the most widely used means to detect CMV.

672. **(C)** Immune globulin (IG) has not been found to convey passive immunity against mumps. Passive immunity against chickenpox is best achieved by administration of specific IG (varicella-zoster immune globulin). When given after exposure to rubella, immune serum globulin may modify or suppress symptoms but does not prevent infection or viremia. It therefore provides no benefit when administered to pregnant women exposed to rubella. Babies born after such therapy have been demonstrated to have congenital rubella. IG does modify or prevent the development of measles in exposed individuals older than 6 months of age, when the maternal antibody wanes. Hepatitis A epidemics occurring in the food service industry are best prevented by careful hygiene and administration of hepatitis A vaccine to workers.

673. **(C)** Chelating drugs are given as treatment for symptomatic poisoning by lead and other heavy metals. They should not be given prophylactically, since the agents themselves have some possible toxic side effects. These toxic effects may add to those already caused by ingestion of the metals and may actually increase absorption of the metal. For these reasons, advice should be given to workers to seek employment away from exposure to the offending agent while therapy continues.

674. **(E)** Only excision by scalpel allows for accurate microscopic histologic examination of

the specimen. This is essential to establish an accurate diagnosis. If the condition has been previously diagnosed in an individual and the lesion is small and clearly defined, any of the other listed methods of treatment may be considered. Scalpel excision by a competent, experienced surgeon is the safest procedure.

675. **(C)** The engineer in a diesel engine room may be working in an environment in which the noise exposure level exceeds that permitted by the Occupational Safety and Health Administration (OSHA) regulations. Work for 8 hours a day is permitted in noise levels as great as 90 dB A, for 2 hours at 100 dB A, and half an hour at 110 dB A. The noise in a diesel engine room has been rated at 125 dB A. This noise is likely to be continuous. A scraper-loader operator may be working in a noise level of 117 dB A, which again is likely to be continuous. The riveting machine produces a noise level of 110 dB A, but this noise is a rapid repeated impact rather than continuous. A jet airplane at ramp generates 117 dB A, but this is also not continuous. An oxygen torch generates 121 dB A, which again is not likely to be continuous. In each of these occupations, ear protection is essential.

676. **(E)** A wide variety of pulmonary function tests may be performed in well-equipped pulmonary laboratories, but spirometry alone can be performed effectively in a physician's office. The equipment need not be expensive to be reliable, and its use has been required by OSHA for medical surveillance of certain occupational hazards. Most lung diseases will yield abnormal results on spirometry long before the patient complains of symptoms, so the technique can be a useful screening method in these circumstances. As tests of function, spirometry results do not aid in differentiating among various causes.

677. **(C)** Several concepts are important in determining the sensitivity of tests. The percentage sensitivity is the percentage of individuals with the disease (true positives [TP]) detected by the tests. False negatives (FN) are those who have the disease but who were not

detected by the test. The percentage sensitivity is calculated as $TP/(TP + FN) \times 100$. In the example given in the question, the calculation is $100/(100 + 50) \times 100 = 66.7\%$.

	Disease Present	Disease Absent	Totals
Test positive	100 (TP)	100 (FP)	200
Test negative	50 (FN)	350 (TN)	400
Totals	150	450	600

678. **(D)** The percentage specificity of a test is the percentage of those persons without the disease (true negatives, or TN) who were correctly labeled by the test as not diseased. The false positives (FP) are those who were incorrectly labeled by the test as having the disease. The specificity is thus expressed as $TN/(TN + FP) \times 100$. In the example given in the question, the calculation is $350/(350 + 100) \times 100 = 77.8\%$.

679. **(D)** HAV was first isolated in 1973. Since then, it has been demonstrated to be conveyed from person to person chiefly by the fecal–oral route. Outbreaks attributed to food and water supplies are reported frequently. While HAV infections have decreased in young children, they occur more frequently among young adults. A number of infant day care centers have reported outbreaks due to poor handling of diapers. In more advanced developing countries, such as Greece, Taiwan, and parts of China, improved hygiene has reduced outbreaks of hepatitis A disease. Outbreaks in groups of young adults (eg, in summer camps) are common. Outbreaks from raw shellfish have been a common source of HAV.

680. **(C)** The mean, or average, reading is the total of all readings divided by the number of readings, or $x = 2\, x/n$. In the example described in the question, $Z\, x$ equals 639; the number of readings is 9. Therefore the mean is 639 divided by 9, or 71.

681. **(B)** The modal reading is the most popular or most frequently occurring observation in a group of data. This reading is not very adaptable to many statistical calculations, and when the series is small, no modal reading may occur. When drawn in graph form, the determination of unimodal or bimodal distribution may be a helpful concept from which conclusions may be drawn. The distribution in the example that accompanies the question is unimodal.

682. **(D)** The median is the observation that lies in the middle of the series, if the observations are tabulated in numerical order. Half of the observations are lower in numerical value than the median, and the remainder are higher. Clearly, this value is easily identified if the series contains an odd number of readings. Although not very frequently used as a statistic, the median has the advantage of not being affected by extreme observations. For example, if the lowest reading of those in the question had been 55 instead of 61, the median would be unchanged.

683. **(C)** The range is the difference between the highest and lowest readings in a group of observations. The lowest reading is subtracted from the highest. Only one of these two readings is included in the range. If both were to be included, the range would be 20, as there are 20 possible values included in the limits of the data presented in the question. For simplicity, the first method is generally accepted. One disadvantage of the concept of range is that it may increase as the number of observations increases.

684. **(C)** The variance is the sum of the squares of the difference of each reading from the mean. This is a mathematical way of eliminating the opposing effects of negative and positive values. But the variance has a result that is of a different order than the original observations. The variance of 58.75 seems to have little relationship to a series of readings from 61 to 80. In order to determine a value that is the same order as the observations, the SD is calculated as the square root of the variance. This is mathematically represented as

$$SD(x) = \sqrt{V(x)} \cdot V(x) = \Sigma(x - x)^2/(n - 1)$$

Without using a calculator, it can be seen that the nearest correct answer (correct to 1 decimal place) is 7.7.

685. **(D)** Although the difference appears small, differences in crude mortality rates may enable specific deductions to be made. Since the differences seem to occur only in the older population, it is not generally warrantable to assume that living in one country is healthier than another. Of the statements listed, considering that age specific death rates were greater in all age groups except the elderly, only the fact that a greater proportion of the population in Sweden is in the older age groups could account for the difference in crude mortality rate.

686. **(C)** The odds ratio is used when the denominator data are missing. It is calculated using the formula for comparing smokers and non-smokers:

$$\frac{A \times D}{B \times C}$$

In this case, the mathematics is relatively simple: $(75 \times 75) + (25 \times 25)$. By reduction, this is $3 \times 3 + 1 = 9$.

687. **(E)** A true risk ratio cannot be calculated from a case control study.

688. **(B)** For ease of calculation, to illustrate the concept, the numbers in the question were kept simple. If the numbers of controls were increased, the difference would be smaller. The odds ratios are a reasonable estimate when denominator data are missing. Relative risk is determined when denominator data are available. Few case control experiments have denominator data.

689. **(B)** Bias is a systematic error that may be introduced, generally unwittingly, into an investigation. Selection bias is due to systemic differences between those selected and not selected for a study. When selecting all admissions to a community hospital, alcoholics may be overrepresented among hospital pa-

tients and not reflect the community base from which the patients were admitted. Further, the investigator has not chosen a control sample but only potentially patients already in the hospital, which further invalidates any outcome. While other biases may creep into this study, the selection bias is the major problem with the study.

690. **(A)** Cutaneous anthrax is associated with a characteristic skin lesion, which becomes infected by the introduction of the bacillus through the skin. Occasionally, an infected carcass is not identified before butchering. A minor wound on the butcher may become infected. Human anthrax is secondary to the disease in animals, primarily mammals. In humans, the disease has three major clinical forms: cutaneous, inhalational, and gastrointestinal.

691. **(D)** Rodents frequently infest granaries, despite strenuous efforts to control them. Murine (endemic) typhus has its principal reservoir in rodents and is conveyed to humans by flea bites. In the United States, murine or endemic typhus occurs mainly in the Southeastern and Gulf states. It is also common in parts of South America, Africa, and Southeast Asia. The disease generally follows a less severe course than epidemic typhus.

692. **(B)** *Brucella* infections in humans follow a varied and sometimes chronic or recurrent course. Chronic disease is rare in appropriately treated patients. Human infections generally occur through one of three routes: ingestion, direct contact, or inhalation. Cattle sheds become infected after abortion, a manifestation of the disease, or occasionally after normal parturition. Worldwide, ingestion of unpasteurized dairy products is the primary source of infection.

693. **(C)** Lyme disease appears to be increasingly common, having been identified relatively recently. It may be identified some time after the initial illness, which in many ways is a rather vague collection of symptoms. The vector is a tick found on the white-footed mouse, which is the reservoir. Not only ranchers, but any person who spends a significant amount of time in wooded areas is at risk of Lyme disease.

694. **(A)** Local health departments make plans for the entire population in the jurisdiction for which they have responsibility, whether it is a single county, city, or multicounty health department. Their planning is population based. This involves estimating health requirements, matching them with existing resources, and outlining a health strategy based on the deficit or surplus demonstrated.

695. **(B)** A distinction is frequently made between what the patient wants (which would be used if available and money was no object), needs (services determined by professionals to be appropriate), and demands (services that are actually used in the current market situation). Planning for an HMO is based on that segment of the population or "market" for which the HMO is responsible. The population may or may not live in contiguous areas. The planning is designed to identify goals and objectives in institutional terms: What is the market for the services the organization provides, and what is the estimate of future demands? The population need (as opposed to the population demand) is rarely a concern of institutional planners.

696. **(D)** Program planning concerns itself with neither the fiscal need for a particular service nor its marketability. By definition, "the program" (eg, maternal and child health care) will be developed and provided as directed by the state or local government. The planning is directed to carry out program goals for a targeted (select) population (pregnant women and their infants). This type of planning is necessary to implement government or private foundation–sponsored programs.

697–701. **(697-C, 698-B, 699-A, 700-B, 701-A)** Epidemic typhus (classical typhus fever, or louse-borne typhus) has disappeared from most areas of the world but might reappear in conditions of famine, war, or other disasters. There are small areas where it is endemic. The responsible organism, a rickettsia, is conveyed from case to case by the human body louse, *Pediculus humanus corporis*. Malaria, in its various forms (*Plasmodium falciparum, P vivax, P ovale,* and *P malariae*), is spread from human to human by females of the various *Anopheles* group of mosquitoes. Dengue fever has a worldwide distribution in tropical and subtropical areas. In addition to producing the classical fever with severe myalgia (breakbone fever), it can also cause a hemorrhagic fever. The causative agent, a group B arbovirus with four distinct serogroups, is virus-conveyed from case to case by the *Aedes aegypti* mosquito. Colorado tick fever occurs mainly in mountainous areas of the United States within the range of its vector, *Dermacentor andersoni*. The highest incidence is in May and June. Several hundred cases are recorded annually, but it is likely that the actual incidence is much higher. Avoidance of tick bites is the principal control measure. Yellow fever is African in origin but has spread to and remains endemic in equatorial regions of Central and South America. The vector, *A aegypti,* has also spread worldwide, but surprisingly, cases have not been reported in India and Southeast Asia. The illness varies in severity from a mild, nonspecific fever to a more severe condition that causes hepatitis with hemorrhagic and renal manifestations.

702–706. (702-C, 703-A, 704-C, 705-B, 706-E) In the United States, the organization of food and water control is complex. Among the federal control agencies, the EPA is the most recent, and in many ways the most active and powerful. This agency has now set up an elaborate system of regulation and control of the use of pesticides (which until 1970 were the responsibility of the USDA) and has banned the marketing of chlorphenothane (DDT) for use in the home. The FDA has authority to remove food from the market if it contains pesticides (eg, PCBs in fish) in excess of the action levels set by the EPA. The FDA also retains the authority to remove from the market any food with inappropriate additives,

that contains substances harmful to human health, that is stored in unsanitary conditions, that has decomposed, or that is not fit for consumption. The USDA enforces wholesomeness standards that it sets for the production and sale of meat. International control is assisted by the WHO. This agency has mounted control programs for the eradication of communicable disease with conspicuous success in the case of smallpox. It also publishes the International Statistical Classification of Disease (ICD-9).

707–710. (707-B, 708-E, 709-A, 710-D) Knowing the incubation period (average and range) of a pathogen can be important in determining the source of infection in food-borne disease. For example, knowing what food was eaten on the day of an attack of food poisoning may not help in establishing *Clostridium botulinum* as the cause of illness, since its average incubation period is typically 12 to 48 hours but may be as long as 6 days. Obtaining accurate histories of food consumed over this period of time will be difficult. Staphylococci cause food-borne disease by the production of enterotoxin. As no time is required after ingestion for the growth of colonies in the infected host, the incubation period is brief. *Clostridium perfringens*, formerly known as *C welchii,* causes food-borne disease, particularly when meat is prepared in bulk for consumption at a banquet or in an institution. The spores that survive initial cooking may start reproducing during cooling and may persist if subsequent rewarming is not completed to a temperature above the 60°C (140°F) required to kill the organisms. *Salmonella* may also survive in meat and other products if cooking is inadequate and heat does not penetrate below the surface of the food. The organisms multiply in the gut of the infected host, and low infective doses may therefore have longer incubation periods.

711.   (C) PCBs were extensively used in the manufacture of electrical transformers until production was halted in the mid-1970s. The first sign of chronic exposure to these substances is the appearance of an acne-like eruption with inflammatory pustules. Other effects are eye irritation and gastrointestinal disturbance. The substances are persistent, and more than 25% of the population in the United States was discovered to have residues of greater than one part per million (ppm) in adipose tissue. Dietary exposure of the general population has been alleged to occur through milk, eggs, cheese, meat, and fish.

712. **(E)** Organophosphorus compounds have been widely used since the 1950s as insecticides, both in national pest control programs and domestically. They have been responsible for many deaths on a worldwide basis, despite the lives initially saved by control of mosquitoes and malaria. From the point of view of the environmental toxicologist, it was perhaps fortuitous that many pests began to develop resistance to the substances fairly early in the use of these compounds. More recently, concern for environmental control has further limited their use; studies have attributed carcinogenic properties to several of these pesticides.

713. **(A)** Nitrosamines are highly toxic and dangerous to handle when used as solvents. Toxic amounts may be absorbed without warning because danger signals such as specific odor or irritant effects are lacking. The manufacture of rubber, dyes, lubricating oils, explosives, insecticides, and fungicides, as well as the electrical industry, all have associations with these substances. Nitrosamines have animal carcinogenic properties and have been transmitted transplacentally in rats.

714. **(B)** Epoxy compounds are used in the production of resins. They cause irritation of the skin and mucosae and have caused acute pulmonary edema.

715. **(D)** Formaldehyde commercial solutions contain up to 15% methanol. Formaldehyde has numerous industrial applications including, use as a base for urea formaldehyde resins. The odors of products manufactured with formaldehyde products have been responsible for actions against manufacturers of tightly built manufactured homes.

716. **(D)** Ozone is generated by electrical storms and UV light and electric arcs and some forms of fuel combustion. In the stratosphere, it is protective by blocking solar radiation. At 10 ppm, it can cause pulmonary edema and tracheal pain and is believed to cause asthma. Based on animal tests and observations of gases trapped during inversions, an action level of 10 ppm has been set for workplace exposure.

717. **(C)** Hydrogen sulfide produces nausea, headache, and shortness of breath. Because it paralyzes the nasal receptors at a concentration of 150 ppm and cannot be smelled shortly after exposure, it is highly dangerous, with instant death from a concentration as low as 1000 ppm.

718. **(B)** Methane (coal damp) is a frequent cause of death in inadequately ventilated mines and wells. It acts as an asphyxiant as well as being explosive. Miners used to take caged animals, especially birds, with them. The birds succumbed to the asphyxiants (methane and carbon dioxide) sooner than humans.

719. **(A)** Carbon monoxide is widely recognized as a product of incomplete combustion. The amounts produced by cigarette smoking are not insignificant. The gas combines with hemoglobin preferentially to form carboxyhemoglobin. This diminishes the oxygen-carrying capacity of the blood. The resulting anoxia is the major hazard. The onset of symptoms is insidious. Individuals exposed to carbon monoxide may not voluntarily take the action necessary to remove themselves from the toxic fumes.

720. **(E)** Sulphur dioxide is an irritant gas. It causes tearing, mucous membrane irritation, cough, and eventually pulmonary edema. Like other irritant gases, in large quantities, it will damage alveolar and also capillary endothelial cells.

721. **(D)** There has been a great deal of discussion about earlier introduction of mammography for women at younger age ranges. The recommendation of the U.S. Task Force is that mammography be conducted every 1 to 2 years from ages 50 through 69 when there is no history of high risk.

722. **(F)** Routine screening with a Pap smear is recommended for every women who is or has been sexually active. Start when sexual activity is started. If smear is negative, repeat every 3 years.

723. **(G)** Annual fecal occult blood testing or flexible sigmoidoscopy (no periodicity) is recommended for all persons over 50 years of age. No recommendations are made for rectal digital examination due to lack of data.

724. **(C)** Screening with hepatitis B surface antigen (HbsAg) is recommended during the first trimester of pregnancy (during the first prenatal visit) for all pregnant women. The test may be repeated during the third trimester for women who were negative at the first test but are at high risk for acquiring the infection during pregnancy.

725. **(A)** Routine screening for prostate cancer with digital rectal examination. Serum tumor markers (eg, PSA) or transurethral ultrasound is not recommended.

726–730. **(726-A, 727-B, 728-B, 729-A, 730-C)** IG given before exposure or within 14 days of exposure is 75 to 85% effective in preventing symptomatic illness. IG is produced from the plasma of normal adults and does not contain sufficient antibody to prevent hepatitis B infection. Hepatitis B immune globulin (HBIG) is prepared from plasma known to contain high antibody titers for HBsAg and is specific for hepatitis B. Studies of the usefulness of IG in hepatitis C have yielded equivocal results. IG administered to individuals exposed to measles infection who are susceptible to the disease has been shown to be effective if given within 6 days. Recent use of IG is a contraindication to immunization

with rubella vaccine; infants with congenital rubella syndrome have been born to women given IG shortly after exposure. The routine use of IG is contrain-dicated. IG should be administered only if abortion would not be considered under any circumstances. *(Last, 1997, pp 67, 133)*

731–737. **(731-A, 732-D, 733-E, 734-D, 735-C, 736-B, 737-D)** The incubation period for diphtheria is 1 to 7 days. The incubation period for chickenpox is 10 to 21 days, average 14. Infectious mononucleosis, caused by the Epstein–Barr virus, has an estimated incubation period of 30 to 50 days. The incubation period following infection by the mumps virus is usually 16 to 18 days but, like chickenpox, may vary from 12 to 25 days. Pertussis has a shorter incubation period, *usually* 7 to 10 days, with a variation of 4 to 21 days. The usual period from contamination with tetanus spores to clinical symptoms is generally 6 to 8 days. For rubella, the incubation period is from 14 to 21 days, but usually ranges from 16 to 18 days. *(Last, 1997, pp 74, 76, 78, 89, 90, 141)*

738–748. **(738-I, 739-B, 740-D, 741-E, 742-G, 743-A, 744-F, 745-C, 746-J, 747-H, 748-A)** Giardiasis may cause a chronic diarrheal syndrome, with malabsorption and weight loss. It is found in 20% of homosexual males. Its distribution is worldwide, particularly where hygienic standards are not high. It also occurs sporadically in high-risk individuals. Streptococcal pyoderma, including erysipelas and impetigo, has been demonstrated to precede acute glomerulonephritis. Even when appropriate antibiotics are given in adequate dosage and duration for these conditions, renal damage may still result. *Mycoplasma* infections are particularly common in families with younger children. They are frequently imported to the family by school-aged children, leading to a low-grade fever and persisting tracheobronchitis in the parents, or more acutely, an atypical pneumonia. *Bordetella pertussis* is the organism that gives rise to pertussis or whooping cough. In an unprotected child, the classic inspiratory stridor or whoop is pathognomonic. More serious cases can result in pneumonia or atelectasis. *E coli* was first reported as a cause of watery diarrhea in nurseries in the 1940s. Although nursery epidemics with enteropathogenic serotypes had decreased in recent years in the United States, the increase of infant–child day care centers has resulted in their relatively frequent occurrence. Furunculosis is most frequently caused by coagulase-positive staphylococcal infections. The public health significance of this largely relates to the hazards of skin infections in food handlers and subsequent staphylococcal toxin in the food, leading to staphylococcal intoxication food-borne disease. *H pylori* is a frequent part of the normal flora of the intestinal tract. It is also known as *Campylobacter pylori*. Epidemiologic studies have associated the organism with gastric ulcer, but not with duodenal ulcer. *H influenzae*, together with the pneumococcus, is one of the two most common causes of acute otitis media. It is one of the most common antecedents of deafness in the world. *C perfringens*, with rare exceptions, is transmitted in a meat dish prepared in bulk. Under propitious circumstances for the organism, especially upon cooling of the food, bacterial multiplication can be very rapid. Symptoms begin to occur in the affected population in about 12 hours. Epidemic typhus is a rickettsial illness. Man is the host and long-term reservoir. The vectors are body lice (*Pediculis humanus corporis*) The rickettsia are not present in human excretions and cannot be transmitted by person-to-person contact. Toxic shock syndrome is an acute multisystem illness due to infection with *S aureus*. Most reported cases have occurred in previously healthy young women.

749–753. (749-H, 750-C, 751-B, 752-A, 753-F) Asbestosis is a pneumoconiosis-causing chronic lung disease. Additionally, asbestos passes through the alveoli into the pleura and peritoneum, giving rise to mesothelioma. In addition to cigarette smoking as a major etiologic factor in bladder cancer, occupational risks are frequently additive. For example, benzidine-derived dyes have been recognized as potential human carcinogens. Ura-

nium miners have an excessive mortality rate from lung cancer. Ores containing uranium include all of its decay products. Radon diffuses out of the rock into the mine atmosphere. Many workers, including those exposed to natural sunlight, are exposed to excess UV radiation. Also included are arc welders and those who use the radiation for its germicidal properties, such as physicians. In addition to causing eye injuries, chronic UV exposure can lead to premalignant and malignant lesions of the skin. Radium is known to cause bone sarcomas. Although rarely used in industry today, women who were employed to paint dials of watches were recognized to be at risk. Radium implants, formerly used for therapy, have now been almost completely replaced.

754–755. (754-A, 755-C) The following table was constructed using the data in the question. The false positives were the 4995 in the population who truly had a negative HIV, but the test incorrectly labeled them as having the disease. Conversely, only two people had false-negative tests.

	Disease		
Test	Present	Absent	Totals
Positive	98 (sensitivity)	4995	5093
Negative	2	94,905 (specificity)	94,905
Totals	100 (prevalence)	99,900	100,000

756–760. (756-A, 757-B, 758-C, 759-B, 760-B) Three types of prevention have been identified, depending on when intervention is made: primary, secondary, and tertiary prevention. Primary prevention includes preventing exposure to risk factors of disease and reduction of risk factors in those exposed. Secondary prevention refers to early detection (screening) and prompt treatment of disease in asymptomatic individuals. Tertiary prevention refers to limitation of the effects of disease and disability, where disease had already occurred and left residual damage.

761. (B) In a randomized, controlled trial, the determination of treatment group assignment is left to chance. The procedure maximizes the probability that the two groups are similar in important background characteristics. Thus, it avoids self-selection of study subjects to different exposure groups.

762. **(A)** In a cross-sectional study design, it is generally difficult to ascertain the antecedent-consequent aspects of the hypothesized relationship. In other words, since the exposure and outcome are measured at a given point in time, it is difficult to determine which came first.

763. **(C)** A cohort study classifies study subjects by exposure status and follows them forward in time to determine development of disease. More than one disease can be targeted as outcomes of interest.

764. **(D)** A case-control study defines cases and controls and retrospectively assesses the frequency of exposure. Multiple exposures can be assessed in connection with a specific disease.

765. **(E)** The design of a cohort study requires a follow-up of a group of subjects who are susceptible but free of the disease of interest at the beginning of the study period.

766. **(D)** In a prospective cohort design, a group of subjects at risk of developing disease are followed over a specified period of time. This design permits the direct calculation of incidence by dividing the number of subjects who developed the disease of interest during the follow-up period by the population or person-time at risk. In contrast, incidence cannot be calculated directly from the other observational study designs (cross-sectional, case-control).

767. **(B)** The odds ratio for those who drink 5+ cups of coffee relative to those who drink 0 cups is calculated as follows: $(60 \times 32)/(9 \times 65) = 3.3$.

768. **(A)** Calculating the odds ratio for each coffee drinking category using 0 cups per day as reference gives odds ratios of 1.7, 2.4, and 3.3 for the 1 to 2, 3 to 4, and 5+ categories, re-

spectively. These results suggest that the risk of pancreatic cancer increases with rising levels of coffee consumption.

769. **(B)** The health survey was conducted in a defined population at a particular date. With this information, the prevalence of conjunctivitis can be determined, but not the incidence. Measuring incidence requires information on new occurrences of the disease from a follow-up study.

770. **(B)** By definition, sensitivity is the probability of testing positive if the disease is truly present. It indicates the percentage of persons with the disease of interest who have positive test results.

771. **(C)** Positive predictive value estimates the probability of disease in those who have positive test results. It indicates the percentage of persons with positive test results who actually have the disease of interest.

772. **(E)** Additional information on prevalence is needed to calculate the positive predictive value.

773. **(B)** The randomized, controlled trial is the best study design to test the efficacy of a new drug, because the design permits random assignment of study subjects into treatment groups and is not influenced by the investigator's or patient's preference. All the other study designs listed are observational and are less suitable in testing the efficacy of a drug.

774. **(D)** The incidence rate of CHD in smokers (IRe) is calculated by dividing the number of cases of CHD by the person-years at risk calculated from all smokers:

$$IR_e = \frac{\text{No. of new cases}}{\text{Person-years}} = \frac{160}{1000 \times 10 \ yr} \times 1000 \ pyr = 16/1000 \ pyr$$

775. **(A)** The incidence rate of CHD in nonsmokers (IRo) is calculated by dividing the number of cases of CHD by the person-years at risk calculated from all nonsmokers:

$$IR_o = \frac{\text{No. of new cases}}{\text{Person-years}} = \frac{60}{1000 \times 10 \; yr} \times 1000 \; pyr = 6/1000 \; pyr$$

776. **(C)** The rate ratio (RR) is calculated by dividing the incidence rate of CHD in smokers by the incidence rate in nonsmokers:

$$RR = \frac{IR_e}{IR_o} = \frac{16/1000 \; pyr}{6/1000 \; pyr} \times 1000 \; pyr = 2.7$$

777. **(A)** The 10-year rate difference (RD) is calculated by subtracting the incidence in the unexposed (IRo) from the incidence in the exposed (IRe).

778. **(E)** The attributable risk percent (AR%) is calculated as follows:

$$AR\% = \frac{IR_e - IR_o}{IR_e} \times 100 = 62.5\%$$

779. **(C)** The problem can be represented by the following table:

	Breast Cancer	
Abortion	**Yes**	**No**
Yes	15	10
No	85	190
Total	100	200

The odds of exposure among cases is calculated by dividing the probability that a case was exposed by the probability that a case was not exposed: $(15/100)/(85/100) = 15/85 = 0.176$.

780. **(D)** The odds of exposure among controls is calculated by dividing the probability that a control was exposed by the probability that a control was not exposed: $(10/200)/(190/200) = 10/190 = 0.053$.

781. **(E)** The odds ratio (OR) for exposure is calculated by dividing the odds of exposure for cases by the odds of exposure for controls: $OR = (15/85)/(190/200) = 3.35$.

782. **(B)** A z transformation is needed to use the standard normal distribution as follows:

$$z = \frac{X - \mu}{\sigma} = \frac{130 - 120}{10} = 1.00$$

We know from the characteristics of the normal distribution that the area above an SD of 1.00 is approximately 16%. Thus, 16% of the subjects have a systolic blood pressure above 130 mm Hg.

783. **(A)** As shown in the previous question:

$$z_1 = \frac{X_1 - \mu}{\sigma} = \frac{100 - 120}{10} = -2.00$$

$$z_2 = \frac{X_2 - \mu}{\sigma} = \frac{140 - 120}{10} = +2.00$$

Since the area between −2 and +2 is 0.95, 95% of the subjects have a systolic blood pressure between 100 and 140 mm Hg.

784. **(A)** The illness described is consistent with hemolytic uremic dyndrome associated with *E coli* O157:H7 infection. *E coli* O157:H7 is the most common strain found of the enterohemorrhagic *E coli* (EHEC) group. Although its most common reservoir is thought to be in cattle, it has been found in other livestock. The usual mode of exposure is contamination of beef. The problem is compounded significantly when beef is ground and mixed in bulk. Testing and elimination programs do not appear sensitive enough to eliminate exposure, although active research in the area continues. In addition, there are many other outbreaks associated with fresh vegetables, bean sprouts, and unpasteurized juices. It is hypothesized that these are due to contamination with human or animal waste. Since the organism is killed by heating, thorough cooking of ground beef products and washing of produce intended to be served fresh is the most practical intervention. Currently, this remains the most practical advice to give the public.

785. **(B)** The actual causes of death were tabulated in a historic paper by McGinnis and Foege in 1993. Of 2,100,000 deaths, the top three contributors to mortality were tobacco

(400,000), diet and inactivity (300,000), and alcohol (100,000). *(Bodenheimer and Grombach, p 136)*

786. **(D)** Since the 1980s, inflation in medical costs had been double digit. These costs were largely carried by employers who provide health care coverage for employees, purchasers of group plans, and governmental providers of care such as Medicaid and Medicare. President Clinton's Health Security Act was intended to correct this, but it was perceived as too regulatory and was not passed. Some officials advocated a one-payor (government) system as a solution, but this received even less support. After failure of passage of the Health Security Act, employers and other large-scale purchasers turned to managed care concepts to control the double-digit inflation. This has apparently succeeded. Althoug the number of providers is increasing, it is not related to increasing costs.

787. **(C)** This is because the insurance company charges premiums to groups based on its experience with their use of health care services. The opposite approach is community rating, which charges one premium to all groups. The premium is set so that with some groups, the company loses money; with others, it makes money. Premiums based on community rating in this instance might be $300 for each individual regardless of his or her group. Obviously, some groups will subsidize others. Since community rating redistributes funding from the healthy to the sick, it makes health insurance more affordable to chronically ill groups. *(Bodenheimer and Grumbach, pp 10–11)*

788. **(E)** The patient has a positive reaction to PPD. This indicates tuberculosis infection, but not necessarily clinical disease. Since conversion is recent (she had a negative test last year), the risk of progressing to disease is relatively large compared to the risk of hepatotoxicity from preventive treatment with isoniazid. Such preventive treatment is 65 to 80% effective in preventing progression to active disease.

789. **(E)** The food item having the largest difference in attack rates is tuna salad. There are several reasons that there is an attack rate for those not eating the tuna salad. One is people's inability to recall exactly what they ate (recall bias). This gets worse as more time passes from the event. The other is the possibility of a background rate of disease. These people may have acquired the disease from another source. *(Wallace and Doebbeling, p 264)*

790. **(A)** Medicaid and Medicare began under federal legislation in 1966. Medicaid is a state-run program funded with federal and state tax dollars. It was established to provide medical services to the poor, with special consideration to pregnant women and small children. Medicare is a federal program, completely financed and run by the federal government. Its purpose is to provide medical care to citizens over 65. Blue Cross/Blue Shield is a private insurance that must be purchased; the Robert Wood Johnson Foundation is a large foundation that provides grants; and the WIC program is a food supplement program for needy mothers and children. *(Bodenheimer and Grumbach, p 213)*

791. **(A)** Transmission of rabies virus by a bat bite has been well documented, and in many areas of the country, bats are known to harbor rabies virus. There are also well-documented cases of human rabies due to viral strains found in bats, but without a good history of being bitten. Therefore, presumptive treatment is recommended in the case of a bite (and in some cases a possible bite) when the bat cannot be recovered and tested. Lacrosse encephalitis, distemper, and tularemia are not known to be transmitted by bats. Tetanus is unlikely, because a child this age has probably been immunized.

792. **(B)** Manufacturing, storage, and shipping problems do occur. However, they have not been related to nationwide failures. It is more likely that the vaccine in use is not completely protective against the prevalent viral strain. The WHO monitors influenza outbreaks worldwide. Based on strains present in outbreaks, and especially in the Pacific

Rim, WHO makes a recommendation every spring on the antigens to use for the fall immunization campaign. Manufacturing then begins. Although their track record is good in this regard, antigen changes in influenza may reach the United States undetected or ahead of schedule. (*Wallace and Doebbeling, p 110*)

793. **(B)** Testing for the presence of coliform bacteria is a standard bacterial test of water quality. Since coliform bacteria are ubiquitous in nature, their presence means only that the water has been contaminated with water from the ground surface or the septic system. It is only an indicator. Coliform bacteria are not the principal agents of disease. It is the other agents introduced into the water by the contamination that create the risk. The problem should be resolved before using the well water. A common cause of contamination is poor well construction, resulting in surface water moving down the outside of the well casing and into the water source. (*Wallace and Doebbeling, p 745*)

794. **(E)** The U.S. Congress passed the Safe Drinking Water Act (SDWA) in 1974 and amended it in 1986. Prior to this, the Public Health Service provided recommendations that were adopted by states. The SDWA created maximum contaminant levels and established a process for setting their values. The SDWA placed most large public drinking water systems under some form of federal regulation. (*Wallace and Doebbeling, p 741*)

795. **(D)** Crude mortality rates for a population are calculated using total deaths divided by total population. Differences in the age compositon of the population can make an enormous difference in crude mortality rates, since the elderly have a much higher mortality rate. Adjusting for age computes a hypothetical "adjusted" rate for each country based on their own age-specific mortality rates, but using standard population. The technique is called age adjusting or standardization. It is used in other rate studies as well. For instance, the crude mortality rate for MI would be different between a largely middle-aged population and an older one. Age adjusting will allow comparison.

796. **(B)** Although clinical trials can determine which treatment works best, they cannot determine the cost of this success. Unfortunately, they do not take into account costs and ultimate benefits, which would be the role of a cost–benefit study. If properly constructed, with study and control groups randomly drawn from the general population, the results should be applicable to the general population. In addition, they usually determine what works best by measurement of a clinical endpoint. In many cases, the treatment may achieve its objective, but the change in parameters may not be significant.

797. **(E)** It is true that mammography in older women is technically easier and probably more sensitive. However, the burden of cost and mortality resulting from screening women less than 40 was the real reason. For first mammograms of women aged 40 to 49, cancers were diagnosed at half the rate of the aged 50- to 59-year-old group, yet twice as many follow-up diagnostic tests were performed. Simply put, the cost in terms of dollars, mortality from testing, and mortality from radiation exposure were not considered to be worth the benefit. (*U.S. Preventive Services Task Force, pp 73–84*)

798. **(B)** The U.S. infant mortality rate for 1997 was 7.1 infant deaths/1000 live births.

799. **(D)** In 1997, the white infant mortality rate was 6.0 infant deaths/1000 live births. The black infant mortality rate was 13.7 infant deaths/1000 live births. This is approximately twice the white infant death rate. These are provisional numbers, supplied in the fall of 1998.

800. **(H)** Surveillance is the "ongoing systematic collection, analysis, and interpretation of health data." In this case, the system, once established, passively collects data for analysis. It means, literally, to watch over. (*Wallace and Doebbeling, p 741*)

801. **(C)** In this case, a system is lacking an automatic system for the collection of data; the data are actively solicited and cases recruited. This technique is much more suited to fast-breaking situations and to rare diseases of possible grave public health significance.

802. **(D)** Surveys are systematic interviewing of a sample population. They are extremely useful in obtaining information on the prevalence of conditions, use of health care resources, and the behaviors that influence health.

803. **(B)** An event like this is a full investigation. The investigators will use the full array of public health skills. Usually, they follow the 10 classic steps of an epidemiologic investigation:

1. Determine the existence of an epidemic.
2. Confirm the diagnosis.
3. Define and count the cases.
4. Orient the data in terms of time, place, and person.
5. Determine who is at risk of having the health problem.
6. Develop and test an explanatory hypothesis.
7. Compare the hypothesis with the proven facts.
8. Plan a more systematic study.
9. Prepare a written report.
10. Propose measures for control and prevention.

804. **(F)** In this case, the problem is identified and several solutions are at hand. All that remains is to pick an approach and provide the mechanism to implement it. This is the policy development side of public health. While at the highest levels it may not be public health workers that choose a policy option, the choice will certainly be affected by the information and analysis provided by public health professionals. *(Wallace and Doebbeling, p 31)*

805. **(B)** This activity is secondary prevention since it identifies individuals with a risk factor for a disease and attempts to prevent the disease. It is important to note that the disease itself is not yet present, only the risk factor for its development. In this case, the risk factor for development of atherosclerotic vessel disease was high cholesterol, and the subjects of the intervention did not yet have any symptoms.

806. **(A)** Primary prevention applies interventions to groups of individuals before they have disease and before they are identified as having risk factors. For instance, programs aimed at reducing atherosclerotic vessel disease by urging people to eat less fat are primary prevention. If the same program were aimed at people who already had risk factors such as hypercholesterolemia or a family history of coronary artery disease, it would be considered secondary prevention.

807. **(C)** Tertiary prevention is the correction of a diseased state. In this case, the patient already had developed disease from smoking. Cessation of tobacco use is simply treating the disease. In this sense, most medical therapy is tertiary prevention.

REFERENCES

Last JM, ed. *Maxcy-Rosenau's Textbook of Public Health & Preventive Medicine,* 13th ed. East Norwalk, CT: Appleton & Lange; 1992.

Hill BA. *Principles of Medical Statistics,* 8th ed. Oxford University Press; 1966.

LaDou I. *Occupational Medicine,* 2nd ed. Stamford, CT: Appleton & Lange; 1997.

Last JM. *Public Health and Human Ecology,* 2nd ed. Stamford, CT: Appleton & Lange; 1997.

U.S. Preventive Services Task Force. *Guide to Clinical Preventive Services,* 2nd ed. DHHS; 1996.

Zenz C. *Occupational Medicine,* 3rd ed. Editors. Dickerson BO, Horvath EP. Mosby, St. Louis; 1994

Dawson-Saunders B, Trapp RG, *Basic and Clinical Biostatistics,* 2nd ed. Appleton & Lange; 1994.

Greenburg RS, Daniels SR, Flanders WD, Eley JW, Boring JR, *Medical Epidemiology,* 2nd ed. Appleton & Lange; 1996.

Subspecialty List: Preventive Medicine

Question Number and Subspecialty

616. Epidemiology/Infectious disease
617. Epidemiology/Infectious disease
618. Occupational health/Toxicology
619. Chronic disease epidemiology/Secondary prevention
620. Epidemiology/Infectious disease/Host
621. Primary prevention/Infectious disease
622. Epidemiology/Infectious disease
623. Primary prevention/Infectious disease
624. Occupational health/Primary prevention
625. Chronic disease epidemiology/Secondary prevention
626. Primary prevention
627. Community epidemiology/Food hazards
628. Community epidemiology/Food hazards
629. Community epidemiology/Population distribution
630. Community epidemiology/Water hygiene
631. Descriptive epidemiology
632. Community epidemiology/Water hygiene
633. Community epidemiology/Lead poisoning prevention
634. Ethics/Occupational health
635. Ethics/Primary care
636. Analytic epidemiology
637. Public health law
638. Public health law
639. Primary prevention/Infectious disease
640. Public health law
641. Primary prevention/Infectious disease
642. Health administration
643. Health administration (disaster management)
644. Health administration
645. Health administration
646. Health administration
647. Biostatistics

648. Community epidemiology/Food hazards
649. Biostatistics
650. Biostatistics
651. Epidemiology/Infectious disease
652. Public health law
653. Epidemiology/Definition
654. Biostatistics
655. Epidemiology/Descriptive
656. Epidemiology/Descriptive
657. Epidemiology/Descriptive
658. Biostatistics
659. Biostatistics
660. Biostatistics
661. Biostatistics
662. Biostatistics
663. Biostatistics
664. Biostatistics
665. Biostatistics
666. Biostatistics
667. Epidemiology/Vector analysis
668. Epidemiology/Infectious disease
669. Descriptive epidemiology
670. Analytic epidemiology
671. Community epidemiology/Water hygiene
672. Epidemiology/Infectious disease
673. Public health toxicology/Lead poisoning
674. Occupational health/Carcinogenesis
675. Occupational health/Primary prevention
676. Occupational health/Secondary prevention
677. Epidemiology/Descriptive
678. Epidemiology/Descriptive
679. Epidemiology/Infectious disease
680. Biostatistics
681. Biostatistics
682. Biostatistics
683. Biostatistics
684. Biostatistics
685. Descriptive epidemiology

686. Biostatistics
687. Biostatistics
688. Biostatistics
689. Biostatistics
690. Occupational health/Primary prevention
691. Occupational health/Primary prevention
692. Occupational health/Primary prevention
693. Occupational health/Primary prevention
694. Health administration
695. Health administration
696. Health administration
697. Epidemiology/Vector analysis
698. Epidemiology/Vector analysis
699. Epidemiology/Vector analysis
700. Epidemiology/Vector analysis
701. Epidemiology/Vector analysis
702. Health administration
703. Health administration
704. Health administration
705. Health administration
706. Health administration
707. Epidemiology/Incubation periods
708. Epidemiology/Incubation periods
709. Epidemiology/Incubation periods
710. Epidemiology/Incubation periods
711. Occupational health/Toxicology
712. Occupational health/Toxicology
713. Occupational health/Toxicology
714. Occupational health/Toxicology
715. Occupational health/Toxicology
716. Occupational health/Toxicology
717. Occupational health/Toxicology
718. Occupational health/Toxicology
719. Occupational health/Toxicology
720. Occupational health/Toxicology
721. Primary prevention
722. Primary prevention
723. Primary prevention
724. Primary prevention
725. Primary prevention
726. Primary prevention
727. Primary prevention
728. Primary prevention
729. Primary prevention
730. Primary prevention
731. Epidemiology/Incubation periods
732. Epidemiology/Incubation periods
733. Epidemiology/Incubation periods
734. Epidemiology/Incubation periods
735. Epidemiology/Incubation periods
736. Epidemiology/Incubation periods
737. Epidemiology/Incubation periods
738. Epidemiology/Agent identification
739. Epidemiology/Agent identification
740. Epidemiology/Agent identification
741. Epidemiology/Agent identification
742. Epidemiology/Agent identification
743. Epidemiology/Agent identification
744. Epidemiology/Agent identification
745. Epidemiology/Agent identification
746. Epidemiology/Agent identification
747. Epidemiology/Agent identification
748. Epidemiology/Agent identification
749. Occupational health/Toxicology
750. Occupational health/Toxicology
751. Occupational health/Toxicology
752. Occupational health/Toxicology
753. Occupational health/Toxicology
754. Analytic epidemiology
755. Analytic epidemiology
756. Secondary prevention
757. Secondary prevention
758. Secondary prevention
759. Secondary prevention
760. Secondary prevention
761. Epidemiologic study designs
762. Epidemiologic study designs
763. Epidemiologic study designs
764. Epidemiologic study designs
765. Epidemiologic study designs
766. Epidemiologic study designs
767. Analytic epidemiology
768. Analytic epidemiology
769. Analytic epidemiology
770. Analytic epidemiology
771. Secondary prevention
772. Secondary prevention
773. Epidemiologic study designs
774. Analytic epidemiology
775. Analytic epidemiology
776. Analytic epidemiology
777. Analytic epidemiology
778. Analytic epidemiology
779. Analytic epidemiology
780. Analytic epidemiology
781. Analytic epidemiology
782. Biostatistics
783. Biostatistics
784. General public health knowledge
785. General public health knowledge

786. Health administration
787. Health administration
788. Tertiary prevention
789. Disease outbreak investigation
790. Health administration
791. General public health knowledge
792. Disease outbreak investigation
793. Environmental health
794. Environmental health
795. Age standardization
796. Clinical decision analysis

797. General public health knowledge
798. General public health knowledge
799. General public health knowledge
800. General public health knowledge
801. General public health knowledge
802. General public health knowledge
803. General public health knowledge
804. General public health knowledge
805. General public health knowledge
806. General public health knowledge
807. General public health knowledge

CHAPTER 7

Practice Test 1
Questions

DIRECTIONS (Questions 1 through 31): Each of the numbered items or incomplete statements in this section is followed by answers or by completions of the statement. Select the ONE lettered answer or completion that is BEST in each case.

Questions 1 and 2

A 68-year-old man comes to the emergency department with complaints of watery diarrhea, crampy abdominal pain with distension, and low-grade fever of 3 days' duration. He underwent coronary artery bypass surgery 10 days ago and was discharged on postoperative day 5 on an oral first-generation cephalosporin for wound cellulitis that has since resolved. Physical exam reveals a temperature of 100°F, pulse 95, blood pressure (BP) 110/60, respiratory rate 12, and a mildly distended abdomen with mild left-lower-quadrant pain with guarding, no rebound tenderness, and heme-positive stool on rectal exam. Pertinent laboratory tests reveal an elevated blood urea nitrogen (BUN) and creatinine, and white blood count (WBC) of 25,000.

1. Which of the following tests is most likely to yield a definitive diagnosis?

    (A) chest and abdominal x-rays
    (B) stool for ova and parasites
    (C) stool for *Clostridium difficile* toxins
    (D) stool for enterotoxigenic *Escherichia coli*
    (E) computed tomography (CT) scan of the abdomen

2. Which of the following are the most appropriate next steps in management of this patient?

    (A) intravenous (IV) fluids in the emergency department and discharge to home on an oral cephalosporin with instructions to return for increasing symptoms or fever greater than 101.5°F
    (B) IV fluids, admittance to the hospital, and institution of third-generation cephalosporin antibiotics
    (C) IV fluids, admittance to the hospital, discontinuation of cephalosporin, and colonoscopy
    (D) IV fluids, admittance to the hospital, discontinuation of cephalosporin, and institution of metronidazole
    (E) IV fluids in the emergency department and discharge to home on an oral cephalosporin with an appointment to return for an air contrast barium enema

3. A 40-year-old man calls your office asking for a chest x-ray. He is worried because a friend just learned he has lung cancer. Both he and his friend smoke two packs of cigarettes a day. He admits he seldom goes to the doctor unless he has a serious injury. You order an x-ray, and it is normal. What is your best course of action at this point?

    (A) Advise the patient that he really needs a CT scan, since x-rays can miss early cancers.

    (B) Reinforce his concern by showing him pictures of victims of lung cancer and emphysema.

    (C) Congratulate the patient on the normal study, and advise him to have an x-ray every 6 months for purposes of early detection.

    (D) Cultivate the patient's confidence by not nagging him about smoking. Instead, order a battery of screening tests for heart disease and colorectal cancer.

    (E) Schedule an office visit to learn more about him, advise him to quit smoking, and offer your assistance.

4. A 1-day-old infant has persistent vomiting. He has not had any stools. He was born at term and has not had any respiratory difficulties. A nasogastric tube is easily placed into his stomach. An abdominal film is ordered and is shown in Figure 7–1. What is the most likely diagnosis for this infant?

    (A) adrenogenital syndrome
    (B) pyloric stenosis
    (C) duodenal atresia
    (D) esophageal atresia with distal tracheo-esophageal atresia
    (E) cystic fibrosis

Questions 5 Through 7

A 22-year-old college student is evaluated by a psychiatrist for the onset of paranoid delusions, command auditory hallucinations, and an overwhelming sense that his thoughts are being drawn out of his brain by "negative electromagnetic waves." There is no prior psychiatric history. His parents,

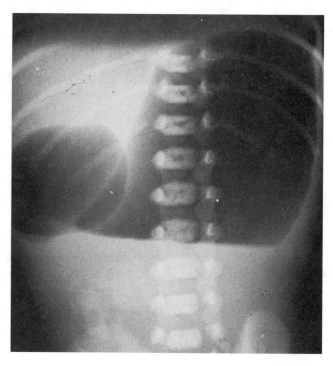

Figure 7–1. Duodenal atresia. Gas-filled and dilated stomach as well as a gas-filled and dilated duodenum show the classic "double bubble" appearance of duodenal atresia. No distal gas is present.

who accompany him, report that 2 months ago he had moved back home with them, isolated himself in his room, and became increasingly careless about his personal appearance. He was described as a quiet but friendly person with several good friends. In both high school and college (except for the last 2 or 3 months), he was a good student and seemed to enjoy his studies as well as participated in soccer and track. It seemed to his parents that he was worried about graduation and fears of finding a job. The patient denied the use of illicit drugs. It was noted that a paternal uncle had a diagnosis of schizophrenia.

5. Which of the following would be the best initial drug to treat this man?

    (A) buspirone
    (B) bupropion
    (C) fluvoxamine
    (D) clomipramine
    (E) quetiapine

6. The sense that thoughts were being drawn out of his brain by "negative electromagnetic waves" is an example of

   (A) projection
   (B) loose association
   (C) delusion
   (D) hallucination
   (E) heightened sensitivity to environmental stimuli

7. Which of the following supports the possibility of a good prognosis for this man?

   (A) uncle with schizophrenia
   (B) history of good achievement in school
   (C) being single
   (D) insidious onset
   (E) no clear precipitating factors

8. Which of the following study designs is most subject to bias?

   (A) a randomized, controlled trial
   (B) a prospective cohort study
   (C) a case-control study
   (D) they are all equally subject to bias
   (E) none of these designs are subject to bias

9. A 59-year-old woman with four adult children had 3 days of vaginal bleeding 1 month ago, the first episode of vaginal bleeding since menopause at age 43 years. She has a history of alcoholic cirrhosis. Her body mass index (BMI) is 32 kg/m². She has taken a combination estrogen–progestin for hormone replacement therapy (HRT) since the age of 44. She currently has three sexual partners. Her pelvic exam is normal and her Pap smear is subsequently read as normal. The most appropriate next step is

   (A) office endometrial biopsy
   (B) colposcopy
   (C) transvaginal ultrasonography
   (D) serum Ca-125 measurement
   (E) vaginal hysterectomy

10. The risk factor for endometrial carcinoma in this woman is

    (A) high parity
    (B) early menopause
    (C) BMI > 26 kg/m²
    (D) multiple sexual partners
    (E) estrogen and progestin replacement therapy

11. A side effect of methotrexate is

    (A) congestive heart failure
    (B) peripheral neuropathy
    (C) bone marrow depression
    (D) hemorrhagic cystitis
    (E) conduction hearing loss

12. Which of the following is a side effect or toxic effect of cisplatin?

    (A) renal toxicity
    (B) leukopenia
    (C) atopic dermatitis
    (D) hemorrhagic cystitis
    (E) decreased visual acuity

Questions 13 Through 16

A 22-year-old man presents to the physician's office with the complaint of a new nodule in the neck noted 1 month ago. He is the oldest of five children ranging in age from 8 to 22. His family history is pertinent for thyroid carcinoma, hypertension in his paternal grandparents, and an unknown type of tumor in the abdomen of his father, now deceased. On exam, he has a normal appearance and body habitus. He is afebrile, with a BP of 145/90 and pulse 70. Neck exam reveals a firm, 2-cm thyroid nodule. Fine-needle aspiration of the nodule reveals thyroid carcinoma.

13. Which of the following is the most likely type of thyroid carcinoma?

    (A) papillary
    (B) follicular
    (C) Hürthle cell
    (D) medullary
    (E) anaplastic

14. Screening for which disease must be undertaken prior to treatment of the thyroid carcinoma?

   (A) an adrenocorticotropic hormone (ACTH)-producing tumor
   (B) Zollinger–Ellison syndrome
   (C) pituitary adenoma
   (D) pheochromocytoma
   (E) ganglioneuroma

15. Which of the following is the minimal treatment for the patient's thyroid carcinoma?

   (A) ipsilateral subtotal lobectomy
   (B) ipsilateral lobectomy and isthmectomy
   (C) subtotal thyroidectomy and isthmectomy
   (D) total thyroidectomy
   (E) total thryoidectomy and parathyroidectomy

16. Screening for abnormalities in which proto-oncogene should be offered to his siblings?

   (A) myc
   (B) ret
   (C) ras
   (D) myb
   (E) erbB

17. An infant recently had a sweat chloride test because her private physician was concerned about her having cystic fibrosis. The test was positive. She has been referred to you for further diagnostic testing and counseling. She is the first child of a married couple. No one in either family has ever been diagnosed with this disease. Which of the following advice would you include in your initial session with this patient and her family?

   (A) The sweat chloride test is a screening test, but further tests should be done to confirm the diagnosis.
   (B) Pulmonary complications are severe and serious but fortunately are uncommon.
   (C) Glucose intolerance is common in the first year of life.

   (D) Current therapy does not provide a cure for this disease but can prolong life considerably.
   (E) The disease is clearly genetic but does not follow a definite autosomal or recessive pattern.

Questions 18 and 19

A 30-year-old man complains to his internist that he is always worrying about the quality of his work as a manager at a local electronics store. He tends to be somewhat irritable, even with his customers. In spite of reassurances from his colleagues, he feels edgy most of the time, has trouble falling asleep, and is tired much of the time. He claims to have been uncomfortable like this for most of the past year. He denies the use of caffeine or illicit drugs. A recent physical exam was essentially normal.

18. The most likely diagnosis is

   (A) generalized anxiety disorder
   (B) panic disorder
   (C) adjustment reaction
   (D) phobic disorder
   (E) dysthymia

19. Of the following, which drug would be most quickly effective in relieving this man's symptoms?

   (A) buspirone
   (B) imipramine
   (C) thioridazine
   (D) lorazepam
   (E) carbamazepine

20. A Puerto Rican woman, treated for depression, is reported to be pulling out her hair. In evaluating her, you note that her eye lashes are missing and her head hair is very thinned, with patches of no hair evident. She repetitively pulls on her hair, but at least for the moment appears not to pull any out. She reports that she has engaged in this behavior for almost a year. This condition is known as

   (A) catatonic schizophrenia—excited form
   (B) trichotillomania

(C) ghost sickness

(D) mal de ojo

(E) autism

21. Which of the following statements about pac-litaxel (Taxol) is true?

(A) It is extracted from the roots of the western yew.

(B) Myelosuppression is the major dose-limiting effect.

(C) It acts by preventing microtubule as-sembly.

(D) It is used to treat advanced cervical cancer.

(E) Nausea and vomiting are uncommon side effects.

22. Labor is induced with a dilute IV oxytocin in-fusion at 42 weeks' gestation in a 29-year-old woman whose pregnancy was uncompli-cated. Her pelvis is adequate. Following a vaginal birth, she receives a bolus injection of 20 units of oxytocin intrave-nously. Which one of the following is a pos-sible complica-tion of oxytocin?

(A) hypertension

(B) uterine atony

(C) hypernatremia

(D) hypotension

(E) hyperkalemia

23. Dysfunctional uterine bleeding can be char-acterized by which of the following state-ments?

(A) It tends to occur several years after menarche.

(B) It may be severe enough to lead to anemia.

(C) It is usually associated with dysmenor-rhea.

(D) It is thought to result from the unop-posed effect of progesterone in the en-dometrium.

(E) It should be treated with antiestrogens.

24. Which of the presentations is more consistent with a pathologic grief reaction?

(A) complaints regarding exhaustion or lack of strength

(B) feelings of increased emotional distance

(C) preoccupation with guilt and personal responsibility

(D) increased activity without feelings of loss

(E) feelings of irritability, hostility, and anger

Questions 25 and 26

A 37-year-old woman presents to the physician's office with a 2-week history of right breast pain. The pain is localized to the nipple areolar complex and surrounding skin and associated with redness and swelling and does not change with the men-strual cycle. On exam, vital signs are normal, and there is induration, erythema, and tenderness in-volving the nipple areolar complex of the breast, with a subareolar mass. Axillary exam reveals slightly tender ipsilateral nodes. She declines mam-mography due to the tenderness, but ultrasound exam suggests the presence of a subareolar com-plex cystic structure.

25. Which of the following is the most likely di-agnosis?

(A) inflammatory carcinoma of the breast

(B) periductal mastitis with abscess

(C) Paget's disease of the nipple

(D) Mondor's disease (thrombophlebitis)

(E) intraductal papilloma

26. Which of the following is the most appropri-ate next step in management?

(A) modified radical mastectomy

(B) lumpectomy with axillary node dissec-tion, followed by radiation therapy

(C) incision and drainage with biopsy of the cyst

(D) antibiotics and repeat evaluation in 1 week

(E) excisional biopsy

27. A 24-year-old G_2P_2 woman engages in un-protected intercourse on the fourteenth day of her menstrual cycle. Two days later, she requests emergency contraception. Which of the following is effective contraception?

    (A) one triphasic oral contraceptive tablet daily for 21 days starting on cycle day 16
    (B) methotrexate, 50 mg/m² intramuscularly (IM)
    (C) diethylstilbestrol (DES), 5 mg orally one time
    (D) norethindrone, 10 mg twice daily for 2 days
    (E) Ovral, two tablets given twice, 12 hours apart

28. A thin, white 53-year-old woman who had her last menstrual period 2 years ago complains of hot flashes for 1 year, vaginal dryness, and sleep loss from night sweats. You offer hormone replacement with combination estrogen–progesterone therapy, explaining that it will

    (A) increase her risk of endometrial carcinoma
    (B) increase her risk of breast cancer
    (C) increase orgasmic ability
    (D) increase bone mineral density
    (E) increase her risk of colon cancer

29. A 12-month-old infant, previously in good health, develops an illness characterized by 3 days of fever followed by defervescence and the development of a maculopapular rash on the trunk. No other signs or symptoms are present. The most likely diagnosis is

    (A) erythema infectiosum (Fifth disease)
    (B) Kawasaki disease
    (C) roseola infantum (exanthem subitum)
    (D) rubeola (measles)
    (E) scarlet fever

Questions 30 and 31

30. Premenstrual dysphoric disorder (premenstrual syndrome [PMS]) can be described by which of the following statements?

    (A) With close examination, symptoms characteristically are found throughout the menstrual cycle.
    (B) Nonmenstruating women cannot, by diagnostic definition, have this disorder.
    (C) Affected women seeking treatment usually are younger than 25 years of age.
    (D) Diagnosis by *Diagnostic and Statistical Manual of Mental Disorders,* 4th edition (DSM-IV) criteria requires that a woman's work or social function be impaired.
    (E) Some affected women experience pain and physical distress without any emotional discomfort.

31. The most effective treatment of choice for premenstrual dysphoric disorder is

    (A) alprazolam
    (B) diuretics
    (C) progestogens
    (D) fluoxetine (Prozac)
    (E) none of the above

DIRECTIONS (Questions 32 through 38): For each item, select the ONE best lettered option that is most closely associated with it. Each lettered heading may be selected once, more than once, or not at all.

For each patient with gastrointestinal bleeding, select the most likely diagnosis.

    (A) diverticulosis of the colon
    (B) ulcerative colitis
    (C) Meckel's diverticulum
    (D) ischemic colitis
    (E) aortoenteric fistula
    (F) peptic ulcer
    (G) carcinoma of the colon
    (H) esophageal varices
    (I) gastric ulcer

32. A 60-year-old man is brought to the emergency department following a fainting episode at home. He complains of bright red blood per rectum for the last 6 hours. He denies abdominal pain or vomiting. Exam re-

veals a pulse of 110; BP of 95/50; and no significant heart, lung, or abdominal findings. He has gross blood on rectal exam.

33. A 56-year-old woman presents to the emergency department following an episode of melenotic stool 48 hours ago. She underwent resuscitation at another facility prior to transfer. She has no current complaints. The melena has not recurred. Past surgical history is pertinent for appendectomy at age 25 and abdominal aortic aneurysm repair 2 years ago. She has a 30-pack year smoking history and drinks alcohol socially on weekends. Upper gastrointestinal (UGI) endoscopy to the duodenal bulb is normal, as well as colonoscopy.

34. A 65-year-old woman presents to the emergency department complaining of severe fatigue and weakness over the last week. Past history is pertinent for hypertension, diabetes, and coronary artery disease. Medications include a calcium channel blocker, insulin, and daily aspirin. She has a 40-pack year smoking history and drinks a moderate amount of alcohol. Exam reveals pulse of 90, BP of 105/65, and unremarkable heart and lung findings. She has fullness and mild tenderness in the right lower quadrant. Blood tests reveal a hematocrit of 21.

35. A 65-year-old man is transferred to the emergency department from an outside facility for evaluation of hematemesis and melena. Past history is pertinent for recently discovered cholelithiasis, for which he has not yet received a surgical consult. He has complained of abdominal pain for the last 3 to 4 weeks and has been taking ibuprofen four times daily for 3 weeks as well as alcohol for the pain. Exam reveals a pulse of 100 and BP 100/60 following resuscitation. Abdominal exam reveals tenderness in the right upper quadrant and epigastrium. Rectal exam reveals melenotic stool.

36. A 50-year-old man presents to the emergency department following an episode of hematemesis. Past history is pertinent for a 40-pack year smoking history and chronic alcoholism. Exam reveals a pulse of 120, BP

90/60, and an unremarkable heart and lung exam. Skin exam reveals spider angiomata and palmar erythema. Abdominal exam reveals a nontender abdomen that is distended.

37. A 35-year-old man presents to the emergency department with abdominal pain; hematemesis; and black, tarry stools. He complains of abdominal pain for 2 weeks, for which he has taken antacids with partial relief. Past history is pertinent for hypertension, 20-pack year smoking history, and occasional alcohol intake. Exam reveals a pulse of 110, BP 95/60, tenderness in the epigastrium, and melenotic stool on rectal exam.

38. A 35-year-old woman presents to the emergency department with a 1-week history of bloody diarrhea. She complains of intermittent abdominal pain for 1 month that is now constant and weight loss of 10 pounds. Past history is unremarkable. Exam reveals a temperature of 101°F, pulse 85, and BP 110/60. Heart and lung exam is unremarkable. Abdominal exam reveals diffuse abdominal tenderness.

DIRECTIONS (Questions 39 through 108): Each of the numbered items or incomplete statements in this section is followed by answers or by completions of the statement. Select the ONE lettered answer or completion that is BEST in each case.

39. A 25-year-old nullipara consults you because she has suddenly stopped menstruating. On questioning her, you find that she recently lost 19 lb soon after she started long-distance running. The most appropriate first step in her evaluation is measurement of

(A) serum thyroid-stimulating hormone (TSH) concentration
(B) serum prolactin concentration
(C) human chorionic gonadotropin (hCG) concentration
(D) serum estradiol-17β concentration
(E) serum testosterone concentration

40. Which of the following is a contraindication to taking oral contraceptives?

(A) obesity

(B) previous pregnancy-induced hypertension

(C) uncomplicated diabetes mellitus

(D) cigarette smoking

(E) migraine headaches

41. The parents of an infant born at term are concerned about the possibility of their child having developmental dysplasia of the hip. Which of the following historical factors would make this diagnosis more likely?

(A) The baby is a boy.

(B) The baby was delivered in the breech position.

(C) The baby was delivered vaginally.

(D) The baby is their third child.

(E) The family is African-American.

42. A 25-year-old man is hospitalized after weeks of worsening psychosis. He is begun on the antipsychotic drug thiothixene. Five days later, he develops a fever of 39.8°C. In addition, he has become delirious and is lying stiffly in his bed and is uncommunicative. His family reports he had been physically well at the time of admission. The admission physical exam confirmed this. The diagnosis of most immediate concern at this point is

(A) worsening psychotic state

(B) pseudoparkinsonism reaction

(C) ruptured cerebral aneurysm

(D) unsuspected opioid dependence

(E) neuroleptic malignant syndrome

43. A 24-year-old woman has clear evidence of having bipolar disorder. An adequate trial of lithium therapy has proved unsuccessful. Which of the following drugs would be most reasonable for her psychiatrist to prescribe next?

(A) chlorpromazine

(B) carbamazepine

(C) alprazolam

(D) amitriptyline

(E) phenelzine

Questions 44 Through 46

A 22-year-old, previously healthy, 176-lb man was rescued from a house fire, after being trapped in a small bedroom of the house for several hours. When brought to the emergency department, he is noted to be combative and disoriented. His lungs are clear to auscultation bilaterally. His respiratory rate is 30/min, BP 100/70, and heart rate 115/min. He has sustained 15% second- and third-degree burns on the lower extremities, with a circumferential full-thickness injury below the right knee.

44. The most appropriate initial step in management is

(A) sedation with IV midazolam

(B) IV morphine for analgesia

(C) administration of 100% oxygen by face mask

(D) debridement of the lower-extremity burns

(E) IV fluid bolus of 20 mL/kg

The patient improves and is transferred to the intensive care unit for further management.

45. Appropriate initial fluid resuscitation would be

(A) IV dextrose/0.5 normal saline at 150 mL/hr

(B) IV lactated Ringer's at maintenance rate per hour, with boluses of albumin as required

(C) IV lactated Ringer's at twice maintenance rate per hour

(D) 4800 mL of lactated Ringer's, given at 200 mL/hr

(E) IV maintenance fluids plus an additional 4800 mL of lactated Ringer's, one half given over the first 8 hours and the remainder given over 16 hours

Within several hours of admission, the patient begins to complain of pain in the right foot. He is noted to have swelling of the foot and ankle, decreased capillary refill of the right toes, and decreased sensation.

46. The treatment of choice is

(A) elevation of the affected extremity

(B) initiation of antibiotics

(C) hyperbaric oxygen

(D) administration of 100% oxygen by face mask

(E) escharotomy

47. A 55-year-old woman refuses to take hormone replacement therapy because she fears that she will develop breast cancer. You discuss the use of a selective estrogen receptor modulator (SERM) such as raloxifene (Evista). Which of the following statements is supported by data?

(A) Bone mineral density is increased after 24 months.

(B) High-density lipoprotein (HDL) concentrations are increased within 6 months.

(C) Hot flashes are relieved.

(D) Endometrial thickness increases after 12 months.

(E) Urinary incontinence is improved after 6 months.

48. A 15-year-old girl comes to the emergency department 4 hours after ingesting aspirin. After obtaining the history, you estimate that she has ingested approximately 150 mg/kg of aspirin. Her physical examination is entirely normal. Which of the following treatments would be most useful in her management?

(A) induced emesis

(B) administration of N-acetylcysteine

(C) administration of a cathartic

(D) administration of IV fluid to increase urine output

(E) no medical intervention is necessary

49. Which of the following is required as part of the pre-lithium workup?

(A) erythrocyte sedimentation rate (ESR)

(B) electroencephalogram (EEG)

(C) TSH, serum triiodothyronine (T_3) and thyroxine (T_4)

(D) liver function tests

(E) dexamethasone suppression test

50. A 50-year-old woman presents with weakness of her right hand, accompanied by a tingling sensation upon awakening each morning. She is found to have hypesthesia of the thumb, index, and middle fingers, along with atrophy of the thenar muscles. The most likely diagnosis is compression of the

(A) digital nerve to the thumb

(B) median nerve in the hand

(C) median nerve in the carpal tunnel

(D) median nerve by the pronator teres

(E) median nerve in the axilla

51. A 24-year-old multiparous woman experiences severe postpartum hemorrhage immediately after vaginal delivery. IV pitocin and IM ergot preparations have failed to stop the bleeding. The uterus is firm. Inspection of the vagina and cervix reveals no lacerations. The most appropriate next step is

(A) infusion of fresh frozen plasma

(B) hypogastric artery ligation

(C) intrauterine infusion of warm saline

(D) hysterectomy

(E) uterine packing

52. A 2-year-old toddler refuses to move his left arm and is holding it flexed at the elbow, with the forearm pronated. His father had been swinging him by the forearms; there is no other history of trauma. The most likely diagnosis is

(A) fractured clavicle

(B) Salter type IV fracture of the distal humerus

(C) dislocation of the radial head

(D) torus fracture of the distal radius

(E) contusion of the ulnar nerve

53. A 14-year-old boy comes to the clinic for a checkup. His only concern is that he has developed acne. On physical exam, he has moderate facial acne and is Tanner stage 3. Which of the following is the next step in his management?

    (A) Advise him to wash his face vigorously four times per day.
    (B) Advise him that it should resolve as he continues to progress through puberty.
    (C) Ask him to decrease his intake of chocolate, starches, and oily or fried foods.
    (D) Reassure him that no treatment is necessary unless he develops cystic acne.
    (E) Treat him with topical benzoyl peroxide and tretinoin.

54. According to Erikson, the successful resolution of the identity crisis in adolescence depends on

    (A) successful participation in cohesive groups
    (B) choice of a successful social ideology
    (C) success in maintaining rigorous moral standards
    (D) identification with appropriate personal, familial, and social models
    (E) success in academics and early work experiences

55. In 1990, a study was conducted to determine the relationship between outdoor air pollution and bronchitis in postal workers employed during the period 1970 to 1980. Information on the occurrence of bronchitis since employment and other relevant factors were gathered from the medical records of 2500 postmen delivering mail outdoors as well as those of 500 comparable post office employees who had worked indoors. The risk of bronchitis was found to be higher among those working outdoors. The design of this study is

    (A) an ecological study design
    (B) a historical cohort design
    (C) a cross-sectional design
    (D) a prospective cohort design
    (E) a randomized, controlled trial design

56. A 19-year-old student at a rural state university is admitted to a hospital with rapid onset of fever, headache, photophobia, and a stiff neck. The student soon develops an extensive purpuric skin rash and becomes obtunded. Gram stain of the cerebrospinal fluid (CSF) shows numerous gram-negative diplococci. Within 3 days, two other students are admitted with fever, headache, and stiff neck. Gram stains of their CSF also show gram-negative diplococci. One of the students had attended a seminar with the first student. The third has no known relationship with the others. You are the public health officer for the area, and school officials are calling you for advice. There are 2 months of school left. The best recommendation you can make is

    (A) administer rifampin, 500 mg twice daily for 2 days, to all students and faculty
    (B) close the school and send the students home
    (C) conduct a mass immunization for meningococcal disease
    (D) identify the source of infection using a quick case-control study
    (E) conduct a mass media campaign on the signs and symptoms of meningitis

Questions 57 and 58

A 26-year-old, previously healthy man is brought to the emergency department with a stab wound to the fifth left intercostal space in the midclavicular line. He is found to have a pulse of 140/min, systolic blood pressure of 80 mm Hg, and respiration of 20/min. His trachea is midline, heart sounds appear distant, and breath sounds are equal bilaterally.

57. The most likely diagnosis is

    (A) transected descending aorta
    (B) cardiac tamponade
    (C) massive left hemothorax
    (D) tension pneumothorax
    (E) phrenic nerve paralysis

58. The most appropriate next step in management is

(A) insertion of a left chest tube

(B) emergency department thoracotomy

(C) pericardiocentesis

(D) rapid infusion of an IV fluid bolus

(E) intubation and assisted ventilation

59. An infant is born to a mother treated late in pregnancy for primary syphilis. After birth, the infant is evaluated for evidence of congenital syphilis. Which of the following statements is true?

(A) Mean infant birth weight is increased because of fetal hydrops.

(B) Congenital syphilis is more common when the mother had late syphilis versus primary syphilis.

(C) The stillbirth rate is significantly increased.

(D) Evidence of congenital syphilis is usually present at birth.

(E) The false-negative rate of serologic tests for syphilis is increased in human immunodeficiency virus (HIV)-infected women.

60. A patient had an uncomplicated cesarean section 6 days previously. She has been on a regimen of ampicillin, gentamicin, and clindamycin for 5 days, but still has temperature spikes of 39.4°C (103°F). Physical exam is normal. Her fever is most likely caused by

(A) a pelvic abscess

(B) septic pelvic thrombophlebitis

(C) endometritis

(D) pyelonephritis

(E) breast engorgement

Question 61

Over the course of an evening, 10 individuals present to an emergency department complaining of abrupt onset of severe nausea, vomiting, and abdominal cramps. Many were prostrate with sweats and dizziness. Some of the individuals developed diarrhea. On examination, they were afebrile. All of them noted the onset of symptoms within 1 to 3 hours of eating at the same restaurant, and all of them had eaten minced barbecue from the restaurant buffet. The health department conducted an inspection the next day.

61. Which of the following findings would be most likely associated with the illness?

(A) a history of vomiting and diarrhea from the food handler preparing the barbecue

(B) inadequate reheating of previously refrigerated food

(C) an infected cut on the hand of a food handler who prepared the barbecue

(D) an outbreak of gastroenteritis among restaurant staff 1 week ago

(E) the meat for the barbecue came from a supplier previously implicated in an *Escherichia coli* O157:H7 outbreak

62. A 17-year-old female is brought to the emergency department because she ingested vitamins that contained iron. Which of the following symptoms might you see early in the course of acute iron poisoning?

(A) bleeding diathesis

(B) gastrointestinal hemorrhage

(C) liver failure

(D) prolonged QT interval

(E) respiratory failure

63. A 12-year-old girl with malaise, fatigue, sore throat, fever, hepatosplenomegaly, and generalized lymphadenopathy is diagnosed as having Epstein–Barr virus–related mononucleosis. Which of the following complications is most likely in this patient?

(A) azotemia

(B) chronic active hepatitis

(C) encephalitis

(D) leukopenia

(E) pancreatitis

64. A 55-year-old woman is referred for psychiatric consultation for depression. She is 60 days post–bone marrow transplant. Her husband says that she "just cries," barely says anything, sleeps very restlessly if at all, and has lost interest in him and their children as well as in her housework and hobbies. The oncologist who referred her wants you to "give her something for her depression." Of the following, what is the next appropriate step?

(A) prescribe sertraline
(B) prescribe lorazepam
(C) interview the woman
(D) have a family conference
(E) electroconvulsive therapy (ECT)

65. Which of the following statements about suicide among children is true?

(A) Its frequency is stable nationwide.
(B) Impulsive children are the most likely victims.
(C) Physically abused children are less likely to commit suicide.
(D) Children younger than 14 years do not act on suicidal thoughts.
(E) It is a rare cause of death among adolescents.

66. A 30-year-old, previously healthy woman slips on the ice while crossing the street and strikes her head on the pavement. Bystanders report that she has loss of consciousness for 2 minutes, following which she is lucid but complaining of a headache. She is taken to a nearby emergency department. Over the next few hours, the patient develops a decreased level of consciousness, a dilated right pupil, and left hemiparesis. The most likely diagnosis is

(A) right occipital intracranial hematoma
(B) right subdural hematoma
(C) right epidural hematoma
(D) left epidural hematoma
(E) subarachnoid hemorrhage

67. A 32-year-old, previously healthy man is a victim of a drive-by shooting, sustaining a gunshot wound to the left lower extremity. The entrance wound is located over the medial aspect of the calf, with an exit wound over the anterior pretibial region. Neurovascular exam of the extremity is normal. There is associated soft-tissue injury from the blast effect and a severely comminuted tibial fracture demonstrated on radiographs. Appropriate management of this injury includes

(A) local wound irrigation, closure of the soft-tissue defect, closed reduction, and immobilization in a long-leg cast
(B) local wound irrigation with antibiotic solution, closed reduction, and immobilization in a long-leg cast, with continued local wound care through an anterior cast window
(C) tetanus prophylaxis, IV antibiotics, and operative wound irrigation and debridement, with application of an external fixation device
(D) tetanus prophylaxis, IV antibiotics, operative wound irrigation with closure of the soft-tissue defect, closed reduction, and immobilization in a long-leg cast
(E) tetanus prophylaxis, IV antibiotics, long-leg splint for immobilization, and operative intervention during elective surgical schedule

68. A 19-year-old primipara at 38 weeks' gestation has a blood pressure of 150/106, hyperreflexia, and 3+ proteinuria. Which of the following statements is correct?

(A) The risk of eclampsia increases with increasing systolic blood pressure.
(B) Delivery of the infant is the treatment for this woman.
(C) A beta blocker is contraindicated in pregnancy.
(D) The risk of placenta previa is increased in this woman.
(E) Perinatal mortality is increased slightly in hypertensive pregnant women.

69. After a 12-hour first stage, a 45-minute second stage, and a 10-minute third stage of labor, a healthy primigravid woman delivers a 7.9-lb boy with Apgar scores of 9 at 1 minute and 10 at 5 minutes. Which of the following statements about labor is correct?

   (A) Labor is defined by the presence of regular uterine contractions at an interval of 5 minutes or less.

   (B) The first stage begins with the onset of regular uterine contractions and ends with full dilatation of the cervix.

   (C) The first stage of labor is prolonged in this patient.

   (D) The second stage is from complete cervical dilation to the delivery of the placenta.

   (E) The third stage of labor begins after delivery of the placenta and ends when the episiotomy is repaired.

Questions 70 and 71

A 16-year-old girl with a history of ulcerative colitis managed with steroid therapy presents to the emergency department with a 36-hour history of nausea, crampy abdominal pain, and severe bloody diarrhea. On examination, the patient is febrile and pale, with a blood pressure of 90/60 mm Hg and heart rate of 130/min. Her abdomen is distended and diffusely tender. A complete blood count (CBC) demonstrates a leukocytosis with a left shift. The patient receives IV fluid resuscitation and nasogastric tube decompression.

70. Further therapeutic interventions should include

   (A) 6-mercaptopurine
   (B) azothioprine
   (C) opioid antidiarrheals
   (D) colonoscopic decompression
   (E) high-dose IV steroids and broad-spectrum antibiotics

71. After 48 hours, there is no clinical improvement. The next step in management is

   (A) colonoscopic decompression
   (B) cyclosporine
   (C) subtotal colectomy and ileostomy and Hartmann's procedure
   (D) colectomy with ileal pouch–anal anastomosis
   (E) subtotal colectomy with ileorectal anastomosis

72. A 19-year-old G_1 whose last menses began 9 weeks ago comes to the emergency department because of heavy vaginal bleeding and lower abdominal cramping for 3 hours. Her blood pressure is 146/96, and her pulse rate is 84 beats/min. A lower abdominal mass is palpable halfway between her symphysis and umbilicus. The cervix is closed, and there is active bleeding through the cervical os. On bimanual examination, the uterus is approximately 16-weeks size. Fetal heart tones could not be heard, and a fetus is not seen by abdominal and transvaginal ultrasonography. Her serum hCG concentration is 80,000 mIU/mL, significantly higher than normal for a 9-week pregnancy. The most likely diagnosis is

   (A) multiple gestation
   (B) tubal pregnancy
   (C) blighted ovum
   (D) singleton pregnancy in a myomatous uterus
   (E) hydatidiform mole

73. A 5-month-old child has a history of 2 days of rhinorrhea and 1 day of fever and worsening cough. She has been well prior to this time and has not previously had similar symptoms. On physical exam, she has inspiratory stridor. Which of the following should be considered in the differential diagnosis?

   (A) acute bronchiolitis
   (B) acute laryngotracheobronchitis
   (C) a foreign body in the upper airway
   (D) laryngomalacia
   (E) peritonsillar abscess

74. A 2-week-old infant is brought to the emergency department with vomiting for 1 day. On physical exam, the baby is very lethargic, is poorly perfused, and appears moderately dehydrated. His electrolytes are sodium, 115; potassium, 6.0; and carbon dioxide 15. His glucose is 40. Which of the following is the most likely diagnosis?

    (A) congenital adrenal hyperplasia
    (B) duodenal atresia
    (C) gastroenteritis
    (D) pyloric stenosis
    (E) tracheoesophageal fistula

75. Which of the following laboratory findings is best associated with heavy alcohol drinking?

    (A) increase in gamma-glutamyl transpeptidase (GGT)
    (B) decrease in GGT
    (C) decreased serum glumatic oxaloacetic transaminase (SGOT)
    (D) decrease in triglycerides
    (E) none of the above

76. The most widely accepted and useful test for the assessment of intelligence in children is the

    (A) Stanford–Binet Test
    (B) Metropolitan Achievement Test
    (C) Wechsler Intelligence Scale for Children
    (D) Bellevue–Wechsler Scale
    (E) Vineland Social Maturity Scale

Questions 77 and 78

A premenopausal woman complains of a thick, white, malodorous discharge. The pH is less than 4.5. There is no amine odor when potassium hydroxide is added to the discharge on a slide. There are no clue cells on wet smear. The microscopic appearance of the discharge is shown in Figure 7–2.

77. The cause of the discharge is

    (A) *Gardnerella vaginalis*
    (B) *Trichomonas vaginalis*
    (C) *Chlamydia trachomatis*
    (D) *Candida albicans*
    (E) *Treponema pallidum*

78. Appropriate treatment for the discharge seen in Figure 7–2 is

    (A) oral metronidazole
    (B) oral ketoconazole
    (C) IM ceftriaxone
    (D) oral doxycycline
    (E) oral clindamycin

79. A 16-year-old girl comes to the clinic for a checkup. Her parents are concerned about her weight. Over the past year, she has lost 20 pounds. She has not been ill. She is an excellent student and active in many after-school activities. On physical exam, she is emaciated, hypothermic, and bradycardic. Which of the following is the most likely diagnosis?

    (A) anorexia nervosa
    (B) bulimia
    (C) hyperthyroidism
    (D) diabetes mellitus
    (E) depression

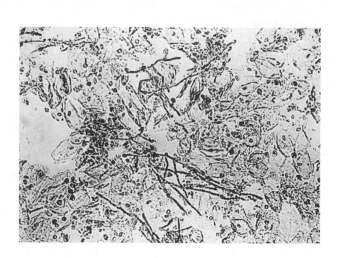

Figure 7–2.

80. A child is diagnosed with acute lymphoblastic leukemia (ALL). Which of the following is a favorable prognostic factor in ALL in childhood?

    (A) age > 7 years
    (B) female gender
    (C) initial WBC of 10,000
    (D) presence of a mediastinal mass
    (E) platelet count of 100,000

81. Which of the following would be the most effective first step in managing a threatening person?

    (A) demanding that the person sit before talking with him
    (B) standing directly over and to the side of the person as a show of strength
    (C) asking the person to explain the reasons for his or her anger
    (D) acknowledging the person's anger and fear
    (E) threatening to call security if the person does not control himself

82. A 60-year-old female with no previous psychiatric history is seen by her family physician at the request of her family. She has experienced a severe weight loss, a loss of interest and enjoyment in her various activities, and has quit her job as a teachers' aide. She appears cachectic, older than her stated age, lethargic, and withdrawn. She responds to no questions. According to the family, her symptoms began shortly after the death of her husband about 8 months ago. An appropriate diagnosis at this time is

    (A) major depression
    (B) pathological grief reaction
    (C) pancreatic cancer
    (D) hypothyroidism
    (E) none of the above

Questions 83 Through 85

A 19-year-old woman has never menstruated, although breast growth began about the age of 11 years. Pubic hair first appeared 6 to 12 months later. She has a 22-year-old maternal cousin who also has primary amenorrhea. This 19-year-old has a blood pressure of 106/68 and a pulse rate of 68/min. Her breasts are developed to Tanner stage 5, but pubic hair is sparse (Tanner stage 2). There is no cervix seen by speculum exam, and a uterus cannot be palpated, despite an adequate bimanual examination.

83. The most appropriate next step in evaluating the cause of her amenorrhea is

    (A) pelvic ultrasound
    (B) CT scan of her pituitary
    (C) laparoscopy
    (D) serum estradiol
    (E) karyotype

84. The most likely diagnosis of this patient's amenorrhea is

    (A) anorexia nervosa
    (B) gonadal dysgenesis
    (C) müllerian agenesis
    (D) testicular feminization
    (E) 17α-hydroxylase deficiency

85. The pathophysiology of this patient's condition is

    (A) congenital absence of Leydig cells
    (B) congenital absence of ovarian follicles
    (C) congenital abnormality of the preoptic hypothalamus
    (D) congenital deficiency of steroid 21-hydroxylase
    (E) congenital abnormality of testosterone receptors

86. Which of the following neuroleptic-induced conditions may be significantly worsened by treatment with benztropine?

    (A) parkinsonism
    (B) oculogyric crisis
    (C) laryngeal dystonia
    (D) tremors
    (E) urinary retention

87. Which of the following factors is associated with an increased risk of occult pneumococcal bacteremia in children?

    (A) no change in temperature after acetaminophen
    (B) WBC < 15,000
    (C) low socioeconomic status
    (D) temperature > 39°C (102.2°F)
    (E) age > 2 years

88. Which of the following statements regarding tuberculous meningitis in children is correct?

    (A) A CSF protein concentration greater than 1 g/100 mL generally indicates ventricular obstruction.
    (B) With proper therapy, the prognosis is excellent even for patients with advanced disease.
    (C) A negative tuberculin skin test effectively rules out the diagnosis.
    (D) The onset of signs and symptoms is acute in most cases.
    (E) Cranial nerve involvement is rare.

Questions 89 Through 91

A 38-year-old married woman, the mother of two children and a medical social worker, is hospitalized with a diagnosis of breast cancer. She is anticipating surgery and then possible radiation and chemotherapy. Since arriving, she has been demanding, hostile, and uncooperative. She complained bitterly to the nurses about their insensitivity and rudeness. Her husband tried to reassure the nurses that "really, she is not like this at all," but then he left when his wife told him to "get out!" The nursing staff requested a psychiatric consult to medicate this "unreasonable, uncontrolled woman."

89. This woman's behavior is most likely

    (A) a borderline personality disorder
    (B) PMS
    (C) regression and acting out
    (D) metastasis to the brain, giving rise to behavioral changes
    (E) major depression with agitation

90. The nurses' anger is best described as an example of

    (A) acting out
    (B) transference
    (C) countertransference
    (D) reaction formation
    (E) splitting

91. The major goal of a psychiatrist evaluating this woman would be to

    (A) determine the need for restraints
    (B) determine the need to transfer her to another hospital
    (C) set firm limits to her shouting and complaining
    (D) help her identify and talk about her fears
    (E) get specific information about specific nurses in order to file a grievance

Questions 92 and 93

A 27-year-old woman complains of progressive facial hirsutism and menstrual intervals that vary from 26 to 90 days. Her hirsutism and oligomenorrhea began shortly after menarche at the age of 13 years. She takes no medications with androgenic effects. Her family history is negative for hirsutism or oligomenorrhea. Her blood pressure is normal. She has no galactorrhea, and her pelvic exam is normal except for a male pubic hair pattern. Her vagina contains rugae, and abundant clear mucus is present in the cervical canal.

92. The most appropriate diagnostic test is

    (A) a pelvic ultrasound
    (B) measurement of serum dehydroepiandrosterone (DHEA) concentration

(C) an ACTH stimulation test

(D) a dexamethasone suppression test

(E) measurement of serum follicle-stimulating hormone (FSH)

93. The tests in question 92 that were obtained were normal. In addition, her serum prolactin concentration is 13 ng/mL (normal, < 20). The most likely diagnosis is

(A) polycystic ovary syndrome

(B) attenuated 21-hydroxylase deficiency

(C) pituitary adenoma

(D) Sertoli–Leydig cell tumor

(E) adrenal adenoma

Questions 94 and 95

A 19-year-old man with onset of psychotic symptoms, including bizarre delusions and hallucinations, the belief that someone is controlling his mind, and increased isolation, is brought to the psychiatric hospital for treatment.

94. Which of the following neurochemical systems is most likely involved?

(A) cholinergic

(B) gamma-aminobutyric acid (GABA)

(C) dopamine

(D) norepinephrine

(E) glutamate

95. Which of the following drugs will affect the system to help ameliorate the psychotic symptoms?

(A) haloperidol

(B) fluvoxamine

(C) imipramine

(D) divalproex

(E) doxepin

96. The largest source of estrogen in women with the polycystic ovary syndrome is

(A) ovarian estrogen secretion

(B) extraglandular aromatization of DHEAS

(C) adrenal estrogen secretion

(D) extraglandular aromatization of androstenedione

(E) extraglandular aromatization of testosterone

97. Acrodermatitis enteropathica is characterized by which of the following?

(A) zinc deficiency

(B) autosomal dominant inheritance

(C) hypergonadism

(D) onset shortly after birth in breast-fed babies

(E) constipation

98. An 18-month-old boy presents with a 2-day history of intermittent vomiting and irritability. On physical exam, he looks uncomfortable, has right-lower-quadrant fullness, and a "currant jelly" stool in his diaper. Which of the following is the most likely diagnosis?

(A) constipation

(B) gastroenteritis

(C) intussusception

(D) Meckel's diverticulum

(E) volvulus

99. A 3-day-old infant is brought to the clinic because she is constipated. She was born at term and went home within 24 hours. She has not had any stools since she was born. She has been breast feeding well and has not had any vomiting. Her mother thinks that her abdomen is bloated. On physical exam, her weight is equal to her birth weight. Her abdomen is distended, and there are no other abnormal findings. Which of the following is the most likely diagnosis?

(A) duodenal stenosis

(B) esophageal atresia

(C) functional constipation

(D) Hirschsprung's disease

(E) breast-feeding failure

100. A 6-month-old boy is brought to the clinic with a 1-day history of rectal bleeding. He has not had any pain or discomfort and has had no other symptoms. On physical exam, he looks well. His abdominal exam is normal. The diaper that the parents brought in is filled with dark red blood. Which of the following is the most likely diagnosis?

(A) anal fissure
(B) intussusception
(C) Meckel's diverticulum
(D) milk allergy
(E) volvulus

101. A 3-year-old boy is scheduled for a tonsillectomy. As part of his preoperative evaluation, coagulation studies are obtained. They are normal except for an increased bleeding time and a prolonged partial thromboplastin time (PTT). Which of the following is the most likely diagnosis?

(A) idiopathic thrombocytopenia purpura
(B) von Willebrand's disease
(C) classic hemophilia
(D) deficiency in factors II, VII, IX, and X
(E) deficiency in factor IX

102. A 1-week-old infant is brought to the emergency department with a 1-day history of fever. He has also been irritable and been eating less than usual. On physical exam, he has a temperature of 39°C. He is irritable and inconsolable. Which of the following diagnostic studies should be done?

(A) CBC
(B) CBC, blood culture
(C) CBC, blood culture, urinalysis (UA)
(D) CBC, blood culture, UA, urine culture
(E) CBC, blood culture, UA, urine culture, spinal tap

103. The appropriate diagnostic studies are obtained. Which of the following organisms is

most likely to cause systemic infection in this infant?

(A) group A *Streptococcus*
(B) group B *Streptococcus*
(C) *Hemophilus influenzae*, type B
(D) *Listeria monocytogenes*
(E) *Staphylococcus aureus*

104. Which of the following organisms is most likely to cause acute cervical adenitis in an 8-month-old child?

(A) group A *Streptococcus*
(B) group B *Streptococcus*
(C) *Hemophilus influenzae*, type B
(D) *Pasteurella multocida*
(E) *Streptococcus pneumoniae*

Question 105

An unmatched case-control study of the relationship between colon cancer and exposure to ionizing radiation reported the following data:

Colon Cancer

Ionizing rad	Cases	Controls	Total
Yes	11	35	46
No	50	209	259
Total	61	244	305

105. These results indicate that

(A) the lifetime risk of colon cancer in the total population is approximately 20%
(B) among those without colon cancer, the odds of ionizing radiation exposure are about 1 to 5
(C) among those who were exposed to ionizing radiation, the estimated risk of colon cancer is 23.9%
(D) the relative risk of colon cancer associated with exposure to ionizing radiation is approximated by an odds ratio of 1.3
(E) the risk of colon cancer in the control group is 79.5%

106. A 9-year-old girl with a history of intermittent wheezing for several years is brought to the pediatrician. The child has not been on medications for some time. Physical examination reveals a febrile child who is agitated and has perioral cyanosis. Intercostal and suprasternal retractions are present. The breath sounds are quiet, and wheezing is audible bilaterally. Which of the following is the most appropriate initial intervention?

(A) Prescribe IV aminophylline.
(B) Obtain a chest film.
(C) Prescribe nebulized cromolyn sodium.
(D) Obtain a CBC and blood culture.
(E) Prescribe nebulized albuterol.

107. A 4-year-old girl is brought to the office 2 days after she was bitten by her neighbor's cat. The bite is on her hand and occurred when she was teasing the cat. On physical exam, there are two closed puncture sites with erythema and induration around the wound. Which of the following organisms is most likely to cause the infection in this wound?

(A) *Rochalimaea henselae*
(B) *Eikenella corrodens*
(C) *Pasteurella multocida*
(D) *Francisella tularensis*
(E) *Spirillum minus*

108. The most common measure of central tendency that is most sensitive to extreme values in a sample is the

(A) median
(B) mean
(C) mode
(D) standard deviation
(E) standard median

109. A 36-year-old alcoholic patient has cirrhosis and pancreatic insufficiency due to recurrent pancreatitis. He complains of night blind-

ness, decreased ability to taste food, and dry skin with hyperpigmentation. These complaints suggest deficiency of

(A) copper
(B) zinc
(C) selenium
(D) chromium
(E) manganese

Questions 110 Through 112

A 52-year-old schoolteacher presents to the emergency department for evaluation of a tender, swollen, red left thigh. She just returned from spring break, during which she drove for 9 hours one way to visit her parents. She is a smoker whose only medications are estrogen and progesterone. Her vital signs, including respiratory rate, are normal. Other than her leg, her exam is unremarkable.

110. What is the best initial step in her evaluation?

(A) ventilation–perfusion (VQ) scan
(B) pulmonary angiography
(C) duplex scanning of her left leg
(D) venogram
(E) pulse oximetry

111. After finding that she has thrombosis of the left femoral vein, she is admitted for IV heparin treatment. After 5 days of therapy, her platelets are noted to be 45,000. Admission platelets were 375,000. You make the diagnosis of heparin-induced thrombocytopenia. Which of the following is true about this syndrome?

(A) It usually occurs within hours after beginning heparin.
(B) Risk usually is dose-dependent and increases with higher doses.
(C) It usually produces marked thrombocytopenia with counts less than 20,000.
(D) There is an IgA antibody that binds to a complex of heparin and platelet factor 4.
(E) Risk is higher with use of porcine rather than bovine heparin.

112. Which of the following is the most common complication?

    (A) bleeding
    (B) arterial thrombosis
    (C) deep venous thrombosis (DVT)
    (D) stroke
    (E) skin necrosis

113. If a clinical trial shows that drug A is more efficacious than drug B, with a *P* value of 0.02, which of the following statements best describes the results?

    (A) There is a 2% probability that the results are false.
    (B) There is a 2% probability that the difference observed occurred by chance.
    (C) The probability of drug B's being superior is 2%.
    (D) The probability of type II error is 2%.
    (E) The study had sufficient statistical power.

Questions 114 and 115

A 65-year-old woman presents to the physician's office for evaluation of depression. Past history is pertinent for passage of a kidney stone 1 month ago. Physical exam is unremarkable. Screening blood tests reveal a calcium of 12.8 and albumin of 4.0. Parathyroid hormone (PTH) assay reveals an elevated value of 328.

114. Which of the following is the most likely etiology of her symptoms?

    (A) parathyroid adenoma
    (B) parathyroid hyperplasia
    (C) multiple endocrine neoplasia type I (MEN I)
    (D) MEN IIa
    (E) parathyroid carcinoma

115. Which of the following tests is indicated prior to surgery (ie, neck exploration)?

    (A) high-resolution real-time ultrasonography
    (B) CT scan

    (C) magnetic resonance imaging (MRI)
    (D) radionuclide scanning
    (E) none

116. According to Piaget's Cognitive Developmental Stages, the critical achievement of the sensorimotor period of development is the completion of

    (A) object permanence
    (B) object constancy
    (C) transitional objects
    (D) preoperational reasoning
    (E) concrete operations

117. A 28-year-old normal-appearing woman has a 21/21 translocation. Her risk of having a child with Down syndrome is

    (A) 1%
    (B) 5%
    (C) 25%
    (D) 50%
    (E) 100%

Questions 118 and 119

An 18-year-old primigravid woman is at 26 weeks' gestation. Cervical culture is positive for *Chlamydia trachomatis*.

118. The most appropriate antibiotic is

    (A) dicloxacillin
    (B) doxycycline
    (C) ampicillin
    (D) vancomycin
    (E) erythromycin

119. Appropriate treatment of this 18-year-old woman's sexual partner is

    (A) dicloxacillin
    (B) doxycycline
    (C) ampicillin
    (D) vancomycin
    (E) erythromycin

Questions 120 and 121

A 37-year-old woman is being evaluated for possible multiple sclerosis (MS). She began noting paresthesias in both legs intermittently several months ago and now has symptoms of urinary incontinence.

120. What physical finding is characteristic of MS?

   (A) memory loss

   (B) constipation

   (C) internuclear ophthalmoplegia

   (D) intention tremor

   (E) bilateral upgoing toes

121. What is the best initial step in establishing the diagnosis?

   (A) brain CT scan

   (B) brain MRI

   (C) EEG

   (D) visual evoked potentials

   (E) auditory evoked potentials

Questions 122 Through 124

A 41-year-old man reports that he washes his hands 50 times a day. In the evening, he will check the doors, windows, and stove at least a dozen times before retiring for the night. He is fearful of the number 3; for example, he will not write out a check with a 3 in the number, and he will not stop his car if the odometer number ends in 3.

122. The most likely diagnosis for the man described above is

   (A) paranoid disorder

   (B) paranoid schizophrenia

   (C) schizotypal personality disorder

   (D) obsessive–compulsive disorder

   (E) presenile dementia

123. Of the following drugs, which is recommended as a first choice to control this man's symptoms?

   (A) fluvoxamine

   (B) alprazolam

   (C) buspirone

   (D) haloperidol

   (E) lithium

124. The man wants to know if he can be treated nonpharmacologically. Successful therapeutic intervention would most likely be accomplished by

   (A) ECT

   (B) behavioral therapy

   (C) hypnosis

   (D) short-term dynamic psychotherapy

   (E) none of the above

Questions 125 and 126

A 3-day-old term infant presents with progressive vomiting and abdominal distension. On questioning the nursery staff, they report that the child passed meconium at 48 hours but only after receiving a glycerin supository. He has not tolerated oral feeds, and urine output has decreased over the preceding 12 hours.

125. Which of the following diagnostic and/or therapeutic interventions are essential prior to transporting the child to the regional pediatric hospital?

   (A) nasogastric tube decompression and IV fluid resuscitation

   (B) blood and urine cultures, followed by initiation of broad-spectrum antibiotics

   (C) barium enema

   (D) plain abdominal radiographs

   (E) sweat chloride determination

126. On arrival at the receiving pediatric hospital, the most appropriate approach to establishing the diagnosis would be

   (A) anorectal manometry

   (B) abdominal ultrasound

   (C) plain radiographs, followed by a barium enema, and subsequent rectal biopsy if indicated

   (D) plain radiographs, followed by a UGI contrast study

   (E) rectal biopsy

Answers and Explanations

1–2. **(1-C, 2-D)** Antibiotic-associated colitis often occurs in the elderly, after exposure to antibiotics, and is caused by enterotoxins produced by *Clostridium difficile*. Whereas abdominal x-rays and CT scanning can demonstrate abnormal findings, detection of toxin in the stool will yield a definitive diagnosis. The appropriate treatment of patients with dehydration and abdominal symptoms would be IV fluids and admittance to the hospital for monitoring of their disease, discontinuation of the antibiotics that precipitated the disease, and institution of metronidazole. Barium enema should be avoided since it may precipitate complications. Whereas proctoscopy may be helpful, colonoscopy may precipitate perforation and should be avoided. (*Greenfield et al, pp 1172–1180*)

3. **(D)** The single most effective intervention a physician can make in smoking cessation is delivering an unambiguous, nonjudgmental, informative statement on the need to quit smoking. It is especially helpful to deliver this message consistently over successive visits. Physicians can help establish a "quit date," prepare the patient for withdrawal symptoms, and supply positive reinforcement on successive visits. Nicotine products may be useful for many smokers withdrawing from tobacco products. It is surprising how often clinicians fail to counsel smoking patients to stop using tobacco products. (*U.S. Preventive Services Task Force, p 602*)

4. **(C)** Duodenal atresia presents with vomiting on the first day of life. The diagnosis is sus-

pected when the abdominal film shows the "double bubble" sign shown in Figure 7–1. The surgical repair is usually successful and the prognosis is excellent. Pyloric stenosis typically manifests after the second to third week of life, and the vomiting grows progressively worse as the pyloric muscle hypertrophies. The obstruction is rarely present at birth. Adrenogenital syndrome presents with vomiting at birth or shortly thereafter. Electrolyte abnormalities are a major issue. Esophageal atresia is excluded by passing a nasogastric tube into the stomach. Cystic fibrosis does not present with vomiting unless meconium ileus is present at birth. (*Rudolph, pp 1054–1055, 1068–1072, 1526–1532, 1775–1778*)

5. **(E)** This young man has psychotic symptoms. Of the medications listed, quetiapine is the only antipsychotic. This is a benzodiazepine with high affinity for serotonin types 2 and 6 (5-HT$_2$ and 5-HT$_6$), moderate affinity for dopamine type 2 (D$_2$) receptors, and lower for dopamine type 1 (D$_1$) and lower still for dopamine type 4 (D$_4$). It has been found effective for various psychotic disorders and is fairly new among the antipsychotic agents. Buspirone is a non-benzodiazepine anxiolytic agent. Bupropion is an antidepressant drug recently experiencing renewed use in smoking cessation programs. Fluvoxamine, an antidepressant (selective serotonin reuptake inhibitor [SSRI]), and clomipramine, an antidepressant, have been of particular value in the treatment of obsessive–compulsive disorder. (*Kaplan and Sadock, pp 1079, 1001, 1004, 1105*)

6. (C) The sense that thoughts are drawn out of one's brain by "negative electromagnetic waves" is a delusion, a false belief that cannot be changed by logical argument. Other responses noted here may also be found in this young man's disorder. Projection is attributing to another person or thing one's own impulses or feelings. In loose associations, thoughts shift without any apparent connection to one another. Hallucinations are sensory experiences not associated with any real external stimuli. Heightened sensitivity to environmental stimuli, while occurring in most people at some time in their lives, has gone beyond what is reasonable in this young man. (Kaplan and Sadock, pp 221, 282–284; Stoudemire, Clinical Psychiatry, pp 148–150)

7. (B) A history of good achievement in school suggests good premorbid functioning, which in turn supports the possibility of a good prognostic outcome. All the other items weigh toward poor outcome when one is assessing prognosis. One needs to factor in all the various indicators, positive and negative, that point to the eventual outcome. This is critical in providing hope for the patient as well as for making reasonable future plans. (Kaplan and Sadock, p 468)

8. (A) Bias is a systematic error in any study that leads to a distortion of the results. The distortion is greatest in observational studies in which randomization is not possible, increasing the chance that the study groups will differ with respect to important characteristics. Among observational studies, however, the prospective cohort study design is least susceptible to bias because information about the risk factor (exposure) is determined prior to the observation of disease status. (Last JM, Maxcy-Rosenau-Last Public Health & Preventive Medicine, pp 24–27)

9. (A) An office endometrial biopsy is the appropriate initial step to evaluate postmenopausal bleeding because it will detect more than 90% of endometrial cancers. While cervical cancer may cause postmenopausal bleeding, there is usually a visible and friable cervical lesion. A Pap smear detects only about 50% of endometrial cancers. With a normal pelvic exam and Pap smear, colposcopy is unnecessary. Measurement of endometrial thickness by ultrasonography is a screening test reserved for those women in whom an office endometrial biopsy is technically impossible. While elevated levels of Ca-125 may occur in endometrial cancer, it is more likely to be elevated in ovarian cancer. A vaginal hysterectomy is contraindicated with undiagnosed postmenopausal bleeding. (Mishell et al, pp 873–899)

10. (C) Nulliparity may be the result of chronic estrogenic anovulation and is a risk factor for endometrial cancer. Conversely, a woman with four children is presumed to have ovulatory menses; parous women with ovulatory menses have a lower risk of endometrial cancer. Late menopause (and/or early menarche) increases the risk of endometrial cancer slightly. Age, obesity, and hepatic disease increase the extraglandular production of estrogen, principally estrone, and increase the risk of endometrial cancer. A BMI over 26 kg/m² is considered obese, and a BMI over 31 kg/m² is considered morbid obesity. As a chronic source of increased estrogen unopposed by progesterone, the risk of endometrial cancer increases three- to sixfold over time. Multiple sexual partners may be a risk factor for cervical cancer but is not a risk factor for endometrial cancer. Menopausal hormone replacement with estrogen alone also increases the risk of endometrial cancer by a factor of two- to tenfold. Estrogen plus progestin replacement after menopause reduces the risk of endometrial cancer to that of women not taking hormone replacement. (Speroff et al, pp 611–612)

11. (C) Bone marrow depression is the most serious toxic effect of methotrexate. Other toxic effects include megaloblastic anemia, diarrhea, stomatitis, vomiting, vasculitis, and pulmonary fibrosis. Myocardial damage leading to heart failure, peripheral neuropathy, hemorrhagic cystitis, and hearing loss are not side effects of methotrexate, but may occur with other chemotherapeutic agents. (DiSaia and Creasman, pp 519–523)

12. **(A)** Dose-related and cumulative renal insufficiency is the major dose-limiting toxicity of cisplatin. The main route of excretion of cisplatin is through the kidneys, and good hydration may help minimize potential tubular damage. Other toxic reactions include myelosuppression and neurotoxicity. Dermatitis, cystitis, and decreased visual acuity are not toxic effects of cisplatin. Cisplatin is commonly used to treat ovarian cancer. *(DiSaia and Creasman, pp 519–523)*

13–16. **(13-D, 14-D, 15-D, 16-B)** Medullary carcinoma of the thyroid (MCT) appears in three clinical settings: sporadic, as a component of multiple endocrine neoplasia type IIa (MEN IIa) or MEN IIb. A family history of thyroid carcinoma with or without pheochromocytoma is invariably present as part of the MEN IIa syndrome. Patients with MEN IIb have a marfanoid habitus and characteristic facies with ganglioneuromas. Patients with MEN syndrome must be evaluated for possible pheochromocytomas before treatment of the thyroid carcinoma. Total thyroidectomy is essential and represents the minimal treatment in patients with MEN IIa disease. Total parathyroidectomy results in hypoparathyroidism and should be avoided. Genetic screening for ret proto-oncogene mutations is highly sensitive and specific. Prophylactic thyroidectomy is recommended for patients with proven mutations consistent with MEN IIa. *(Greenfield et al, pp 1304–1305)*

17. **(D)** Glucose intolerance is very common in patients with cystic fibrosis, and about 10% of adolescent and older patients will develop clinical diabetes mellitus. The diabetes associated with cystic fibrosis resembles maturity-onset diabetes more than juvenile diabetes mellitus, in that ketoacidosis is rare, and satisfactory clinical control usually can be achieved with low-dose insulin. The sweat test is too labor intensive to be practical as a mass screening test for the general population. However, because of its accuracy, it is the diagnostic test of choice. Pulmonary complications are serious and also, unfortunately, very common. Cystic fibrosis clearly is an autosomal recessive disorder. Treatment programs aimed at symptomatic control of pulmonary, gastrointestinal, and other manifestations can significantly prolong life, although they certainly do not amount to a cure. *(Rudolph, pp 1640–1650)*

18–19. **(18-A, 19-D)** Described here is a man with excessive anxiety and worry for a period greater than 6 months. Additionally, he is irritable, tired most of the time, and has a sleep disturbance—all criteria of a generalized anxiety disorder. There are no physical complaints, thus excluding somatization disorder, and neither does he indulge in common substances that cause anxiety (ie, caffeine and illicit drugs). There are no discrete episodes of sympathetic discharge as seen in panic disorder, nor discrete focus of fear of a specific place or object as seen in phobic disorder. For a diagnosis of adjustment reaction, one would expect a specific stressor to be described. For dysthymic disorder, symptoms would be present for the greater part of 2 years, and in addition to those described in the case example, depressed mood would be a predominant characteristic.

Of the medications listed, lorazepam would relieve this man's symptoms most quickly, as would most other benzodiazepines. Buspirone, also an anxiolytic, would be effective but would require 1 to 2 weeks' treatment until some relief was obtained. Tricyclic antidepressants such as imipramine have also been of value in treating this disorder. Both thioridazine, an antipsychotic, and carbamazepine, used as a mood stabilizer, are not indicated for the specific use as an anxiolytic agent. In treating generalized anxiety disorder with a benzodiazepine, particular care must be given to avoid chronic use of these agents, which can lead to tolerance, thus resulting in increased dosage and dependency. Reduction of anxiety symptoms may also inadvertently prevent patients from addressing underlying psychodynamic issues and conflicts in psychotherapy. *(APA, pp 434–449; Kaplan and Sadock, pp 623–627)*

20. **(B)** Trichotillomania is an impulse control disorder characterized by recurrent compulsive pulling out of one's hair from any area of the body. The symptoms described here give no support for a diagnosis of catatonic (nor any) schizophrenia. Ghost sickness and mal de ojo are culture-bound syndromes. Ghost sickness is seen in members of American Indian tribes and is characterized by a preoccupation with death and the deceased. Associated symptoms include bad dreams, weakness, hallucinations, feelings of futility, and others. Mal de ojo ("evil eye") is seen in Mediterranean cultures. Persons with this disorder experience disturbed sleep, crying without apparent cause, diarrhea, and vomiting. It is usually seen in children. Autism is seen in children and is characterized by a profoundly abnormal and impaired ability to interact socially with others. *(APA, pp 618–620, 846–847)*

21. **(B)** Taxol is frequently used in the treatment of advanced epithelial ovarian cancers. Originally, it was derived from the bark of the western yew tree, but can now be chemically synthesized. It is a mitotic spindle inhibitor, but acts in a manner different from other such inhibitors. Taxol promotes assembly of microtubules and stabilizes them, thus preventing depolymerization and cell duplication. Myelosuppression is the major toxic effect that limits the utility of Taxol, and other typical side effects of chemotherapy, such as alopecia, nausea, vomiting, and peripheral neuropathies, are also seen. *(DiSaia and Creasman, pp 519–523)*

22. **(D)** A bolus IV injection of oxytocin to cause myometrial contraction and minimize postpartum blood loss may cause a rapid fall in arterial blood pressure. Doses of 20 units or less rarely cause symptomatic hypotension. Hypertension is not a complication of oxytocin. Excessive doses of oxytocin during labor may cause overstimulation of the myometrium, myometrial tetany, and possibly fetal distress. Prolonged oxytocin administration can have an antidiuretic hormone (ADH) effect and produce renal reabsorption of free water. This can lead to hyponatremia and hypokalemia. *(Cunningham et al, pp 340–341)*

23. **(B)** Dysfunctional uterine bleeding is thought to result from the unchecked proliferation of the endometrial lining, with eventual sloughing of underperfused portions. The proliferation is due to stimulation by estrogen from immature ovarian follicles that do not ovulate and therefore do not experience transformation into a corpus luteum and do not produce progesterone, which would check endometrial proliferation and induce transformation into a secretory phase. Anovulatory cycles are common 1 to 2 years after menarche, making this problem common in young adolescents. The bleeding characteristically is irregular, painless, and can be heavy enough to produce anemia. Patients with repeated cycles characterized by dysfunctional bleeding may receive treatment with progesterone replacement to mimic a luteal phase for several months until fully mature ovulatory cycles are established. *(Rudolph, pp 61–62)*

24. **(D)** Acute grief is a definite syndrome with psychological and somatic symptoms. It may present immediately after a crisis, or onset may be delayed. The clinical presentation is remarkably consistent in all individuals. Common features of grief reactions include sensations of somatic distress, feelings of diminished strength or physical exhaustion, feelings of mild depersonalization or derealization, recurrent dreams or ruminations about the death itself or the deceased person, feelings of guilt and personal responsibility for the loss, diminished desire for interpersonal contact, mood lability, and irritability. Morbid or pathological grief reactions represent distortions of the normal response to personal loss. These distorted reactions may present as overactivity without a sense of loss, acquisition of physical symptoms belonging to the deceased, onset of a new medical condition, conspicuous alteration in social adjustment, extreme deterioration in mood and character, and frank depression or psychosis. *(Kaplan and Sadock, pp 69–71)*

25–26. **(25-B, 26-C)** The presentation of a painful swelling involving the nipple areolar complex associated with erythema and subareolar cystic structure in a young woman are the typical findings of periductal mastitis and abscess. The organisms responsible for the disease are staphylococcal species and anaerobes. The diagnosis can be confused with inflammatory carcinoma, whose presentation includes peau d'orange, a solid mass, and other findings that usually involve larger areas of skin of the breast rather than localized to the nipple areolar complex. Paget's disease of the nipple is characterized by an eczematoid lesion; Mondor's disease usually affects the peripheral breast and represents superficial thrombophlebitis; and intraductal papilloma is usually nonpalpable and presents with a nipple discharge without inflammatory changes. The treatment of the abscess is incision and drainage with biopsy of the wall of the cavity to confirm the diagnosis. Antibiotics are often administered as adjunctive therapy, but usually do not suffice as the only therapy. Mastectomy, lumpectomy, and excisional biopsy are not appropriate therapies. (*Greenfield et al, p 1377*)

27. **(E)** High doses of estrogen effectively prevent conception if given within 72 hours after intercourse. Although the exact mechanism of action is unknown, this treatment appears to prevent implantation. Any oral contraceptive taken in the usual manner of one tablet daily is ineffective because sufficiently high blood levels of estrogen are not reached. DES must be given twice daily for 5 days to be effective. The possibility of a pre-existing pregnancy should be eliminated, as high doses of estrogen can be teratogenic. Progesterone alone (eg, norethindrone) is not proven to prevent unwanted pregnancies. Methotrexate is ineffective until after implantation, which does not occur until 7 to 9 days after conception. (*Speroff and Darney, pp 123–126*)

28. **(B)** A recent meta-analysis of 55 studies concluded that estrogen replacement increases the risk of breast cancer by 35%. The addition of a progestin does not appear to reduce this risk. Although estrogen given alone increases the risk of endometrial adenocarcinoma three- to eightfold, estrogen replacement given with adequate progesterone supplementation actu-

ally decreases the likelihood of developing endometrial carcinoma. At least 70 mg of medroxyprogesterone acetate (Provera, Cycrin) monthly is necessary to prevent an increased risk of endometrial cancer. Culture and attitude, plus the availability of a suitable sexual partner, is more responsible than estrogen deficiency for the decline in sexual activity and response after menopause. Estrogen replacement will stabilize bone mineral density but will not increase it. Evidence is increasing that estrogen replacement decreases the risk of colon cancer. (*Speroff et al, pp 583–649*)

29. **(C)** Roseola infantum (also known as exanthema subitum) is a common disease of childhood. It is seen predominantly in infants between the ages of 6 and 24 months and typically causes temperatures as high as 38.9 to 40.5°C (102 to 105°F) for 3 to 5 days without accompanying symptoms. Physical examination is frequently normal but may reveal mild pharyngeal injection, suboccipital lymphadenopathy, or a bulging anterior fontanel. Defervescence then occurs, followed closely by the development of a truncal maculopapular rash, which fades after 2 to 3 days. It is most often caused by human herpes virus-6. It is the appearance of a rash *after* the cessation of fever that differentiates roseola infantum from other infectious exanthems. Measles is characterized by a generalized red, blotchy rash in a febrile individual with cough, coryza, conjunctivitis, and photophobia. The typical fine red papular rash of scarlet fever usually appears at the height of fever. Kawasaki disease is characterized by conjunctivitis, oral lesions, cervical adenitis, fever for 5 days, palmar or plantar erythema, and desquamation from the fingers or toes. The accompanying red rash is nonspecific. The rash in erythema infectiosum is a bright red rash on the cheeks (slapped cheek), followed by a reticular rash on the extremities. (*Rudolph, pp 654–655, 664, 931–932*)

30–31. **(30-D, 31-E)** Included in the DSM-IV is a syndrome known as premenstrual dysphoric disorder, which is popularly referred to as premenstrual syndrome or PMS. By DSM-IV criteria, this disorder is diagnosed if during the week or so before menses emotional and behavioral distress is significant enough to disrupt occupational, social, or interpersonal functioning. For the remainder of the menstrual cycle, affected women should be free of symptoms; if not, other psychiatric disturbances, such as depression, should be considered. Most women who seek help for late luteal-phase dysphoric disorder are older than 30 years of age. The cause of this disorder has yet to be elucidated. Various pharmacologic treatments have been tried, including alprazolam, fluoxetine (Prozac), progestogens, and diuretics; their effectiveness has been variable, and none have been consistently reliable. (APA, pp 715–717; Kaplan and Sadock, pp 528–529)

32. **(A)** The leading cause of massive bleeding per rectum in the older population is angiodysplasia and diverticulosis of the colon. The absence of abdominal findings suggests these possibilities rather than an inflammatory process. (Schwartz et al, pp 1034–1035)

33. **(E)** A sentinel, or herald, bleed is common in patients with an aortoenteric fistula. The key point in the history is prior aneurysm repair with a graft. The location of the fistula is the third or fourth portion of the duodenum, so UGI endoscopy to the duodenal bulb would miss the lesion. Immediate operation is indicated since these patients will suffer a subsequent life-threatening bleed. (Schwartz et al, pp 1034–1035)

34. **(G)** Colon carcinoma may be the source of chronic blood loss that often presents with fatigue and orthostasis, particularly from a right-sided lesion. Abdominal fullness and tenderness is suggestive of a large, right-sided colon cancer. (Schwartz et al, pp 1034–1035)

35. **(I)** Bleeding from acute gastric ulcer may occur and become life-threatening, especially in the elderly taking nonsteroidal anti-inflammatory drugs (NSAIDs). Immediate operation is indicated following resuscitation. (Greenfield et al, pp 783–784)

36. **(H)** Varices account for 10% of UGI bleeding and are suggested in patients with an alcohol history and exam findings suggestive of cirrhosis. (Schwartz et al, pp 1032–1033)

37. **(F)** Peptic ulcer disease is the most common cause of acute UGI hemorrhage. Duodenal ulcers occur slightly more frequently than gastric ulcers. Brisk hemorrhage occurs from the gastroduodenal artery from a posterior penetrating ulcer in the duodenal bulb. (Greenfield et al, pp 1162–1164)

38. **(B)** The features of ulcerative colitis include age of onset usually between 15 and 40 years, bloody diarrhea, abdominal pain, and fever. Bloody diarrhea is the major symptom in 25% of patients. (Greenfield et al, pp 1093–1097)

39. **(C)** The most common cause of secondary amenorrhea in reproductive-age women is pregnancy. Therefore, a pregnancy test should be the first step in the evaluation of secondary amenorrhea. Sudden weight loss and increased physical activity may cause secondary amenorrhea. Hypothyroidism and hyperprolactinemia can also cause secondary amenorrhea. Serum estradiol concentrations are less useful in assessing the cause of amenorrhea than measurement of FSH. A decresed estradiol concentration occurs with either hypothalamic–pituitary failure or ovarian failure. A decreased serum FSH concentration indicates hypothalamic–pituitary failure, whereas an elevated FSH concentration indicates ovarian failure. A serum testosterone concentration is appropriate only if the amenorrhea is accompanied by signs of androgen excess (eg, hirsutism, deepening of the voice, clitoral enlargement, etc). (Speroff et al, pp 435–441)

40. **(D)** There are relatively few contraindications to the use of oral contraceptives. Smoking in women over the age of 35 years is a contraindication, as is smoking more than 15 cigarettes per day in women younger than 35. An obese but otherwise healthy woman can use a low-dose oral contraceptive. If she is obese in association with androgen excess (eg, polycystic ovary syndrome), use of oral

contraceptives may actually be useful as an adjunct for weight loss. Contraceptive suppression of excess ovarian androgen production may suppress appetite and make control of caloric intake more manageable. Oral contraceptives are not contraindicated in women with diabetes mellitus, unless they have superimposed vascular complications. Even patients who have had eclampsia do not show increased evidence of hypertension when using oral contraceptives. Women with migraine headaches may take oral contraceptives. A small percentage of women whose migraine headaches cluster around the time of menstruation may have relief of their migraines with oral contraceptives. *(Speroff et al, pp 742–744)*

41. **(B)** Developmental dysplasia of the hip (DDH), formerly called congenital dislocation of the hip, is a relatively common problem, with a frequency of 1.5 to 10 per 1000 live births. Genetic factors appear to have a major role, with the disorder being especially prevalent among certain ethnic groups. It is common in Northern Italy and Japan and among Navajo Native Americans, but rare in African-Americans and Chinese. Girls are affected six to eight times more often than are boys. However, nongenetic factors also play a part. Uterine crowding and mechanical problems in the uterus appear to predispose to DDH. For example, DDH is more common with breach presentation and more common in firstborn children. Type of delivery is not related to the incidence of DDH. *(Rudolph and Hoffman, pp 2136–2137)*

42. **(E)** Neuroleptic malignant syndrome (NMS) is a rare, potentially fatal complication of the use of antipsychotic medication. Symptoms typically include high fever, delirium, and rigidity, and they usually develop within a week of starting a new drug or raising the dosage of the currently prescribed drug. Once NMS is suspected, the antipsychotic drug should be stopped and emergency supportive measures begun. Mortality from NMS has been reported to be as high as 20%. *(Kaplan and Sadock, pp 958–959)*

43. **(B)** A recent development in the pharmacologic treatment of affective disorders, especially bipolar disorder, has been the use of anticonvulsant drugs. The first to be tried, carbamazepine (Tegretol) often is the next line of treatment for bipolar disorder for persons unresponsive to lithium therapy. Carbamazepine has various side effects, although most are dose related and can be avoided by judicious clinical practice. The most worrisome side effects are aplastic anemia and agranulocytosis, which occur very rarely but in an idiosyncratic manner. *(Kaplan and Sadock, pp 1008–1013)*

44–46. **(44-C, 45-E, 46-E)** This patient has carbon monoxide poisoning, first requiring oxygen. Initial fluid resuscitation in burn injury is isotonic crystalloid. Colloid is not recommended in the first 24 hours because of the profound capillary leak associated with the early injury phase. The most common formula for fluid resuscitation in burn injury is the Parkland formula. This is based on body weight and percentage of body surface area (BSA) burned; that is, 4 mL × body weight (kg) × %BSA = mL resuscitation fluid/first 24 hours. One half of this amount is given in the first 8 hours after the burn, with the remainder over the next 16 hours. This fluid is given in addition to the patient's maintenance fluid requirements. Patients with circumferential burn injury are at risk of developing compartment syndrome. Burn wound edema increases the enclosed compartment pressure above systemic perfusion pressures, resulting in tissue ischemia. The patient will have pain in the affected extremity, especially with passive stretch. The limb will demonstrate signs of decreased distal perfusion, including pallor, decreased sensation, and motor weakness. Compartment pressure is relieved with emergency escharotomy. Elevation of the extremity is not appropriate as it will further diminish distal perfusion. Supplemental oxygen by mask is an ineffective means of increasing oxygen delivery because of diminished perfusion to the affected limb. *(Sabiston, pp 227–232; Greenfield et al, pp 426–434)*

47. **(A)** Raloxifene is a new SERM that acts as an estrogen in some systems and as an antiestrogen in others. Currently, it is approved by the Food and Drug Administration (FDA) only for treatment of osteoporosis. Bone mineral density is increased approximately 3% after 24 months. Raloxifene exerts no effect on HDL cholesterol concentrations but does lower total cholesterol and low-density lipoprotein (LDL) cholesterol concentrations. Evidence that there is a cardioprotective effect in humans is currently mixed. It acts as an antiestrogen in the hypothalamus; as a result, approximately 25% of women who take raloxifene experience hot flashes (vs. approximately 18% receiving a placebo). It also acts as an antiestrogen in the reproductive tract. Endometrial stripe thickness does not increase in response to raloxifene, and there is no change from an atrophic endometrium with its use. There is no evidence that raloxifene has any effect on incontinence, although its antiestrogenic effect in the genital tract would suggest that it will not improve urinary incontinence. (*Delmas et al, pp 1641–1647*)

48. **(D)** Aspirin is well absorbed from both the stomach and small intestine. Removal from the body involves both hepatic and renal pathways. Treatment is indicated when the ingested dose exceeds 100 mg/kg, and intensity of therapy is guided by the severity of the ingestion as estimated by serum salicylate levels in relationship to time since ingestion. Therapeutic intervention is aimed at limiting absorption of aspirin from the gastrointestinal tract (effectively accomplished by gastric lavage and administration of activated charcoal) and enhancing renal excretion of the drug. Maintenance of high urine flow aids rapid clearance, and alkalinization of the urine results in an ionized form of the drug that is poorly reabsorbed from the renal tubule, thus increasing excretion. *N*-acetylcysteine has no place in the treatment of aspirin poisoning. It is, however, quite effective in preventing the hepatotoxicity associated with severe acetaminophen overdose. Induced emesis is rarely used in the emergency department since it tends to delay the administration of activated charcoal. Several studies have not shown any benefit from the addition of cathartics to charcoal in the management of acute aspirin ingestions. (*Ellenhorn et al, pp 210–221*)

49. **(C)** Because of its effects on multiple body systems, including but not limited to renal, hematologic, and thyroid systems, appropriate baseline studies must precede the start of lithium therapy. The minimal tests to be done include serum creatinine, with electrolytes, thyroid function tests, and a complete blood count with differential. Additionally, because of its cardiac effect, an electrocardiogram (ECG) is indicated. Any woman thought to be pregnant should have a pregnancy test. (*Stoudemire, Clinical Psychiatry, pp 536–537; Kaplan and Sadock, p 1053*)

50. **(C)** Carpal tunnel syndrome is secondary to compression of the median nerve at the wrist. This compression neuropathy affects women more often than men. The patient may experience weakness of the hand, which is typically worse at night and relieved by shaking the hand upon awakening. There is hypesthesia in the median nerve distribution, and when long-standing, there may be atrophy of the thenar muscles. Management includes wrist splinting, anti-inflammatory agents, steroid injection, and avoiding repetitive movement of the hand and wrist. Surgical decompression may be required if nonoperative measures do not relieve symptoms. Compression of the digital nerve of the thumb produces paresthesias limited to the affected digit. The motor branch of the median nerve may be compressed in the palm secondary to direct trauma. Median nerve compression by the pronator teres is usually associated with forearm pain in addition to paresthesias in the nerve distribution. (*Sabiston, pp 1479–1482; Greenfield et al, pp 2155–2156*)

51. **(B)** The major sources of blood supply to the uterus are the uterine arteries, which arise from the hypogastric (internal iliac) arteries. These may be ligated surgically or embolized with newer radiographic techniques. Hysterectomy may be necessary if these maneuvers fail. The primary hemostatic mechanism

postpartum is myometrial contraction. Infusion of fresh frozen plasma is appropriate only with evidence of a clotting deficiency. Intrauterine infusion of warm saline and uterine packing have been used, but with no proven efficacy. These should not be used to control postpartum hemorrhage. (*Rock and Thompson, pp 86–84*)

52. **(C)** Dislocation of the radial head, also known as "nursemaid's elbow," is a very common condition of young children between the ages of 1 and 4 years. It is caused by sudden traction on the forearm, resulting in dislocation of the radial head from the capitulum of the humerus. The child holds the affected arm in flexion at the elbow with the forearm pronated. X-rays reveal no abnormalities. Treatment is by swift supination of the forearm; further treatment is usually not necessary with the first occurrence. (*Oski et al, p 1037*)

53. **(E)** Acne is a skin disorder with its onset in puberty, when testosterone derived from the gonads and adrenal glands stimulates sebaceous gland activity. This results in the formation of sebum, which contains triglycerides, squalene, wax esters, sterol esters, and phospholipids. *Propionibacterium acnes,* an anaerobic pleomorphic skin organism, produces a lipase that releases free fatty acids from the sebum mixture, including highly irritating medium-chain triglycerides. Individuals prone to acne appear to have an increased turnover of abnormally cohesive keratinized cells in the sebaceous duct; these accumulate, plug the duct, and inhibit the release of sebum to the skin surface. Acne tends to persist until the late teens or early twenties. Too frequent or too vigorous face washing can be irritating to the skin and actually worsen the acne. Diet appears to be of little importance in the etiology of acne. The treatment goals are to decrease the risk of scarring and to alleviate the psychological stress during these critical years of social and sexual development. Adolescents with mild to moderate acne usually respond to topical treatment. Therapy sould be individualized, but benzoyl peroxide and tretinoin is a rea-

sonable combination for initial therapy. (*Rudolph, pp 924–925*)

54. **(D)** According to Erikson, the stage of adolescence is marked by the search for identity. Adolescents identify with heroes, loved friends, social groups, and ideologies. The successful resolution of the identity crisis depends on the psychosocial capacity of the youngster to experiment with new roles and models. Therefore, their availability and appropriateness are essential to normal adolescent development. New roles and models are best experimented with and assimilated through participation in peer-related groups. Often, these associations will express a common sentiment or goal for the group—a social or political viewpoint, academic success, athletic proficiency, or competency at a task. (*Kaplan and Sadock, p 234; Wedding, pp 48–49*)

55. **(B)** In a historical cohort study, the cohort is formed in the past, classified by exposure status, and followed forward in time to determine the development of disease. This study is not ecological in design, because information on individual subjects was collected. It was not a cross-sectional design, because new occurrences of bronchitis since employment were used to calculate risk. It was not a randomized, controlled trial, because the investigator did not have anything to do with who works inside or outside of the post office. It was not a prospective cohort design, because the cohort was defined in the past. (*Last JM,* Maxcy-Rosenau-Last Public Health & Preventive Medicine, *pp 25, 1092–1093*)

56. **(C)** A mass immunization program is indicated. Preventive treatment with rifampin is usually limited to close contacts such as household members, day care center contacts, and people exposed to the patient's oral secretions. Sending students home 2 months early will only redistribute exposed persons. A case-control study will be difficult, since there are so many exposure variables and it will take time to do. An education campaign can help with early detection, not with prevention. Immunizations will be more effective. Most of the sporadic outbreaks in this

country are due to serotype C meningococcus, which is covered by the vaccine. Rates of asymptomatic carriage are high, and it may be impractical to eliminate all carriage in a population. It is not clear why a general population with many carriers may suddenly erupt with several cases of disease. Preventing disease through vaccination remains the best method in the face of an outbreak. *(Wallace and Doebbeling, p 206)*

57–58. (57-B, 58-C) Cardiac tamponade results from rapid accumulation of fluid in the pericardial sac, compromising cardiac filling and resulting in decreased cardiac output. The clinical findings of tachycardia, hypotension, and distant heart sounds in the presence of penetrating chest trauma should alert the physician to this diagnosis. Patients may also demonstrate jugular venous distension from decreased venous return to the right heart, and a diminished pulse pressure. Penetrating trauma with an entry wound in this location (fifth intercostal space midclavicular line) would be unlikely to injure the descending aorta. From anatomic landmarks, the left atrium and left ventricle are directly in the path of penetration. A massive hemothorax or tension pneumothorax would be associated with respiratory compromise, decreased breath sounds on the side of injury, and tracheal shift to the contralateral side. Phrenic nerve paralysis would affect diaphragmatic function and lead to altered ventilatory mechanics secondary to paradoxical movement of the hemidiaphragm. Pericardiocentesis is both diagnostic and therapeutic and should be the first step in management. Aspiration of as little as 10 to 20 mL may improve the patient's hemodynamic status. Once stabilized, the patient should be transferred to the operating room for definitive management of the underlying penetrating cardiac injury. This patient does not have respiratory compromise and would therefore not require assisted ventilation or chest tube insertion. The patient's hypotension may not respond to IV fluid bolus, but requires urgent pericardial decompression to improve venous return and cardiac output. Emergency department thoracotomy is reserved for patients with

penetrating chest trauma who arrive in the emergency department with measurable vital signs and subsequently suffer cardiopulmonary arrest. The thoracotomy permits open cardiac massage, and attempt at manual control of blood loss from the site of injury, in preparation for rapid transfer to the operating room. *(Sabiston, p 310; Greenfield et al, pp 328–329)*

59. (C) Reported rates of stillbirth in mothers with syphilis were 14 to 34%, a dramatic increase compared to the 0.7% in the general population. Mean birth weights are decreased significantly in infected mothers. This is the result of both preterm labor and intrauterine growth restriction. Women with primary or secondary syphilis are more likely to transmit infection to their fetus than are those with late or latent syphilis. Most infants with early congenital syphilis do not develop evidence of active disease for 10 to 14 days after birth. Despite the possiblility of immune suppression in HIV-infected women, serologic tests for syphilis are accurate in mother and infant. *(Sweet and Gibbs, pp 150–161)*

60. (B) Septic pelvic thrombophlebitis should be suspected in women with postpartum fever that fails to respond to broad-spectrum antibiotics, and whose physical exam is normal. CT scan or MRI of the pelvis may disclose pelvic vein phlebitis. The clinical impression that anticoagulant doses of heparin result in a rapid defervescence is not supported by convincing clinical data. Infectious causes of postpartum fever usually respond to broad-spectrum antibiotics within 48 to 72 hours. A pelvic abscess is usually easy to palpate on bimanual exam and may be anterior or posterior to the uterus. Subinvolution of the uterus, increased uterine tenderness, and increased postpartum bleeding with a foul lochia are the signs of postpartum endometritis. Pyelonephritis should also have responded to antibiotics within 48 to 72 hours. Breast engorgement may cause a fever within 24 to 48 hours postpartum, but the fever resolves without antibiotics. *(Cunningham et al, pp 547–558, 563)*

61. **(C)** The most likely illness is staphylococcal food poisoning, resulting from contamination by a food handler. Often, the handler has evidence of an infection. The victims exhibit classic symptoms of abrupt, often violent nausea, vomiting, abdominal cramps, and prostration. They frequently feel feverish and perspire, but they are not febrile. Diarrhea is frequent, but not the dominant complaint. The illness is caused by a heat-stable enterotoxin produced from *Staphylococcus aureus*. Regarding the food handler, *S aureus* is a common organism found in mucocutaneous infections. In outbreaks like this, infected lesions on food handlers can sometimes be found. Transmission is usually from an infected food handler to foodstuffs that are prepared ahead of time and then held at suboptimal temperatures, which allows the organism time to replicate and produce enterotoxin. Since the toxin is heat stable, rewarming the food and keeping it hot on a serving table will not neutralize it. The toxin is preformed when ingested, so there is no incubation time required in the victim. Therefore, onset is usually rapid. *(Last JM, Maxcy-Rosenau-Last Public Health & Preventive Medicine, p 195; Kelly, pp 513, 1359–1360)*

62. **(B)** The clinical symptoms of iron toxicity are divided into stages. In a significant ingestion, the first stage begins immediately after the ingestion and lasts 6 to 24 hours. Vomiting, diarrhea, abdominal pain, pallor, lethargy, and hypotension can be seen. These result from the direct toxicity to the GI tract and GI hemorrhage can occur. Liver failure and an associated coagulopathy can occur but not typically until 12 to 24 hours after the ingestion. Arrhythmias and respiratory symptoms are not seen with iron ingestions. If a patient does not develop symptoms within 6 hours of ingestion, it is unlikely that iron toxicity will develop. *(Ellenhorn et al, pp 1558–1562)*

63. **(C)** Numerous complications of Epstein–Barr virus–associated mononucleosis have been described. Hematologic complications are hemolytic anemia and thrombocytopenia. Neurologic complications include aseptic meningitis, encephalitis, optic neuritis, Guillain–Barré syndrome, transverse myelitis, and Bell's palsy. Splenic rupture is rare but potentially fatal. Often, it follows mild trauma. Although liver involvement is not uncommon acutely, chronic active hepatitis has not been described. Pancreatitis and azotemia have not been described. *(Rudolph et al, pp 639–640)*

64. **(C)** Interviewing the patient is critical to determining her needs. Ideally, this would be with her alone. Patients frequently will provide important information about themselves. They may not if a family member is present. All other options listed are premature. Prescribing sertraline, lorazepam, or ECT require a thorough evaluation of the patient's history, symptoms, psychosocial situation, etc. before determining a course of action. A family conference may be of real value, but should follow interview of the patient. *(Kaplan and Sadock, pp 240–242)*

65. **(B)** Suicidal ideation should be taken seriously, regardless of the age of the individual. Young children can become severely suicidal. Although suicide is rare before the age of 14 years, the frequency at which youngsters kill themselves is rising. It is the impulse-ridden child who more likely commits a fatal or serious suicide gesture, especially when the home environment, often the critical respite for the overwhelmed child, is itself in chaos (eg, from parental separation or divorce, death of a spouse or child, financial disaster). For example, children who experience parental violence in the home are at greater risk for making a suicide attempt if they have been physically abused, whereas those who have witnessed parent-to-parent violence are more inclined to manifest assaultive behaviors themselves. Unfortunately, suicide is increasing in incidence and is among the leading causes of death in the adolescent population. *(Kaplan and Sadock, pp 1250–1254)*

66. **(C)** An epidural hematoma most commonly occurs in the temporoparietal region as a result of hemorrhage from the middle meningeal artery. There may be an initial brief loss of consciousness secondary to a concussive event, followed by a variable lu-

cid interval. As the hematoma expands and exerts a mass effect, there is a deteriorating level of consciousness, with tentorial herniation and eventual midbrain compression. The patient develops an ipsilateral dilated fixed pupil and contralateral hemiparesis. Therefore, this patient with a dilated right pupil and left hemiparesis has a *right* epidural hematoma. An occipital intracranial hematoma will present with visual defects. A subdural hematoma develops from injury to the dural venous sinuses, with an acute subdural hematoma presenting with signs of rapidly increasing intracranial pressure and herniation. Subarachnoid hemorrhage is associated with a severe headache and photophobia, without a significant alteration in level of consciousness. *(Sabiston, pp 1359–1360)*

67. **(C)** This is an open fracture, and management constitutes an orthopedic emergency. Tetanus prophylaxis is indicated because the soft-tissue injury is a tetanus-prone wound. An open fracture is associated with a high risk of osteomyelitis. Systemic antibiotics should be started in the emergency department and continued postoperatively. Optimal local wound irrigation and debridement is achieved under general anesthesia. This fracture is severely comminuted and most likely unstable. Fracture stabilization can be accomplished with internal fixation or application of an external fixation device. The soft-tissue defect associated with an open fracture should not be closed primarily. It may require further debridement. With aggressive local wound care, delayed closure may be possible if the wound remains clean. Local wound irrigation and debridement may be limited by patient discomfort. The addition of antibiotics to the irrigation solution is of no additional benefit. Closed reduction would not be possible in this patient, because the fracture is severely comminuted. Furthermore, a long-leg cast will not provide adequate immobilization of the unstable fracture fragments. *(Sabiston, pp 1399–1400; Niederhuber, pp 708–709)*

68. **(B)** The triad of hypertension, hyperreflexia, and proteinuria in pregnancy establishes the diagnosis of preeclampsia. The etiology is still unknown, and the only accepted treatment at term pregnancy is delivery of the infant. The risk of eclampsia is not proportional to the increase in systolic or diastolic pressure, and has been reported to occur at the time of normal blood pressure readings. Beta blockers are not contraindicated in pregnancy, although angiotensin-converting enzyme (ACE) inhibitors are contraindicated. Beta-blocking drugs effectively lower blood pressure, and are most effectively used when the pregnant woman is early in the third trimester and prolongation of pregnancy is desired. The risk of abruptio placenta, not the risk of placenta previa, is increased in hypertensive pregnant women. Perinatal mortality is significantly increased in pregnant women with hypertension and proteinuria. In one study, it was increased threefold in women whose diastolic blood pressures were 105 torr or higher. *(Cunningham et al, pp 694–718)*

69. **(B)** Classically, there are three stages of labor. The first stage begins with the onset of regular uterine contractions that cause cervical dilation and ends with complete dilatation of the cervix. The first stage can be divided into a latent phase and an active phase. In a primigravida, the length of the latent and active phases average 8.6 hours and 4.9 hours, respectively. Both times are shorter in women who have had a child. The second stage begins with complete dilatation of the cervix and ends with delivery of the infant. The third stage begins after delivery of the infant and ends with delivery of the placenta. Subsequent events such as myometrial contractions, inspection of the cervix and vagina, and repair of an episiotomy or laceration are not recognized as a stage of labor. *(Cunningham et al, pp 416–421)*

70–71. **(70-E, 71-C)** This patient presents with an acute exacerbation of ulcerative colitis with systemic toxicity. Toxic megacolon is potentially life-threatening and requires aggressive fluid resuscitation, bowel rest, and systemic antibiotics. High-dose steroids are initiated to treat the colonic inflammation. If there is no clinical improvement after 48 hours of medical therapy, urgent surgery is indicated. Azathioprine and 6-mercaptopurine are immunosuppressive agents that may be beneficial in the treatment of steroid refractory colitis, but they are not indicated in the management of an acute toxic exacerbation. Opioid antidiarrheals are contraindicated, as they may increase colonic distension and increase the risk of perforation. Colonoscopy may also cause increased colonic distension with perforation.

Urgent surgery in a patient with toxic megacolon should consist of colectomy, Hartmann's procedure, and ileostomy. Ileal pouch–anal anastomosis is a lengthy procedure, and is considered only for elective reconstruction. When performed in a systemically ill patient undergoing emergency colectomy of an unprepped colon, there are increased risks of anastomotic complications. Ileorectal anastomosis is no longer appropriate for the management of ulcerative colitis because of the retained diseased rectal mucosa, with concomitant risk of malignancy. (*Sabiston, pp 1008–1009; Niederhuber, pp 312–314*)

72. **(E)** Hypertension before the third trimester, uterine size greater than dates, and the absence of a fetus with a detectable heartbeat after 6 postmenstrual weeks strongly suggests a diagnosis of gestational trophoblastic disease, most likely a hydatidiform mole. A multiple pregnancy is not a consideration because gestational sacs, each containing a fetus, with cardiac activity in each sac, would be seen by transvaginal ultrasonography after 6 postmenstrual weeks. Although the absence of an intrauterine pregnancy is ultrasonic evidence of a tubal pregacy, the ectopic gestational sac is usually seen when the hCG concentration is 10,000 mIU/mL or higher. The presence of a significantly enlarged uterus does not favor a diagnosis of tubal pregnancy. Serum hCG concentrations are lower than expected with a blighted ovum, and the uterus tends to be smaller than the gestational age. The elevated hCG concentration, the hypertension, and the absence of a fetus with a heartbeat is against the diagnosis of a normal intrauterine pregnancy in a woman with a myomatous uterus. Man-

agement of this patient is evacuation of the uterus by suction curettage and serial hCG measurements for one year to be certain that this woman does not subsequently develop choriocarcinoma. (*Mishell et al, pp 998–1002*)

73. **(B)** Any condition that causes narrowing of the upper airway may result in inspiratory stridor. This includes acute laryngotracheobrochitis or croup. This patient has the typical history and exam seen in patients with croup. Laryngomalacia is a condition of unusual softness of the larynx, resulting in inspiratory collapse and stridor. The condition is present early in infancy and usually resolves by 3 to 5 years. Patients with laryngomalacia have chronic stridor. Conditions that cause narrowing of the conducting system of the lower respiratory tract, such as bronchiolitis, result in wheezing. Foreign bodies are more common in children between the ages of 1 and 4 years, when they tend to put things in their mouths. Peritonsillar abscess is seen in older children and adolescents. (*Kliegman, p 127*)

74. **(B)** Congenital adrenal hyperplasia may be caused by many different defects of steroidogenesis. The most common defect, 21-hydroxylase deficiency, accounts for about 95% of these disorders and is transmitted as an autosomal recessive trait. These patients have aldosterone deficiency, which results in hyponatremia, hyperkalemia, and hypotension and shock. They also have glucocorticoid deficiency and therefore have hypoglycemia. The electrolyte abnormalities are the key to the diagnosis. None of the other diseases listed would cause this degree of electrolyte abnormality. (*Rudolph, p 1725*)

75. **(A)** An increase in GGT (> 30 units) is a consistent finding in heavy alcohol drinkers. Seventy percent of individuals with elevated GGT are heavy drinkers. Increases in SGOT, triglycerides, serum glumatic-pyruvic transaminase (SGPT), and uric acid have also been noted, but these are less consistently observed. (*APA, p 200; Kaplan and Sadock, p 397; Stoudemire, Clinical Psychiatry, pp 315–316*)

76. (C) Psychological assessment techniques are, like most tools, useful for a diversity of purposes. Their worth partially depends on the training, competence, and ethical values of the tester. In the hands of a competent clinician, the results of an intelligence quotient (IQ) examination, when correlated with other information from the person's history or present status, are valuable data. In 1896, the French clinician Binet began a project to develop an objective measure by which to quantify individual differences in mental abilities (intelligence). From 1905 to 1908, Binet and Simon introduced a series of standardized IQ tests in which correct responses to items that differed progressively in level of difficulty were correlated with a child's chronological age. In 1916, Terman, at Stanford University, revised the Binet–Simon Intelligence Scale. The Stanford–Binet Test was quickly adopted in the United States for assessing the intelligence of children. Wechsler, as chief psychologist at Bellevue Hospital in New York, introduced the next major development in the history of intelligence testing. Prior to Wechsler, IQ testing was primarily used with children 15 years old or younger. Wechsler developed scales that compared the performance of a child with the performance of his or her own agemates on the same test items. The Bellevue–Wechsler Scale was introduced in 1939. In 1949, this scale was used as the model for a revised test specifically for children (ages 6 to 16 years), the Wechsler Intelligence Scale for Children (WISC). Restandardization of the Bellevue–Wechsler Scale led to the introduction of the Wechsler Adult Intelligence Scale (WAIS) in 1958, with norms for ages 16 to 75 years. The WISC and WAIS are currently the most widely accepted tests of intelligence in use today. The Metropolitan Achievement Test and the Vineland Social Maturity Scale are contemporary standardized tests of school readiness and grade-level achievement and acquisition of culture-based social skills, respectively. *(Kaplan and Sadock, pp 1133–1136)*

77. (D) *Candida* vaginitis is the only local infection in which the vaginal pH is less than 4.5. The absence of clue cells and no amine odor excludes bacterial vaginosis due to *G vaginalis*. *Trichomonas* vaginitis is due to a unicellular, flagellated organism that would demonstrate flagellar motion on a saline wet smear. *Chlamydia* and syphilis present with no diagnostic vaginal discharge. *(Sweet and Gibbs, pp 344, 347–355)*

78. (B) Either oral or vaginal antifungal agents are usually effective in eradication of *Candida* species from the vagina. Metronidazole is used to treat trichomoniasis or bacterial vaginosis. Ceftriaxone is the current treatment of choice for gonorrhea. Oral doxycycline is recommended as cotherapy with ceftriaxone to eradicate concurrent *Chlamydia* infection. Oral or vaginal clindamycin is effective therapy for bacterial vaginosis, giving cure rates comparable to metronidazole (about 95%). *(Sweet and Gibbs, pp 344, 347–355)*

79. (A) Anorexia nervosa is a disorder of unknown cause that primarily affects young women. Its onset most frequently occurs during adolescence and its highest incidence is among white females of Western countries. The clinical picture is predominated by signs of starvation, and obsessive–compulsive traits are often present. Affected individuals are frequently good students who have been characterized as achievers. A loss of 25% or more of total body weight is almost always included in the diagnostic criteria. Hypothermia and bradycardia are seen with severe weight loss. Patients with bulimia tend to binge and then purge. They are often of normal weight. Hyperthyroidism is not common in adolescents but can occur. It can cause weight loss, but this patient does not have other signs of hyperthyroidism, such as tachycardia. Diabetes in adolescents typically is of abrupt onset, with the classic symptoms of polyphagia, polydipsia, and polyuria. Depression can cause weight loss, but patients tend to withdraw from their activities, and the mood changes are the dominant symptom. *(Rudolph et al, pp 42–44, 1766–1768, 1803–1807)*

80. (C) The following factors contribute to a favorable prognosis for children with ALL: age between 3 and 7 years, absence of lymphadenopathy, *female* gender, initial WBC of 10,000, hemoglobin of 7 g/100 mL, and platelet count of 100,000. All of these factors except gender lose their prognostic significance after 2 years of complete and continuous remission. Unfavorable prognostic factors include the presence of a mediastinal mass, Ph[1] chromosome, decreased immunoglobulins, T- or B-cell surface markers on lymphoblasts, more than 25% blast cells in the bone marrow 14 days after treatment, and L2 or L3 lymphoblasts. *(Oski et al, pp 1701–1709)*

81. **(D)** When dealing with a threatening person, it is important to establish an alliance with that person to prevent violent acting out. As much as possible, this requires a quiet, collaborative effort, with the therapist carefully pacing each interaction. Demanding, standing over, and threatening are all confrontive, challenging behaviors that, instead of facilitating control of the situation, may provoke the person to violence. Asking the person the reasons for his or her anger is certainly appropriate; however, as a matter of timing and facilitating a working rapport, an empathic comment made first would be more helpful. *(Stoudemire,* Clinical Psychiatry, *pp 554–556; Tomb, pp 78–81)*

82. **(E)** One "pearl" of clinical wisdom applies here: "In an older person with no previous psychiatric history, suspect an organic etiology to psychiatric symptoms until proven otherwise." At this point in this woman's assessment, further information is needed regarding her physiologic status before arriving at a diagnosis. A thorough physical evaluation and appropriate laboratory work are essential to rule out those medical conditions that masquerade as psychiatric conditions. Two listed here, pancreatic cancer and hypothroidism, can be overlooked, with disastrous consequences. The possibility of a pathological grief reaction is also very strong here. Such a complex situation, which is a psychiatric condition in addition to a medical condition(s), requires well-honed medical acumen. *(Kaplan and Sadock, pp 525–528, 530; Stoudemire,* Clinical Psychiatry, *pp 341–344)*

83. **(E)** A karyotype of peripheral lymphocytes is the most appropriate option of the listed choices. It will be 46,XY in this patient. The normal height, normal breast development, sparse pubic hair, absent cervix and uterus, and a positive family history point to a diagnosis of testicular feminization (androgen insensitivity). In general, a karyotype is a useful early step in the evaluation of primary amenorrhea because 45,X gonadal dysgenesis is the most common cause of primary amenorrhea, and because several causes of primary amenorrhea are associated with the presence of a Y chromosome. Approximately 30% of women with a Y chromosome will develop a gonadal malignancy by the age of 30 years. A pelvic ultrasound is unnecessary if the pelvic exam is reliable in revealing the absence of a cervix and uterus. Breast development signifies the presence of estrogen, which means that the hypothalamic–pituitary–gonadal axis is intact. A CT scan of the pituitary is therefore unnecessary. A laparoscopy is a reasonable procedure to remove the testes once the diagnosis is established but is an inappropriate and unnecessary diagnostic tool. *(Speroff et al, pp 420–422)*

84. **(D)** Women with anorexia nervosa have deficient hypothalamic secretion of gonadotropin-releasing hormone (GnRH) and secondarily decreased secretion of FSH, luteinizing hormone (LH), and ovarian estradiol and progesterone. The presence of breast growth indicates that this woman was exposed to estrogen at some time. The exposure may have been in the past and may have been from exogenous sources. However, anorectic women have a cervix and uterus. The normal height and the presence of breasts excludes gonadal dysgenesis, as these women are never taller than 157.5 cm. (62 inches), and the streak gonads are incapable of estrogen production. Müllerian agenesis is less likely because of the family history, but all other clinical features are consistent with this diagnosis. Since these women have ovaries rather than testes, a test to detect ovulation makes the distinction: a biphasic basal temperature graph or a serum progesterone concentration over 5 ng/mL. Women

with 17α-hydroxylase deficiency have hypertension and are sexually infantile because this steroid enzyme deficiency does not permit normal cortisol, androgen, or estrogen biosynthesis. Deficient cortisol biosynthesis results in increased ACTH secretion, which stimulates an increased adrenal secretion of mineralocorticoids and results in hypertension. (*Speroff et al, pp 404–409, 420–422*)

85. **(E)** The androgen receptors in women with testicular feminization are absent, deficient, or qualitatively abnormal. There are rare instances of male pseudohermaphrodites with testes devoid of Leydig cells. The 46,XY karyotype excludes the possibility of ovarian follicles. The preoptic area of the hypothalamus is a prominent site for GnRH secretion, but hypogonadotropic hypogonadism is not the cause of amenorrhea in this woman. Women with a congenital abnormality of this area of the hypothalamus often lack the sense of smell (Kallmann syndrome). Women with 21-hydroxylase deficiency are hirsute and usually have irregular menses, not primary amenorrhea. (*Speroff et al, pp 404–409*)

86. **(E)** Urinary retention is an anticholinergic side effect to neuroleptics. This condition is exacerbated if treated with the anticholinergics used to effectively treat dopaminergic side effects, such as parkinsonism, oculogyric crisis, laryngeal dystonia, and tremors. (*Kaplan and Sadock, pp 946, 955–961*)

87. **(D)** Occult bacteremia refers to the finding of a positive blood culture in a child who appears well enough to be treated as an outpatient. The response to antipyretics or lack of response does not change the risk for bacteremia. The risk of occult bacteremia correlates statistically with an elevated WBC (15,000) and fever (39°C [102.2°F]). Occult pneumococcal bacteremia is most common between 6 months and 2 years of age, and the incidence declines after the second birthday. Occult bacteremia occurs with essentially the same frequency in all socioeconomic groups. (*Kliegman, pp 982–985*)

88. **(A)** Tuberculous meningitis is characterized pathologically by a thick, gelatinous exudate in the subarachnoid space. The predilection of this material for the base of the brain explains the frequency of cranial nerve findings in afflicted children. Although the concentration of protein in the CSF usually is elevated, levels of 1 g/100 mL or greater generally indicate obstruction of the ventricular system. The tuberculin test is negative in about 10% of patients, especially those with advanced disease. Although the onset may occasionally be acute, signs and symptoms generally begin gradually or insidiously. The prognosis is guarded, and for those who present with advanced neurologic findings such as coma, the prognosis is poor even with appropriate therapy. (*Rudolph, pp 618, 2004*)

89–91. **(89-C, 90-C, 91-D)** A common response to frightening news and a possible life-threatening illness is regression—a return to an earlier form of behavior that is more childlike. It is an attempt to flee overwhelming anxiety and fear. It is a seeking to be cared for and protected. Borderline personality disorder and PMS, though possible, require further investigation, and from the information given are not well-supported diagnoses. Sometimes clinicians, in their own angry countertransference to such patients, may "act out" by labeling the patient with these, since both terms can have a negative connotation. The nurses' anger in this case is an example of countertransference, which are feelings and attitudes of the therapist (medical personnel) toward the patient that may arise from the past or be a reaction to the patient's transference feelings or attitudes toward the therapist. In this case, for example, if the countertransference anger led to angry demands to medicate or to restrain this patient, we would also have an example of "acting out." Although the consulting psychiatrist must be cognizant of the reason for referral "to medicate," he or she must quickly determine what is the real and most therapeutic goal. Given the case scenario, the psychiatrist needs to first determine why this woman is acting the way she is. One would presume that once this woman is encouraged to talk about her angry feelings, she will be able to get to the underlying fears, which might include fear of mutilation, fear for her children, fear of losing her job or her husband's love, and fear of losing life itself. Appropriate medications may be indicated to help this woman deal with her fears and anxieties. (*Stoudemire*, Human Behavior, *pp 54, 79; Wedding, pp 261–262, 265*)

92. **(B)** The initial evaluation of hirsutism should include measurement of serum DHEA, testosterone, and perhaps 17-hydroxyprogesterone. Appropriate tests to evaluate her anovulatory menstrual cycles include serum prolactin and thyroid function. A pelvic ultrasound is appropriate if the bimanual part of the pelvic exam is unsatisfactory: obesity or voluntary guarding. An ACTH stimulation test is appropriate only in those women who may have congenital adrenal hyperplasia, suggested by a positive family history of hirsutism and oligomenorrhea, and significantly increased DHEA levels. One milligram of dexamethasone at 11:00 PM should suppress the next morning's cortisol concentration to less than 5 μg/dL. Failure to do so suggests the possibility of an adrenal tumor, and CT scan of the adrenal glands should be done. Measurement of FSH should be done only if the woman has any climacteric symptoms. (*Speroff et al, p 490*)

93. **(A)** Polycystic ovary syndrome was first described in 1935 by Stein and Leventhal. It is important to understand the features of the disorder as a syndrome that likely has multiple causes. There is growing sentiment to discard the terms polycystic ovary syndrome and Stein–Leventhal syndrome in favor of a more descriptive term, such as chronic estrogenic anovulation. In this way, the disorder can more easily be recognized as one with a spectrum of causes and clinical manifestations. At least 75% of women with chronic estrogenic anovulation will have what has been called polycystic ovary syndrome. The normal DHEA concentration effectively excludes attenuated 21-hydroxylase deficiency and an adrenal adenoma. The normal prolactin concentration tends to exclude a pituitary ade-

noma, although some pituitary tumors do not appear to secrete any hormones. The history of oligomenorrhea and hirsutism since puberty, plus the normal bimanual exam, makes a Sertoli–Leydig cell tumor unlikely. Abrupt cessation of menses, followed by the onset of hirsutism plus unilateral ovarian enlargement, is the usual presentation of a virilizing ovarian tumor. (*Speroff et al, pp 463–467*)

94. **(C)** Of the neurochemical systems listed here, dopamine is considered to play a role in the development of schizophrenia, which seems to be the most likely diagnosis for this young man. It is also believed that serotonin is involved in the development of schizophrenic symptoms. (*Kaplan and Sadock, pp 111–113, 115–116; Andreason and Black, pp 154–162*)

95. **(A)** Haloperidol is an antipsychotic agent that has affinity for dopamine receptors. Fluvoxamine is an SSRI. Imipramine affects norepinephrine and serotonin. Divalproex has a role in the GABA system. (*Kaplan and Sadock, pp 1079, 1089, 1100–1110*)

96. **(D)** Ovarian secretion of estrogen does not increase in women with polycystic ovary syndrome and is equivalent to early–midfollicular phase levels. Aromatization, or conversion of androgens to estrogens, occurs predominantly in adipose tissue. The extent of conversion of DHEA and testosterone to estrogen is low and accounts for little of the extraglandular estrogen formed in adipose tissue. Women with polycystic ovary syndrome secrete increased quantities of androstenedione from their ovaries. In normal-weight women, approximately 1.5% of the androstenedione is converted to estrone in extraglandular sites. To illustrate, androstenedione production in women with polycystic ovaries may double from 3000 μg/day to 4500 μg/day. In obese women, the extent of aromatization may increase from 1.5 to 3% or more. Compared to the 45 μg/day of estrone produced in nonobese ovulatory wo-men (3000 μg/day × 1.5%), women with poly- cystic ovary syndrome may produce 115 μg/ day or more of estrone (4500 μg/day × 3%). (*Speroff et al, pp 463–467*)

97. **(A)** Acrodermatitis enteropathica is an autosomal recessive disorder characterized clinically by dermatitis, alopecia, malabsorption, infections, growth retardation, and, rarely, hypogonadism. Children with this disorder manifest the clinical findings soon after being weaned from breast feeding because of the decreased bioavailability of zinc in cow's milk. Malabsorption is characterized by severe steatorrhea, lactose intolerance, and malnutrition. Some patients are known to develop cutaneous candidiasis, bacterial infections, and eye manifestations, including blepharitis and photophobia. Chronic zinc deficiency is the cause of the disorder. The treatment of choice is the administration of 10 to 45 mg/day of elemental zinc. *(Rudolph et al, pp 373, 888–889)*

98. **(C)** Intussusception, a telescoping of one portion of the gut into another, is the most common cause of intestinal obstruction between the ages of 2 months and 6 years. Typically, there is the onset of severe paroxysmal pain in a previously healthy child. Stools containing both blood and mucus, known as currant jelly stools, are characteristic of this disorder and are passed by 60% of these patients. Constipation can cause abdominal pain and can be palpated in the abdomen if severe enough. It does not cause bloody stools. Patients with infectious gastroenteritis can have blood in their stools, but this patient does not have diarrhea. Meckel's diverticulum causes painless rectal bleeding. *(Kliegman, pp 332–339)*

99. **(D)** Hirschsprung's disease, or congenital aganglionic megacolon, is associated with an absence of ganglion cells in part of the colon. It is the most common cause of intestinal obstruction of the colon and accounts for 33% of all neonatal obstructions. Patients present with constipation as neonates. Duodenal stenosis and esophageal atresia would cause vomiting. Breast-feeding failure can also cause constipation, but this baby has regained her birth weight, so it is obvious that her intake is adequate. Functional constipation does not occur in the first few days of life. *(Kliegman, pp 379–381)*

100. **(C)** Meckel's diverticulum is present in 2 to 3% of the population. Symptoms and signs can occur at any age but usually are manifested in the first 2 years of life. The most common sign is painless rectal bleeding. Anal fissures commonly cause rectal bleeding in infants, but it is a small amount of blood that typically coats the stool. Intussusception can cause bloody stools but usually also causes intermittent abdominal pain. Milk allergy would not occur this acutely. If the patient had a bloody stool with a volvulus, he would be ill-appearing and have abdominal pain. *(Kliegman, pp 332–339)*

101. **(B)** Von Willebrand's disease is an autosomal dominant disorder. Von Willebrand's disease is characterized by a prolonged bleeding time, various abnormalities of the factor VIII complex, and a prolonged PTT. In contrast, the bleeding time is normal in hemophilia and factor IX deficiency, and the PTT is normal in idiopathic thrombocytopenic purpura. Factors II, VII, IX, and X are vitamin K–dependent and may be deficient in a variety of disorders, including liver disease, malabsorption, and altered bowel flora. *(Oski et al, pp 1689–1695)*

102. **(E)** Infants with fever, especially those less than one month of age, are at high risk for serious bacterial infection. Approximately 9% of these infants who look well on exam will have a serious bacterial infection. History and physcial exam alone are not sensitive in detecting these infections. Laboratory evaluation is essential. Bacteremia, urinary tract infection, and meningitis are all possibilities in this age group, and so all of these tests must be done. *(Kliegman, pp 989–991)*

103. **(B)** Group B *Streptococcus* is the most common cause of neonatal sepsis and meningitis in many medical centers. Gram-negative organisms, *L monocytogenes*, and *Salmonella* are also possible, but less common. *H influenzae*, type b, causes invasive disease, but the incidence has decreased dramatically since universal immunization was instituted. *S aureus* would be an unusual organism unless the

infant had some type of break in the skin. *(Kliegman, pp 989–991)*

104. **(A)** Group A *Streptococcus* is the most likely organism. The next most common would be *Staphylococcus aureus*. *H influenzae* and *S pneumoniae* do not cause adenitis. *P multocida* is an organism found in the mouths of cats, which can cause a wound infection after a cat bite. *(Kliegman, p 795)*

105. **(D)** From a case-control study, the incidence (risk) of colon cancer cannot be calculated directly. Thus, choices (A), (C), and (E) should be excluded as possible correct answers. Choice (B) gives the odds of ionizing radiation exposure in those with colon cancer, and so cannot be selected as an answer. Thus, the only correct answer is (D), in which the relative risk of colon cancer associated with exposure to ionizing radiation is approximated by an odds ratio of 1.3. *(Last JM, Maxcy-Rosenau-Last Public Health & Preventive Medicine, pp 25–34)*

106. **(E)** This patient is in severe distress and needs immediate therapy. Inhaled albuterol is the initial treatment of choice. Cromolyn sodium is a drug with efficacy in the prevention of acute exacerbations of allergen- and exercise-induced asthma. It has no bronchodilatory activity and should not be used in the treatment of acute asthma. Aminophylline is rarely used in the acute treatment of asthma, as studies have shown that it does not add to the efficacy of inhaled albuterol. Diagnostic studies may need to be done later when the patient's respiratory distress has been relieved. *(Rudolph et al, pp 464–469)*

107. **(C)** Wounds resulting from animal bites may become infected with the typical skin and soft-tissue infectious agents, *Staphylococcus aureus* and *Streptococcus pyogenes*. Occasionally, they are infected with normal flora of the animal's mouth. Cat bite wounds may become infected with *P multocida*. These infections can be quite severe and may require surgical drainage because the long slender teeth of cats enable deep inoculation of the organism. Dog bite wounds may become

infected with *E corrodens*. Rat bite wounds may result in rat bite fever, of which *S minus* is one causative agent. *R henselae* causes cat scratch disease. *F tularensis* is the etiologic agent for tularemia. *(Oski et al, pp 1208–1209)*

108. **(B)** The mean is the measure of central tendency that is most affected by extreme values. *(Hill, pp 70–84)*

109. **(B)** Several disease states predispose to zinc deficiency, including cirrhosis, alcoholism, poor nutrition, and pancreatic insufficiency. Zinc deficiency can cause growth retardation, hypogonadism, anorexia, impaired sense of taste and smell, diarrhea, alopecia, dermatitis, hyperpigmentation, and poor wound healing. Night blindness due to combined zinc and vitamin A deficiencies improves only if both substances are replenished. Zinc deficiency in cirrhosis is associated with hepatic coma. Adult copper deficiency is also rare and is associated with Keshan's disease, a fatal cardiomyopathy occurring in children. Chromium deficiency causes impaired growth and abnormal lipid, glucose, and protein metabolism. Hypomagnesemia is associated with weight loss, dermatitis, change in hair color, and hypocholesterolemia. *(Fauci, pp 490–492)*

110. **(C)** Deep venous thrombosis is variable in its presentation. A patient may have pain, discoloration, and a palpable cord, but these classic findings are low in sensitivity and specificity. Unilateral leg edema may be the only finding and is the most sensitive indicator of DVT. Duplex scanning is the most sensitive and specific of methods, especially for DVT above the knee, with a sensitivity of 95%, but is less sensitive for clots below the knee. Impedance plethysmography is also an option, but has a high rate of false positives. Venography is the most definitive technique for detection, but is uncomfortable, costly, technically difficult, and may even induce thrombophlebitis. Although she is at risk for pulmonary embolus (PE), her respiratory rate is normal, and there is nothing to suggest PE, so VQ scan, pulmonary angiography, and pulse oximetry are not crucial. *(Goroll, p 209)*

111–112. (111-B, 112-C) Heparin-induced thrombocytopenia (HIT) has been increasing in incidence and is an important immunologic drug reaction because of its potential complications. Evidence suggests that its risk is dose-dependent. The highest risk occurs when heparin is given at full doses, and risk is lower with intermediate-dose heparin (7500 U twice daily). It usually occurs 5 to 15 days into therapy, and thrombocytopenia is moderate (counts range from 25,000 to 100,000). Typically, an IgG antibody (very rarely IgM, but not IgA) binds to heparin. Risk of HIT is higher with bovine rather than porcine heparin. Serious thrombotic complications can occur, both arterial and venous, with venous four times as common. Bleeding is not a common complication. Stroke and skin necrosis can occur, but less commonly. *(Kelly, p 1276)*

113. (B) *P* values express the probability that a difference detected between two populations occurred by chance. This is also called alpha or type I error. This is extremely important in clinical trials, because a difference between the control and study population can be due to either an effect of the study drug or random chance. When the results of a study are called statistically significant, it means that the *P* value is less than the value decided on as acceptable when the study was designed. This is usually $P = 0.05$ or less. *(Hill, p 164; Colton, pp 115–120)*

114–115. (114-A, 115-E) The highest incidence of primary hyperparathyroidism occurs in women over the age of 60. Most patients are asymptomatic and found on screening tests. Those patients with symptoms most often manifest emotional disorders (eg, depression) and hypercalcuria. Five to 10% of patients with first-time renal colic have primary hyperparathyroidism. Most patients with primary hyperparathyroidism have disease limited to one gland rather than multigland disease. MEN syndromes I and IIa manifest parathyroid disease, but are rare and are associated with other endocrinopathies. Carcinoma is rare. Preoperative localization in patients without prior neck exploration is rarely indicated and not cost-effective. In patients with prior neck explorations, imaging studies may be helpful, and individually have comparable sensitivities in the range of 50 to 60%. *(Greenfield et al, pp 1317–1331)*

116. (A) According to Piaget, the ability to develop abstract concepts about objects (animate and inanimate) and a sense of their permanence is achieved through a progressive assimilation and accommodation process. Sensorimotor schemata are coordinated, modified, and reintegrated while infants are interactive with their world. The development of an understanding that objects have an existence and permanence outside themselves signals the completion of the sensorimotor stage and the transition to the preoperational thought stage. Preoperational reasoning and concrete operations are cognitive achievements of later development stages (childhood years). *Object constancy* and *transitional object* are psychoanalytic theoretical constructs, referring to the early development of cognitive and emotional reactions. These concepts have been used to explain how infants begin to develop a sense of self as distinct from others as well as a sense of growing self-sufficiency. *(Kaplan and Sadock, pp 140–141)*

117. (E) The most common parental translocation associated with Down syndrome involves chromosomes 14 and 21. In cases involving 21/21 translocations, no normal gametes will be formed. The gametes will either contain no genetic material from chromosome 21 (resulting in monosomic zygotes which are universally lost in the embryonic stage) or will contain both chromosomes (resulting in a trisomic zygote). Thus, all liveborns will have Down syndrome. *(Creasy and Resnik, pp 24–26)*

118. (E) New guidelines from the Centers for Disease Control and Prevention (CDC) recommend erythromycin for treatment of *Chlamydia* in pregnancy. Tetracyclines are contraindicated in pregnancy. The other antibiotics may be used in pregnancy but are ineffective against *Chlamydia*. When treated with erythromycin, a test of cure 3 weeks later is recommended. *(MMWR, pp 55–56)*

119. **(B)** Doxycycline, 100 mg PO twice daily for 7 days, or azithromycin, 1 g PO in a single dose, is the current recommended regimen for treatment. This would be the treatment of choice for the 18-year-old woman if she were not pregnant. A test of cure is not recommended with either of these treatments, unless symptoms persist or recur. Patients should be instructed to abstain from sexual intercourse until completion of therapy (7 days after single-dose treatment or after completing 7 days of oral therapy). (MMWR, pp 54–55)

120–121. **(120-C, 121-B)** Bilateral internuclear ophthalmoplegia is very characteristic of MS. Careful physical exam reveals evidence of multiple lesions, such as afferent pupillary defect and bilateral upgoing toes. Memory loss may occur later in the course of illness. Autonomic injury may produce constipation, but this is not specific for MS. Intention tremor is a manifestation of cerebellar involvement, but again not specific for MS. Periventricular plaques on brain MRI are characteristic and found in over 90% of patients with known MS. MRI is much more sensitive than brain CT scan and should be the first step. Cerebrospinal fluid is abnormal in 95% of MS patients. Increases in IgG and oligoclonal IgG bands are specific and suggest increased risk of disseminated disease and should also be done. Visual and auditory evoked potentials are abnormal in demyelinated tracts and serve as additional supporting evidence of MS. EEG is not helpful. (Goroll, pp 863–864)

122–124. **(122-D, 123-A, 124-B)** Persons who have significantly disabling obsessions (persistent, intrusive thoughts or impulses) or exhibit disruptive compulsive behavior (stereotyped, purposeful, repetitive behavior that is felt as no longer controllable by the individual) are suffering from obsessive–compulsive disorder (OCD). Obsessive thoughts can be distinguished from psychotic thoughts by the affected person's recognition that these thoughts are their own and have not emanated from an external source. Affected persons typically display few cognitive deficits except those imposed by the concentration and attention demands of the OCD. Treatment of OCD can be multifaceted. Effective pharmacotherapeutic agents include the tricyclic antidepressants, especially clomipramine, and the serotonin reuptake inhibitors, which include fluoxetine, sertraline, paroxetine, and fluvoxamine. These are the drugs of first choice. If these are partially effective, other medications may be added. An anxiolytic (eg, buspirone) or a benzodiazepine (eg, alprazolam or clonazepam) may be tried, especially if anxiety is prominent. Lithium may be added for prominent affective symptoms such as depression. Antipsychotics (eg, haloperidol) may also be used in the event of psychotic symptoms. Behavioral therapy, designed to reduce anxiety, also can be effective. The technique of progressively delaying compulsive responses to anxiety or obsessional thoughts has been helpful in many cases. Group therapy can be useful in providing support, sharing successful intervention techniques, and reducing the fear in persons with OCD that they are crazy. (Andreason and Black, pp 328–333; Kaplan and Sadock, pp 615–617)

125–126. **(125-A, 126-C)** This infant presents with the clinical picture of a bowel obstruction. Initial management should include IV fluid resuscitation and nasogastric decompression. These interventions are essential prior to safe transport of the child to another center for further diagnostic studies. A septic workup, with initiation of antibiotic therapy would only be indicated if there were perinatal risk factors for sepsis. Progressive abdominal distension, vomiting, and delayed passage of meconium is suggestive of Hirschsprung's disease. This infant presents with a clinical picture of a distal bowel obstruction. Plain abdominal radiographs will demonstrate multiple dilated bowel loops. A contrast enema is important to exclude other causes of distal bowel obstruction in the neonate. Hirschsprung's disease is then confirmed with rectal biopsy. Anorectal manometry is a useful diagnostic tool in older children, as it requires the subject's cooperation and communication skills. (Behrman, pp 1070–1072)

REFERENCES

ACOG Technical Bulletin. *Immunization During Pregnancy.* Number 160. October 1991.

Adrogue HJ, Madias NE. Management of life-threatening acid–base disorders. *New Engl J Med* 1998;338:26–34.

Ameli S, Shah PK. Cardiac tamponade. *Card Clin* 1991;9:665–673.

American Academy of Pediatrics. *Report of the Committee on Infectious Diseases,* 24th ed. Evanston: American Academy of Pediatrics; 1997.

American Psychiatric Association (APA). *Diagnostic and Statistical Manual of Mental Disorders,* 4th ed., revised. Washington, DC: American Psychiatric Association; 1994.

Andreason NC, Black DW. *Introductory Textbook of Psychiatry,* 2nd ed. Washington, DC: American Psychiatric Association; 1995.

Bar-Or O. *Pediatric Sports Medicine for the Practitioner,* 1st ed. New York: Springer-Verlag; 1983.

Bartlett JG, Mundy LM. Community-acquired pneumonia. *N Engl J Med* 1995;333:1618–1624.

Behrman RE, Kliegman RM, Arvin AM. *Nelson Textbook of Pediatrics,* 15th ed. Philadelphia: WB Saunders; 1996.

Berkowitz CD. *Pediatrics: A Primary Care Approach.* Philadelphia: WB Saunders; 1996.

Byrne TN. Spinal cord compression from epidural metastases. *N Engl J Med* 1992;327:614–619.

Centers for Disease Control. *Preventing Lead Poisoning in Young Children.* October 1991.

Champion LAA, Schwartz AD, Luddy RE, Schindler S. The effects of four commonly used drugs on platelet function. *J Pediatr* 1976;89:653–656.

Coffey RL, Zile MR, Luskin AT. Immunologic tests of value in diagnosis. I. Acute phase reactants and autoantibodies. *Postgrad Med* 1981;70:163–178.

Colton T. *Statistics in Medicine.* Boston: Little, Brown and Company; 1974.

Committee on Drugs. Treatment guidelines for lead exposure in children. *Pediatrics* 1995;96:155–160.

Creasy RK, Resnik R. *Maternal–Fetal Medicine: Principles and Practice,* 3rd ed. Philadelphia: WB Saunders; 1994.

Cunningham FG, MacDonald PC, Gant NF, et al. *Williams Obstetrics,* 20th ed. East Stamford, CT: Appleton & Lange; 1997.

Dajani AS, Taubert KA, Wilson W, et al. Prevention of bacterial endocarditis: recommendations by the American Heart Association. *JAMA* 1997;277:1794–1801.

DeArce MA, Kearns A. The fragile X syndrome: the patients and their chromosomes. *J Med Genet* 1984;21:84–91.

Diabetes Control and Complications Trial Research Group. The effect of intensive treatment of diabetes on the development and progression of long-term complications in insulin-dependent diabetes mellitus. *N Engl J Med* 1993;329:977–986.

DiSaia PJ, Creasman WT. *Clinical Gynecologic Oncology.* St. Louis: Mosby; 1997.

Dixon AC, Parrillo JE. Managing the cardiovascular effects of sepsis and shock. *J Crit Illness* 1991;6:1197–1214.

Ellenhorn MJ. *Ellenhorn's Medical Toxicology: Diagnosis and Treatment of Human Poisoning,* 2nd ed. Baltimore: Williams & Wilkins; 1997.

Fauci A, Braunwald E, Isselbacher KJ, et al. *Harrison's Principles of Internal Medicine,* 14th ed. New York: McGraw-Hill International Book Co; 1998.

Feigin RD, Cherry JD. *Textbook of Pediatric Infectious Diseases,* 3rd ed. Philadelphia: WB Saunders; 1992.

Fink JN, Fauci A. Immunological aspects of cardiovascular disease. *JAMA* 1982;248:2716–2721.

Fitzpatrick TB, Johnson RA, Polano MK, Suurmond DS. *Color Atlas and Synopsis of Clinical Dermatology,* 2nd ed. New York: McGraw-Hill; 1994.

Gartner LM. Neonatal jaundice. *Pediatr Rev* 1994;15:422–432.

Giammarco R, Edmeads J, Dodick D. *Critical Decisions in Headache Management.* Hamilton, Ontario: BC Decker, Inc; 1998.

Goroll AH, Lawrence AM, Mulley AG. *Primary Care Medicine,* 3rd ed. Philadelphia: JB Lippincott; 1995.

Greenfield LJ, Mulholland M, Oldham KT, Zelenock GB, Lillemoe KD, eds. *Surgery: Scientific Principles and Practice.* Philadelphia: Lippincott-Raven; 1997.

Guyer B, Martin J, MacDorman M, Anderson R, Strobino D. Annual Summary of Vital Statistics-1996. *Pediatrics* 1997;100:905–918.

Hales RE, Frances AJ, eds. *Psychiatry Update: American Psychiatric Association Annual Review,* vol. 6. Washington, DC: American Psychiatry Press; 1987.

Hill BA. *Principles of Medical Statistics,* 8th ed. Oxford University Press; 1966.

Hogan DE. The emergency department approach to diarrhea. *Emerg Clin North Am* 1996;14:673– 692.

Hurst JW. *Medicine for the Practicing Physician.* Stamford, CT: Appleton & Lange; 1996.

Hurwitz S. *Clinical Pediatric Dermatology: A Textbook of Skin Disorders of Childhood and Adolescence.* Philadelphia: WB Saunders; 1981.

Joint National Committee on Prevention, Detection, Evaluation and Treatment of High Blood Pressure. The sixth report. *Arch Intern Med* 1997; 157:2413–2446.

Kaplan HI, Sadock BJ. *Synopsis of Psychiatry: Behavioral Sciences Clinical Psychiatry,* 8th ed. Baltimore: Williams & Wilkins; 1998.

Kelley WN. *Textbook of Internal Medicine,* 2nd ed. New York: JB Lippincott; 1992.

Kligman RM. *Practical Strategies in Pediatric Diagnosis and Therapy.* Philadelphia: WB Saunders; 1996.

Koehler JE. Bartonella infections. *Adv Pediatr Infect Dis* 1996;11:1–27.

Laine L, Suchower L, Connors A, Neil G. Twice-daily, 10-day triple therapy with omeprazole, amoxicillin, and clarithromycin for *Helicobacter pylori* eradication in duodenal ulcer disease: results of three multicenter, double-blind, United States trials. *Am J Gastroenterol* 1998;93:2106–2112.

Last JM, ed. *Maxcy-Rosenau-Last Public Health & Preventive Medicine,* 13th ed. East Norwalk, CT: Appleton & Lange; 1992.

Last JM. *Public Health and Human Ecology,* 2nd ed. Stamford, CT: Appleton & Lange; 1997.

Light RW. Parapneumonic effusions and empyema: current management strategies. *J Crit Illness* 1995;10:832–842.

McAnarney ER, Kreipe RE, Orr DP, et al. *Textbook of Adolescent Medicine.* Philadelphia: WB Saunders; 1992.

The Medical Letter on Drugs and Therapeutics: Drugs for Treatment of Acute Otitis Media in Children. New Rochelle; Medical Letter, Inc; 1994;36:19–21.

Mishell DR Jr., Stenchever MA, Droegemueller W, Herbst AL. *Comprehensive Gynecology,* 3rd ed. St. Louis: Mosby; 1997.

MMWR Morbidity and Mortality Weekly Report. Recommendations and Reports. *1998 Guidelines for Treatment of Sexually Transmitted Diseases.* Volume 47, No. RR-01. January 23, 1998. U.S. Department of Health and Human Services.

Niederhuber JE. *Fundamentals of Surgery.* Stamford, CT: Appleton & Lange; 1998.

Norman ME. Vitamin D in bone disease. *Pediatr Clin North Am* 1982;29:947–971.

Oski FA, DeAngelis CD, Feigin RD, et al. *Principles and Practice of Pediatrics,* 2nd ed. Philadelphia: JB Lippincott; 1994.

Rankin AC, Brooks R, Ruskin JN, et al. Adenosine and the treatment of supraventricular tachycardia. *Am J Med* 1992; 92:655–664.

Relman DA, Schmidt TM, MacDermott RP, et al. Identification of the uncultured bacillus of Whipple's disease. *N Engl J Med* 1992;327:293–301.

Rock JA, Thompson JD. *TeLinde's Operative Gynecology.* 8th ed. Philadelphia: Lippincott-Raven; 1997.

Rowe MI, O'Neill JA, Grosfeld JL, et al. *Essentials of Pediatric Surgery.* St. Louis: Mosby; 1995.

Rudolph AM, Hoffman JIE, Rudolph CD. *Pediatrics,* 20th ed. Stamford, CT: Appleton & Lange; 1996.

Sabiston DC, ed. *Textbook of Surgery,* 15th ed. Philadelphia: WB Saunders; 1997.

Schumacher HR, ed. *Primer on the Rheumatic Diseases,* 10th ed. Atlanta: Arthritis Foundation; 1993.

Schwartz SI, Shires GT, Spencer FC, eds. *Principles of Surgery.* New York: McGraw-Hill; 1994.

Scott JR, DiSaia PJ, Hammond CB, Spellacy WN, eds. *Danforth's Obstetrics and Gynecology,* 7th ed. Philadelphia: JB Lippincott; 1994.

Second Report of the National Cholesterol Education Program Expert Panel on Detection, Evaluation and Treatment of High Blood Cholesterol in Adults. NIH Publication No. 93-3095; 1993.

Speroff L, Glass RH, Kase NG. *Clinical Gynecologic Endocrinology and Infertility,* 5th ed. Baltimore: Williams & Wilkins; 1994.

Stoudemire A, ed. *Clinical Psychiatry for Medical Students,* 2nd ed. Philadelphia: JB Lippincott; 1994.

Stoudemire A, ed. *Human Behavior: An Introduction for Medical Students.* Philadelphia: JB Lippincott; 1990.

Sweet RL, Gibbs RS. *Infectious Diseases of the Female Genital Tract,* 3rd ed. Baltimore: Williams & Wilkins; 1995.

Tancredi LR. Emergency psychiatry and crisis intervention: some legal and ethical issues. *Psychiatry Ann* 1982;12:799–806.

Tecklenburg FW, Wright MS. Minor head trauma in the pediatric patient. *Pediatr Emerg Care* 1991; 7:40–47.

Tomb DA. *Psychiatry,* 5th ed. Baltimore: Williams & Wilkins; 1995.

Traugott L, Alpers A. In their own hands. *Arch Pediatr Adolesc Med* 1997;151:922–927.

U.S. Preventive Services Task Force. *Guide to Clinical Preventive Services,* 2nd ed. Baltimore: Williams & Wilkins; 1996.

Wedding D. *Behavior and Medicine,* 2nd ed. St. Louis: Mosby; 1995.

Yamada T, Alpers D, Owyang C, et al. *Textbook of Gastroenterology.* Philadelphia: JB Lippincott; 1991.

Yen SSC, Jaffe RB. *Reproductive Endocrinology: Physiology, Pathophysiology and Clinical Management,* 3rd ed. Philadelphia: WB Saunders; 1991.

Zinner MJ. *Maingot's Abdominal Operations,* 10th ed., vols. I and II. Stamford, CT: Appleton & Lange; 1997.

Subspecialty List: Chapter 7—Practice Test 1

15. Oncology
16. Oncology
32. Digestive system diseases
33. Digestive system diseases
34. Digestive system diseases
35. Digestive system diseases
36. Digestive system diseases
37. Digestive system diseases
38. Digestive system diseases
44. Trauma
45. Trauma
46. Trauma
50. Nervous system diseases
57. Trauma
58. Trauma
66. Trauma
67. Trauma
70. Digestive system diseases
71. Digestive system diseases
114. Endocrine diseases
115. Endocrine diseases
125. Structural
126. Structural

PSYCHIATRY

5. Intervention
6. Psychopathology
7. Assessment
18. Psychopathology
19. Intervention
20. Psychopathology
24. Psychopathology
30. Psychopathology
31. Intervention
42. Assessment
43. Intervention
49. Intervention
54. Child psychiatry/Development
64. Assessment
65. Child psychiatry/Assessment
75. Assessment
76. Child psychiatry/Assessment
81. Intervention
82. Assessment
86. Intervention
89. Personality theory
90. Personality theory
91. Intervention
94. Neurotransmitters
95. Intervention
116. Child psychiatry/Assessment
122. Psychopathology
123. Intervention
124. Intervention

PREVENTIVE MEDICINE

3. Disease control
8. Biostatistics
55. Biostatistics
56. Disease control
61. Epidemiology
105. Biostatistics
108. Biostatistics
113. Biostatistics

Practice Test 2
Questions

DIRECTIONS (Questions 1 through 36): Each of the numbered items or incomplete statements in this section is followed by answers or by completions of the statement. Select the ONE lettered answer or completion that is BEST in each case.

Questions 1 and 2

A 55-year-old man presents to the physician's office complaining of persistent heartburn of 4 years' duration. He also complains of a chronic cough and regurgitation at night despite raising the head of his bed 30 degrees. He self-medicated intermittently for $3^1/_2$ years with antacids prior to instituting an H_2 blocker, prescribed by another physician 3 months ago, but without significant improvement. His physical exam is normal, and he is referred for upper endoscopy that reveals superficial linear ulcerations of his distal esophagus with 3 cm of epithelial changes consistent with Barrett's esophagus (Figure 8–1, see Color Plate 1). Biopsies reveal esophagitis and high-grade dysplasia of the Barrett's epithelium.

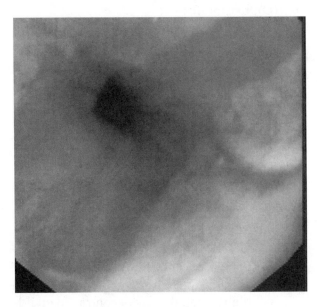

Figure 8–1. Barrett's esophagus. *(Reprinted with permission from Zinner MJ.* Maingot's Abdominal Operations, *10th ed., vol. 1. Stamford, CT: Appleton & Lange, 1997.)*

1. Early treatment with which of the following is most likely to have prevented this condition?

    (A) H_2 blockers
    (B) diet modification
    (C) Nissen fundoplication
    (D) proton pump inhibitor
    (E) regular schedule of antacids

2. Which of the following should be recommended for this patient?

    (A) a short course (3 months) of a proton pump inhibitor and repeat endoscopy
    (B) change to another H_2 blocker and repeat endoscopy in 3 months
    (C) double the dose of the H_2 blocker and repeat endoscopy in 3 months
    (D) Nissen fundoplication
    (E) esophagectomy

3. A 7-year-old girl is brought to the clinic with a 2-day history of right ear pain. She has not had fever, congestion, or other symptoms. On physical exam, she is afebrile. She has pain when you move the pinna. There is drainage in the right ear canal that obscures the tympanic membrane. Which of the following is the most likely diagnosis?

   (A) acute otitis media with perforation
   (B) contact dermatitis
   (C) foreign body in the ear canal
   (D) mastoiditis
   (E) external otitis

4. In 1997, the Public Health Advisory Committee on Immunization Practices changed its recommendation for immunizing children less than 4 years old against polio. The old recommendation was for three doses of oral polio vaccine. The new recommendation was for the first two doses to be injectable polio vaccine, with the remainder oral. This recommendation reflected the fact that

   (A) injectable vaccine is cheaper than oral vaccine due to preparation
   (B) the risk of contracting vaccine-associated paralytic polio from oral vaccine is now higher than the risk of contracting wild-strain polio
   (C) there have been no cases of wild-strain paralytic polio reported in 10 years
   (D) injectable vaccine is more protective than oral vaccine
   (E) injectable polio vaccine is available worldwide

5. A young couple are going on their honeymoon to Mexico and wish to avoid travelers' diarrhea. You advise them to avoid water, ice, salads, and raw vegetables. What organism is the usual culprit?

   (A) *Shigella*
   (B) *Salmonella*
   (C) *Vibrio parahaemolyticus*
   (D) *Escherichia coli*
   (E) *Campylobacter jejuni*

Questions 6 Through 8

The Mini-Mental State Exam is administered to a 65-year-old woman admitted to the hospital following a thwarted suicide attempt. She had walked onto a bridge and was attempting to jump into the river below. A passing motorist stopped her. She successfully completed all aspects of the exam except that she could subtract only to 86 on the serial sevens and could recall only two of three objects named 3 minutes before.

6. Of the following, what is her score on the Mini-Mental State Exam?

   (A) 60
   (B) 26
   (C) 6
   (D) 20
   (E) 30

7. Which of the following does her score indicate about her cognitive functioning?

   (A) no impairment of cognitive functions
   (B) possible impairment of cognitive functions
   (C) definite impairment of cognitive functions
   (D) mild depression
   (E) severe depression

8. The findings on physical exam of this woman included the following: heart rate of 60; thinning, dry hair; thinning of lateral aspect of eyebrows; and slowed deep tendon reflexes. Of the following, which is the most probable diagnosis at this point?

   (A) Pick's disease
   (B) hypothyroidism
   (C) Alzheimer's disease
   (D) hyperadrenalism
   (E) hypoadrenalism

9. A pregnant woman at 31 weeks' gestation complains of fatigue, malaise, and abdominal pain. She has also noticed dark urine and light stools. She admits to the intravenous (IV) use of cocaine on frequent occasions. The

diagnosis of hepatitis B is confirmed by the presence of an elevated

(A) sedimentation rate
(B) alkaline phosphatase
(C) white blood count (WBC)
(D) aspartate transaminase (AST)
(E) blood urea nitrogen (BUN)

10. A 17-year-old girl has moderate dysmenorrhea that began about 1 year after menarche. Physical exam, including the pelvic exam, is normal. Which of the following medications most often provides effective relief for her primary dysmenorrhea?

(A) clomiphene
(B) acetaminophen
(C) bromocriptine
(D) ibuprofen
(E) hydrocortisone

Questions 11 and 12

A young man develops wheezing after eating lobster and presents to the emergency department 15 minutes later with persistent breathing difficulty.

11. What is the most important initial treatment?

(A) oral beta blocker
(B) topical steroid
(C) IV steroid
(D) subcutaneous epinephrine
(E) intramuscular diphenhydramine

12. Which of the following is associated with this type of immediate hypersensitivity?

(A) immunoglobulin A (IgA) binding to mast cells or basophil membranes
(B) delayed skin rash
(C) immediate appearance of symptoms, with self-limited resolution within one half hour
(D) intrinsic asthma
(E) symptoms including laryngeal edema and nausea

13. During a daytime church picnic, a wild fox suddenly appears from the woods and attacks a young woman, biting her several times on the leg. The fox then proceeds to wander around the picnic, attacking brightly colored coolers. A man attempts to catch the fox and is bitten several times on his hands and head in the process. Animal control officers arrive and safely trap the fox. The best course of action is to

(A) observe the fox for 10 days
(B) submit the fox head for rabies testing and treat victims based on results
(C) begin treatment with tetanus antitoxin
(D) begin treatment of bitten victims with rabies vaccine
(E) begin treatment of bite victims with rabies immune globulin and rabies vaccine

Questions 14 and 15

A 20-year-old college student seems very uneasy as you walk in the exam room at the student health office. He tells you he has painful sores on his penis and admits that he has had intercourse with several different coeds in the past several months. The lesions are shown in Figure 8–2.

14. What is the most likely diagnosis?

(A) herpes zoster
(B) syphilis
(C) herpes simplex
(D) condyloma acuminatum
(E) lymphogranuloma venereum

15. The student has lots of questions about this infection. Which of the following is important for him to know about this condition?

(A) He can continue sexual activity while the lesions are present as long as he uses a condom.
(B) Shedding of the organism will cease when the lesions are gone.
(C) Doxycycline is an effective treatment.
(D) He is at very low risk of having a recurrent episode if he uses condoms.
(E) Infection can be transmitted even when he is asymptomatic.

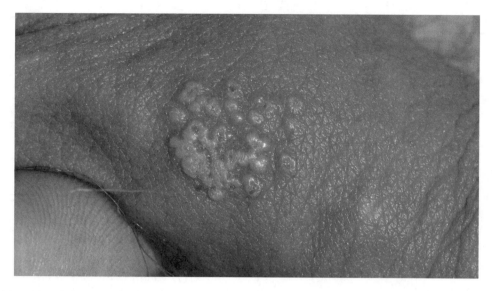

Figure 8–2. Vesicles with early central crusting on a red base. *(Reprinted with permission from Fitzpatrick TB.* Color Atlas and Synopsis of Clinical Dermatology. *New York: McGraw-Hill, 1997)*

16. A 15-year-old boy comes to the emergency department with sudden onset of respiratory distress. He states that he was studying 1 hour ago, when he developed chest pain and dyspnea. He has no history of any previous respiratory problems. On physical exam, he is tachypneic, has moderate retractions, and has decreased breath sounds over the left lung fields. Which of the following is the most likely diagnosis?

    (A) aspiration of a foreign body
    (B) exacerbation of asthma
    (C) empyema
    (D) pneumonia
    (E) pneumothorax

Questions 17 and 18

A 2-week-old boy is brought to your office for a checkup. He has been doing well at home. The results of his newborn screen indicate that he has sickle cell disease (hemoglobin SS disease).

17. Which of the following is the most important next step in his management?

    (A) avoiding heat exposure
    (B) immunizing with pneumococcal vaccine
    (C) prescribing folic acid supplements

    (D) prescribing iron supplements
    (E) prescribing prophylactic penicillin

18. Six months later, this same patient returns to your office with a 3-day history of lethargy and fever. He has also had rhinorrhea and a cough. On physical exam, he is pale, tachycardic, and has a left-upper-quadrant mass. His hemoglobin is 4 g/dL, platelet count is 100,000, and WBC is 15,000 with 50% segmented neutrophils. His reticulocyte count is 15%. Which of the following is the most likely diagnosis?

    (A) acute chest syndrome
    (B) acute splenic sequestration
    (C) aplastic crisis
    (D) intussusception
    (E) vaso-occlusive crisis

19. An apparent increase in survival among cases found by screening, which results from the fact that screening is more likely to pick up those with a long preclinical phase of disease, is termed

    (A) volunteer bias
    (B) berksonian bias
    (C) lead-time bias

(D) diagnostic bias

(E) prognostic bias

Questions 20 Through 22

A 55-year-old man presents to the emergency department with an acute onset of excruciating substernal chest and epigastric pain following a prolonged episode of vomiting. His past history is significant for hypertension, diabetes, and a 30-pack year smoking history. Vital signs show a blood pressure (BP) of 90/60, pulse 100, respiratory rate 18, and temperature 100°F. Exam reveals an ill-appearing man with subcutaneous emphysema and distant breath sounds on the left. A chest x-ray reveals pneumomediastinum and a left hydropneumothorax. A left chest tube is placed and IV fluids are administered with resolution of his hypotension.

20. Which of the following is the most likely diagnosis?

    (A) bronchopleural fistula

    (B) esophageal perforation

    (C) Mallory–Weiss tear

    (D) spontaneous pneumothorax

    (E) gastric perforation

21. Which of the following is the most appropriate diagnostic test?

    (A) computed tomography (CT) scan

    (B) esophagogram

    (C) analysis of the pleural fluid

    (D) esophagoscopy

    (E) tracheobronchogram

22. Which of the following factors has the most influence on outcome?

    (A) choice of antibiotics

    (B) time to definitive treatment

    (C) intensive care management

    (D) early intubation and mechanical ventilation

    (E) history of smoking

Questions 23 and 24

A 52-year-old patient is seen in a walk-in medical clinic complaining of a headache. On exam, his BP is noted to be 210/140. His retina shows hemorrhages and papilledema. Electrocardiogram shows left ventricular hypertrophy (LVH). BUN and creatinine are both elevated, at 56 and 28.

23. On what basis can the diagnosis of malignant hypertension be made?

    (A) the level of systolic BP

    (B) the level of diastolic BP

    (C) headache

    (D) funduscopic changes

    (E) heart size

24. Which of the following provides the best information regarding the prognosis of the malignant hypertension?

    (A) the level of systolic BP

    (B) the level of diastolic BP

    (C) abnormalities of renal function

    (D) future compliance

    (E) heart size

25. Which of the following psychotropic drugs is most likely to produce a severe withdrawal syndrome when suddenly discontinued?

    (A) amitriptyline

    (B) alprazolam

    (C) chlorpromazine

    (D) benztropine

    (E) lithium carbonate

26. The term *ego dystonic* refers specifically to

    (A) ideas suggested by another individual rather than independently derived

    (B) a dissociative state such as psychogenic fugue or amnesia

    (C) the recognition of one's own thoughts as unacceptable

    (D) the belief in one's own hallucinations

    (E) a character style marked by extreme rigidity reflective of a punitive superego

Questions 27 and 28

A healthy 23-year-old woman has her first prenatal visit. She has monthly menses, and her last menstrual period (LMP) began November 13, 1997.

27. Her estimated due date (EDD) is

    (A) July 30, 1998
    (B) August 6, 1998
    (C) August 20, 1998
    (D) August 27, 1998
    (E) November 6, 1998

28. This woman has a pelvic exam at this prenatal visit. Her uterus fills the pelvis but cannot be palpated by abdominal exam alone. How many weeks pregnant (calculated from her LMP) is she?

    (A) 6
    (B) 8
    (C) 10
    (D) 12
    (E) 16

29. A 64-year-old woman is brought to your office by her husband for evaluation of forgetfulness. She also has some word-finding problems and some paranoid delusions about the next door neighbor. Which of the following is most specific for Alzheimer's disease?

    (A) normal score on the Beck Depression Inventory
    (B) poor score on the Folstein Mini-Mental Status Exam
    (C) mild cerebral atrophy on a brain CT scan
    (D) rapid, resting tremor
    (E) decreased bilateral parietal lobe activity on positron-emission tomography (PET) scan

30. Which of the following is true about Alzheimer's disease?

    (A) Pathological findings include neurofibrillary tangles and neuronal degeneration.
    (B) Most cases have a clear familial pattern.

    (C) Cerebral cortical activity of choline acetyltransferase is increased.
    (D) Electroencephalography (EEG) usually shows seizure activity.
    (E) Symptoms begin before the age of 40.

31. The concerned mother of a 13-year-old girl states that her daughter has been sleeping late, easily becomes irritated with her younger brother, and insists on locking her bedroom door. She is doing well in school and is on the middle school soccer team. On physical exam, she is Tanner stage 4 and the rest of her physical findings are normal. Which of the following is the most appropriate next step in her management?

    (A) checking her thyroid function
    (B) obtaining a urine drug screen
    (C) ordering a pregnancy test
    (D) questioning the patient about possible abuse
    (E) reassuring the mother

32. A 12-month-old boy is brought to the emergency department after having a generalized seizure at home. He has also vomited three times and been very irritable. He has never had a seizure previously and in general is in good health. On exam, he has a temperature of 40°C. He is irritable and does not appear to recognize his mother. A cerebrospinal fluid (CSF) sample obtained shows the following: 2000 white blood cells (98% segmented neutrophils), protein of 155, and glucose of 20. Which of the following organisms is most likely the cause of his infection?

    (A) enterovirus
    (B) group A *Streptococcus*
    (C) group B *Streptococcus*
    (D) *Streptococcus pneumoniae*
    (E) *Mycobacterium tuberculosis*

Questions 33 and 34

A 45-year-old woman presents to the emergency department with malaise, fever, chills, anorexia, and nausea of 2 weeks' duration. Her past history is pertinent for a cholecystectomy 5 years ago and chronic diverticulitis of the sigmoid colon, manifesting as recurrent episodes over the last 2 years, for which she has been treated nonoperatively, the last episode occurring 6 weeks ago. On exam, she weighs 198 pounds and is febrile to 101°F, with a BP of 120/80 and pulse of 85, and has mild right-upper-quadrant abdominal tenderness. Laboratory data reveal a WBC of 18,000 and mildly elevated alkaline phosphatase and bilirubin.

33. Which of the following is the most appropriate diagnostic imaging procedure for this patient?

(A) radionuclide gallium scan

(B) abdominal ultrasound

(C) CT scan

(D) radionuclide technetium-99m sulfur colloid liver scan

(E) magnetic resonance imaging (MRI)

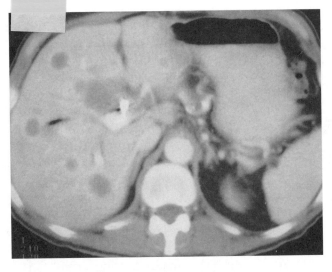

Figure 8–3. Multiple low-density lesions within the liver and characteristic peripheral rim enhancement. *(Reprinted with permission from Zinner MJ.* Maingot's Abdominal Operations, *10th ed., vol. 2. Stamford, CT: Appleton & Lange, 1996.)*

34. An imaging procedure (Figure 8–3) demonstrates multifocal hepatic abscesses of different sizes. Which of the following is the most appropriate course of initial management?

(A) broad-spectrum antibiotics alone

(B) percutaneous drainage alone

(C) surgical drainage alone

(D) broad-spectrum antibiotics and percutaneous drainage

(E) broad-spectrum antibiotics and surgical drainage

35. Which of the following statements is correct regarding conduct disorder?

(A) An estimated 15 to 20% of boys and 2 to 9% of girls under age 18 have the disorder.

(B) Low levels of plasma dopamine beta-hydroxylase have been implicated in some conduct-disordered children.

(C) There is no correlation between parental alcoholism and the emergence of conduct disorder.

(D) Attention deficit disorder cannot, by definition, coexist with a conduct disorder.

(E) The average age of boys is the same as that of girls at the onset of conduct disorder.

36. The freudian concept of the superego is described as

(A) the conscious experience of right and wrong, roughly analogous to the experience of conscience

(B) the unconscious agency that incorporates a moral sense of behavior

(C) the exaggerated perception of one's powers or worthiness

(D) the intrapsychic agency whose action enforces compliance with a personal set of ideals

(E) an innate and unconscious prohibition against sexual expression

DIRECTIONS (Questions 37 through 46): For each item, select the ONE best lettered option that is most closely associated with it. Each lettered heading may be selected once, more than once, or not at all.

For each patient with amenorrhea, select the most likely diagnosis.

(A) anorexia nervosa

(B) endometrial sclerosis

(C) polycystic ovary syndrome

(D) post-pill amenorrhea

(E) pregnancy

(F) premature ovarian failure

(G) prolactin-secreting pituitary tumor

(H) Sertoli–Leydig cell tumor

(I) 17α-hydroxylase deficiency

(J) Sheehan syndrome

(K) testicular feminization syndrome

(L) Turner syndrome

(M) 21-hydroxylase deficiency

(N) true hermaphroditism

37. A 24-year-old nulligravida last menstruated 3 years ago. One month ago, she took medroxyprogesterone acetate for 10 days but failed to bleed vaginally. Her medical history is unremarkable except for chronic schizophrenia, for which she takes an antipsychotic medication. Her blood pressure is normal. She is 165 cm (5 ft 6 in) tall and weighs 59 kg (130 lb). Nipple secretion is present bilaterally. Her vagina is dry, and there is no mucus within the cervical canal. Her pelvic exam and the remainder of her exam are normal.

38. A 19-year-old woman has never menstruated. She has never developed breasts or pubic hair. Physical examination confirms that she has Tanner stage 1 breast development and pubic hair. Her blood pressure is 142/94. Her pelvic exam is normal for a prepubertal female.

39. A 22-year-old woman began to menstruate at the age of 13 years, but has menstruated irregularly at $1^1/_2$- to 5-month intervals since. For the past 6 years, she has noted increasing hair growth on her face, chest, and abdomen. She now shaves every other day. She has no family history of irregular menses or hirsutism. Her blood pressure is normal. She has no galactorrhea. The exam confirms the hirsutism. Her pelvic exam is normal except for a male escutcheon. Her serum dehydroepiandrosterone sulfate (DHEAS) concentration is normal.

40. A 38-year-old woman is now 6 months postpartum, but has not resumed menstruation. She did not breast feed; in fact, she was unable to do so because she did not form milk. Preeclampsia and uterine atony causing an estimated blood loss of 1200 mL within 3 hours after the birth of her child complicated her pregnancy. The uterine atony responded to uterine massage and intramuscular ergot injections.

41. A 16-year-old girl has never menstruated, nor has she developed breasts. She has Tanner stage 2 pubic hair. A trial of oral medroxyprogesterone acetate failed to induce menstruation. She is 150 cm (5 ft) tall and weighs 46 kg (101 lb). Exam confirms the absence of breasts and scant development of pubic hair. A small cervix is seen on speculum exam, and a small uterus is palpated on bimanual examination. Her serum follicle-stimulating hormone (FSH) level is 86 mIU/mL.

42. A 20-year-old woman has never menstruated, but developed breasts to Tanner stage 5 beginning at age 12 years. She has a maternal cousin who has never menstruated. Her blood pressure is normal. Pubic hair is sparse. Her vagina is short, and there is no cervix seen on speculum exam. There is no palpable uterus on bimanual exam.

43. A 31-year-old woman has not menstruated since she had a dilation and curettage (D&C) 6 months ago for an incomplete spontaneous abortion complicated by endometritis.

44. A 35-year-old woman last menstruated 3 months ago. Until then, her menses were monthly and associated with premenstrual symptoms and mild dysmenorrhea. She discontinued oral contraceptives 3 months ago, and her last menses was a withdrawal from the contraceptive. She has noted some breast soreness, fatigue, and increased urinary frequency. Her vaginal epithelium appears slightly cyanotic.

45. A 32-year-old woman ceased to menstruate 1 year ago and has noticed a slight decrease in breast size. Before she stopped menstruating altogether, she recalls that her menses began to occur at irregular intervals at age 26. In the past year, she has noticed short episodes of flushing and perspiration 8 to 10 times daily, which have awakened her at night. She also complains of being tired all the time. Three years ago, a 5-day course of medroxyprogesterone acetate induced a menstrual period; 6 months ago, it did not. Her vaginal epithelium is dry, and there is no mucus within the cervical canal. Her FSH concentration is 53 mIU/mL.

46. A 25-year-old woman had monthly menses until they stopped abruptly 9 months ago. Since that time, she has noted progressive facial hair growth and deepening of her voice. Noteworthy on her physical exam is a prominent male escutcheon and slight enlargement of her clitoris. On bimanual examination, her right ovary has a diameter of approximately 7 cm, while the left ovary is about 4 cm. Her serum DHEAS concentration is normal. Her serum testosterone concentration is elevated, at 183 ng/dL.

DIRECTIONS (Questions 47 through 58): Each of the numbered items or incomplete statements in this section is followed by answers or by completions of the statement. Select the ONE lettered answer or completion that is BEST in each case.

47. Abuse of anabolic steroids is most likely to produce which of the following psychiatric disorders?

   (A) delirium
   (B) mania
   (C) psychosis
   (D) depression
   (E) dementia

48. A 25-year-old male develops low-grade fever, loss of appetite, dark urine, and then jaundice 3 weeks after a month-long humanitarian relief tour requiring extensive back country travel in an underdeveloped country. During the relief effort, he had close contact with young children and lived in the homes of area residents. He relied on locally prepared food and water sources. A laboratory test shows a high titer of immunoglobulin M (IgM) anti-hepatitis A virus (HAV). Which would have been the best method to prevent this from happening?

   (A) administration of a dose of immunoglobulin one week before leaving
   (B) ingesting only foods cooked to high temperature and bottled water
   (C) daily doses of bismuth subsalicylate (Pepto-Bismol) and ciprofloxacin
   (D) administration of a dose of immunoglobulin one week after returning
   (E) prior vaccination with hepatitis A vaccine

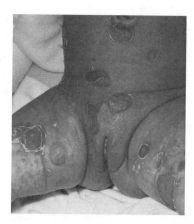

Figure 8–4. Diaper rash. *(Photograph courtesy of M.L. Williams. Reprinted with permission of Yearbook Medical Publishers.)*

49. A 2-month-old infant is brought to the clinic with a diaper rash. Her mother states that it started as a red rash in the diaper area 1 week ago. She treated it with over-the-counter diaper cream, but it continued to spread and then began to peel 2 days ago. On physical exam, she is afebrile, has a diaper rash (Figure 8–4, see Color Plate 2), and otherwise has a normal physical exam. Which of the following is the most likely diagnosis?

    (A) allergic dermatitis
    (B) bullous impetigo
    (C) *Candida* dermatitis
    (D) irritant dermatitis
    (E) seborrheic dermatitis

50. Your next patient is a 4-month-old infant who is returning to have her ear checked. You diagnosed her with otitis media 2 weeks ago, and she has taken amoxicillin for 10 days. She is feeling well, and her mother's only concern is that she has developed a diaper rash over the last 3 days. She has been using emollient creams on it, which have not helped. On her physical exam, there are no abnormal findings except for the rash (Figure 8–5, see Color Plate 3). Which of the following is the most likely diagnosis?

    (A) allergic dermatitis
    (B) bullous impetigo
    (C) *Candida* dermatitis

    (D) irritant dermatitis
    (E) seborrheic dermatitis

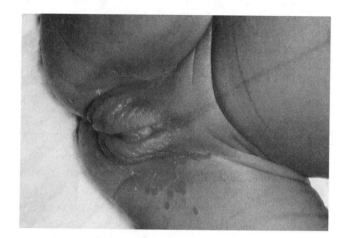

Figure 8–5. Diaper rash. *(Photograph courtesy of Neil S. Prose.)*

Questions 51 and 52

A 33-year-old woman presents to the physician's office with a 2-month history of a left breast mass. The mass is nontender, and there is no associated nipple discharge or skin dimpling. Her past history is unremarkable. Her last menstrual period started 2 weeks ago. Current medications include birth control pills. Family history is positive for breast cancer in a maternal grandmother. Physical exam reveals a 2-cm, firm, well-defined, very mobile, oval mass in the upper outer quadrant of the left breast without regional adenopathy. Mammography shows dense breasts. Ultrasonography demonstrates a well-marginated solid mass (Figure 8–6).

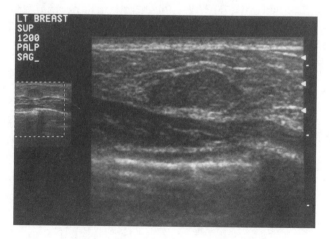

Figure 8–6. Ultrasound of left breast mass.

51. Which of the following is the most likely diagnosis?

   (A) invasive ductal carcinoma
   (B) ductal carcinoma in situ
   (C) fibrocystic changes
   (D) fibroadenoma
   (E) intraductal papilloma

52. Which of the following should be recommended as part of management of the mass?

   (A) discontinuation of birth control pills
   (B) re-exam after the next menstrual cycle
   (C) needle biopsy
   (D) excisional biopsy
   (E) repeat ultrasound in 6 months

53. A 23-year-old female presents to your office with a rash. She reports that she is experiencing low-grade fevers and headache, in addition to the rash. She also relates having noticed a small ulcer in her genital area approximately 6 weeks earlier that has now healed. Upon physical examination, diffuse lymphadenopathy is noted along with the rash pictured in Figure 8–7 (see Color Plate 4). Of the following disorders, which is most likely to be the correct diagnosis?

   (A) leprosy
   (B) secondary syphilis
   (C) chancroid
   (D) acquired immune deficiency syndrome (AIDS)
   (E) tinea

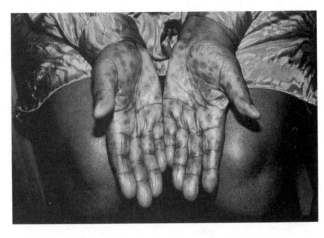

Figure 8–7. Skin rash of 23-year-old female. *(Photograph courtesy of Neil S. Prose.)*

54. A 7-year-old boy is brought to the clinic with a rash. His mother states that the rash has developed over the last several days. It began as a small red bump and has continued to grow (Figure 8–8, see Color Plate 5). He has also had fever, headache, and malaise over the last several days. On physical exam, he has the rash and otherwise has a normal exam. Which of the following is the most likely diagnosis?

   (A) contact dermatitis
   (B) erythema marginata
   (C) erythema migrans
   (D) erythema multiforme
   (E) tinea corporis

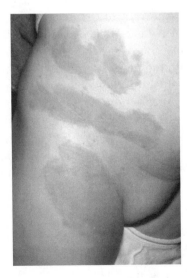

Figure 8–8. Skin rash of a 7-year-old boy. *(Photograph courtesy of M.L. Williams.)*

55. A 7-day-old infant is brought to the clinic with a rash. He was born at term and is the first child in the family. He had no problems at birth and has been doing well at home. On exam, he is afebrile. Other than the rash (Figure 8–9, see Color Plate 6), which is found only on the top of his scalp, his exam is normal. Which of the following organisms is most likely the cause of his rash?

(A) enterovirus

(B) group B *Streptococcus*

(C) herpes simplex virus

(D) *Staphylococcus aureus*

(E) varicella-zoster virus

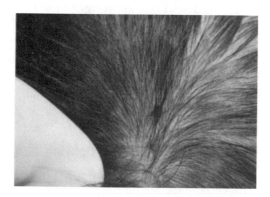

Figure 8–9. Rash of a 7-day-old infant. *(Photograph courtesy of Neil S. Prose.)*

56. A 6-year-old girl is brought to the office with a rash. Her mother states that one week ago she had a fever, headache, and malaise, which lasted for 3 days and then resolved. Now she feels well except for some pruritus with the rash. Her mother has also noted that the rash becomes more prominent when she is outside in the sun. On exam, she has no abnormal findings except for the rash. Her cheeks are intensely red, and on her extremities she has the rash shown in Figure 8–10 (see Color Plate 7). Which of the following is the most likely diagnosis?

(A) erythema infectiosum

(B) Kawasaki disease

(C) measles

(D) roseola

(E) scarlet fever

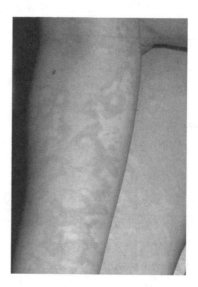

Figure 8–10. Rash of a 6-year-old girl. *(Photograph courtesy of I. Frieden.)*

57. A healthy 28-year-old woman begins prenatal care at 8 weeks' gestation. Her hemoglobin concentration is 13.5 g/dL. The total iron requirement for a normal pregnancy is

(A) 100 to 200 mg

(B) 400 to 500 mg

(C) 800 to 1000 mg

(D) 1400 to 1600 mg

(E) 2000 to 2200 mg

58. A 17-year-old adolescent comes to the clinic for a sports physical. He has no concerns about his health. He is a senior and is looking forward to playing baseball. He states that he is sexually active and has had three partners in the last 6 months. They usually use condoms for birth control. His physical exam is normal except for the lesion shown in Figure 8–11 (see Color Plate 8). On further questioning, he first noted it 2 weeks ago. It has not been bothering him at all, so he did not mention it. Which of the following is the most likely cause of this lesion?

(A) condylomata acuminata infection

(B) herpes simplex infection

(C) staphylococcal infection

(D) trauma

(E) primary syphilis infection

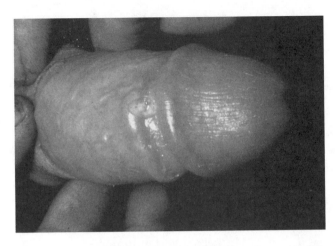

Figure 8–11. Lesion of the penis. *(Photograph courtesy of Neil S. Prose.)*

DIRECTIONS (Questions 59 through 66): Each set of matching questions in this section consists of a list of 4 to 26 lettered options followed by several numbered items. For each item, select the ONE best lettered option that is most closely associated with it. Each lettered heading may be selected once, more than once, or not at all.

Questions 59 and 60

For each of the following children with birth defects, select the most likely diagnosis.

    (A) Beckwith–Wiedemann syndrome
    (B) Cornelia de Lange syndrome
    (C) defects associated with maternal use of coumadin derivatives
    (D) fetal alcohol syndrome
    (E) fetal hydantoin syndrome
    (F) Noonan syndrome
    (G) Prader–Willi syndrome
    (H) Williams syndrome

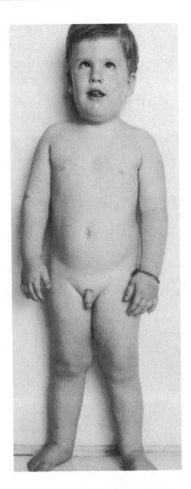

Figure 8–12. A 3-year-old boy with short stature, generalized obesity, almond-shaped eyes, and narrow bifrontal diameter. *(Reprinted with permission from Rudolph AM. Rudolph's Pediatrics, 20th ed. Stamford, CT: Appleton & Lange, 1995.)*

59. A 3-year-old boy was hypotonic at birth. He also has moderate short stature and the physical features shown in Figure 8–12.

60. A 12-month-old boy has a history of failure to thrive and developmental delay. He also has a cleft palate, a ventricular septal defect, and hearing loss. He has the facial features shown in Figure 8–13.

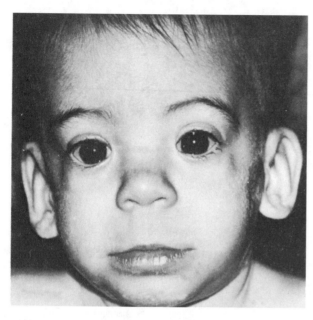

Figure 8–13. A 12-month-old boy with narrow palpebral fissures; short nose with broad, low bridge; and midfacial hypoplasia. *(Reprinted with permission from Rudolph AM. Rudolph's Pediatrics, 20th ed. Stamford, CT: Appleton & Lange, 1995.)*

Questions 61 Through 64

For each clinical setting described below, select the diagnosis that fits.

(A) migraine headache
(B) muscle contraction headache
(C) subarachnoid hemorrhage
(D) subdural hematoma
(E) brain tumor
(F) cluster headache
(G) sinus headache

61. A 42-year-old secretary with pain in her forehead that is worse when she bends over

62. A 32-year-old football coach with the worst headache of his life on the top of his head

63. A 50-year-old alcoholic man with pain around his right eye and excessive tearing

64. A 16-year-old girl with unilateral pain in the frontotemporal area associated with nausea

Questions 65 Through 68

For each patient with rectal bleeding, select the most likely diagnosis.

(A) diverticulosis of colon
(B) ulcerative colitis
(C) Meckel's diverticulum
(D) ischemic colitis
(E) endometriosis
(F) peptic ulcer
(G) carcinoma of colon

65. A 25-year-old woman who had diarrhea, abdominal cramps, and loss of weight of 1 year's duration presents with frequent bloody stools, abdominal pain, fever, and leukocytosis. B

66. A 50-year-old alcoholic man with epigastric pain and tarry black, foul-smelling stools F

67. A 60-year-old previously healthy man presents with massive rectal bleeding. A

68. A 75-year-old woman with recent onset of constipation, small-caliber stools, and intermittent dark red blood per rectum. G

DIRECTIONS (Questions 69 through 96): Each of the numbered items or incomplete statements in this section is followed by answers or by completions of the statement. Select the ONE lettered answer or completion that is BEST in each case.

Questions 69 and 70

A 16-year-old boy comes to the clinic for a sports physical. You have followed him for many years and he has always been healthy. He continues to be healthy and has no concerns. On physical exam, the only abnormality that you discover is an irregular heart rhythm. You order a rhythm strip, which is shown in Figure 8–14.

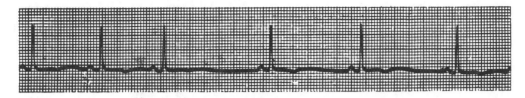

Figure 8–14. Heart rhythm strip of a 16-year-old boy. *(Reprinted with permission from Rudolph AM. Rudolph's Pediatrics, 20th ed. Stamford, CT: Appleton & Lange, 1995.)*

69. Which of the following is the most likely diagnosis?

(A) atrial premature beats

(B) sick sinus syndrome

(C) sinoatrial block

(D) sinus arrhythmia

(E) supraventricular tachycardia

70. After identifying the particular rhythm, you arrange for further testing. Which of the following diagnostic tests would be the most appropriate initial step in caring for this patient?

(A) chest x-ray

(B) echocardiogram

(C) electrocardiogram (ECG)

(D) repeat rhythm strip in 1 week

(E) no further diagnostic tests are necessary

Questions 71 and 72

A 17-year-old previously healthy teenager suffers a direct blow to the upper abdomen during a hockey game. He complains of moderate epigastric pain at the time of the injury. Forty-eight hours later, the boy develops progressively increasing bilious emesis. On arrival in the emergency department, his abdomen is nondistended, with mild tenderness on palpation in the epigastrium and right upper quadrant. Laboratory investigations demonstrate a hematocrit of 36, WBC of 11,000, and an amylase of 235 IU.

71. The most likely diagnosis is

(A) pancreatitis

(B) gastritis

(C) acute cholecystitis

(D) duodenal hematoma

(E) small bowel perforation

72. The treatment of choice is

(A) immediate exploration

(B) nasogastric decompression and parenteral alimentation

(C) retrocolic gastrojejunostomy

(D) antacids and H_2 blockers

(E) cholecystectomy

73. Of the following, which would be the most helpful in the management of the terminally ill patient?

(A) withholding information about prognosis and treatment of side effects so as not to burden the patient

(B) asking the patient how much she or he would like to know about the illness

(C) trusting that families and friends will provide the emotional support the patient needs

(D) administering analgesic medications on a strict schedule so the patient will get the medication regularly

(E) not referring for group therapy, which is of little value for this population

74. Suicide and suicidal behavior can be accurately described by which of the following statements?

    (A) Persons with schizophrenia are most at risk for suicide during periods of acute psychosis.
    (B) Psychosocial risk factors for suicide demonstrate high specificity but low sensitivity.
    (C) Neurobiological correlates of suicidal behavior are as strong in persons with suicidal ideation as in persons who have made a failed suicide attempt.
    (D) Persons failing a suicide attempt tend to be older and less characterologically disturbed than persons who have made a suicide gesture.
    (E) Increased serotonergic function correlates with increased risk for suicide.

75. A healthy, 28-year-old, pregnant woman takes a vitamin with folic acid. The daily amount of folic acid recommended is

    (A) 100 to 200 μg/day
    (B) 250 to 350 μg/day
    (C) 400 to 800 μg/day
    (D) 1000 to 1500 μg/day
    (E) 3500 to 4500 μg/day

76. The benefit of folic acid in pregnancy is

    (A) a reduced risk of macrocytic anemia
    (B) increased birth weight
    (C) decreased blood loss at delivery
    (D) increased blood volume
    (E) reduced risk of fetal anomalies

77. The *Tarasoff* I decision deliberated by the California Supreme Court ruled that

    (A) the state must provide for some form of involuntary hospitalization
    (B) a physician who has reason to believe that his or her patient will kill someone must notify the potential victim
    (C) a person is not criminally responsible for an unlawful act if that act resulted from mental disease or defect

    (D) a person is not competent to stand trial if he is unable to consult with his lawyer
    (E) the harmless mentally ill cannot be confined against their will

Questions 78 and 79

A 53-year-old male with a prior history of a sigmoid colon resection for diverticular disease presents to the emergency department with a 2-day history of crampy abdominal pain and progressive abdominal distension. He has had several episodes of bile-stained vomiting. His last bowel movement was 24 hours prior to presentation. On exam, the patient has moderate abdominal distension, with intermittent high-pitched bowel sounds.

78. Initial management and evaluation of this patient should include

    (A) IV fluids and nasogastric decompression, followed by plain abdominal radiographs
    (B) IV fluids and analgesics
    (C) plain abdominal radiographs
    (D) a barium enema
    (E) a Fleet's enema and stool softeners

79. Over the next 6 hours, the patient does not improve. Plain abdominal radiographs are shown in Figure 8–15. The next step in management would be

    (A) to continue serial examinations and repeat abdominal radiographs in the morning
    (B) insertion of a rectal tube for colonic decompression
    (C) insertion of a Cantor tube for small bowel decompression
    (D) colonoscopy
    (E) urgent exploratory laparotomy

80. A child is able to use a pincer grasp (thumb–first digit) to pick up a raisin. He can stand with support. He says "mama" and "dada." He is shy around strangers. You correctly note that he is developing normally. How old is he?

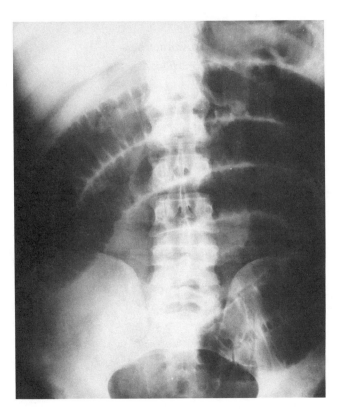

Figure 8–15. Supine abdominal x-ray of a 53-year-old male. *(Reprinted with permission from Zinner MJ. Maingot's Abdominal Operations, 10th ed., vol. 2. Stamford, CT: Appleton & Lange, 1997.)*

(A) 6 months

(B) 9 months

(C) 12 months

(D) 15 months

(E) 18 months

81. A 2-month-old infant is brought to the emergency department after having a seizure at home. The baby has not been ill, and there is no history of trauma. On exam, the baby is afebrile and is very lethargic. You are concerned about the possibility of child abuse. What physical finding would suggest that the child had injuries from violent shaking?

(A) Kernig's sign

(B) neck tenderness

(C) overlapping cranial sutures

(D) positive rooting reflex

(E) retinal hemorrhages

82. A 9-week-old infant has a hemoglobin of 9.2 g/dL. The rest of his complete blood count (CBC) is normal. He has not had any health problems and was born at term without complications. Which of the following statements is true about anemia in infants at this age?

(A) Breast-fed infants commonly develop iron deficiency at this age.

(B) A congenital hemoglobinopathy is likely.

(C) Lead toxicity is a common cause of anemia at this age.

(D) This is likely his physiologic nadir.

(E) Transfusion should be considered for any hemoglobin less than 10 g/dL.

83. A 42-year-old alcoholic woman is admitted to the hospital after suffering a seizure. She is febrile, cachectic, ill-kempt, and has poor oral hygiene. A chest examination is normal; her chest x-ray is shown in Figure 8–16. Which of the following is true regarding this lesion?

(A) often found as multiple lesions

(B) often associated with periodontal disease

(C) often due to aerobes

(D) often due to gram-negative bacilli

(E) second-generation cephalosporin is the drug of choice

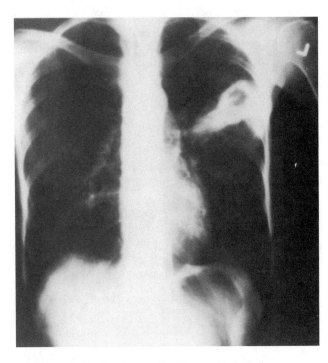

Figure 8–16. Chest x-ray of a 42-year-old alcoholic woman.

84. A 61-year-old man is admitted to the cardiac care unit (CCU) with crushing chest pain and the ECG shown in Figure 8–17. He is agitated, pale, and diaphoretic. Peripheral pulses are weak, and systolic BP is 90 mm Hg. Neck veins are distended, Kussmaul's sign is present, but lungs are clear. There is an S_3 gallop but no murmur. What is the most likely cause of the hypotension?

(A) acute mitral regurgitation

(B) aortic dissection

(C) bacterial endocarditis

(D) right ventricular infarct

(E) pericardial tamponade

Questions 85 and 86

85. A 27-year-old woman presents with cauliflower-like lesions of the external genitalia, vagina, and cervix. They vary in size and are discrete and nontender (see Figure 8–18). The lesions are most likely caused by

(A) herpes simplex

(B) gonorrhea

(C) *Hemophilus ducreyi*

(D) human papillomavirus

(E) *Chlamydia trachomatis*

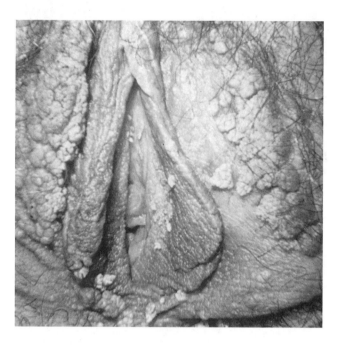

Figure 8–18.

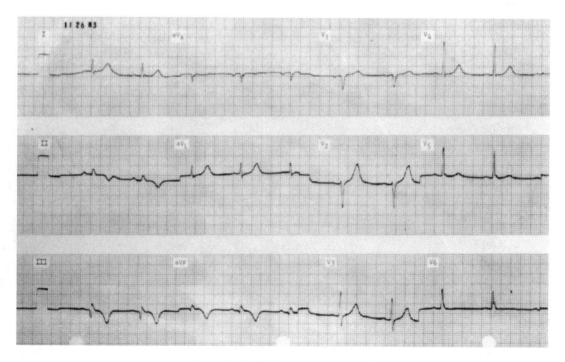

Figure 8–17. ECG of a 61-year-old man.

86. Each of the following is an acceptable treatment for the condition shown in Figure 8–18. Which has the highest efficacy rate?

    (A) podophyllin
    (B) trichloracetic acid
    (C) intralesional interferon
    (D) laser
    (E) excision

87. A 42-year-old woman with 10-week-sized fibroids has a Papanicolaou smear suggestive of a high-grade squamous intraepithelial lesion (HGSIL). Colposcopically directed biopsies and endocervical curettage also show HGSIL. The most appropriate management is

    (A) hysterectomy
    (B) fractional D&C
    (C) cold-knife conization
    (D) cryosurgery of the cervix
    (E) laser ablation of the visible lesion

Questions 88 Through 91

A 55-year-old woman with a long history of schizophrenia is seen for monitoring of her medications. Over the years, she has been on a variety of antipsychotics in both high and low doses. She has usually had a partial response in the reduction of her symptoms. As she talks, she frequently protrudes her tongue and grimaces. Her arms and hands jerk and bizarrely gesticulate as she talks. She is constantly squirming as she sits.

88. The abnormal movements strongly suggest

    (A) an exacerbation of catatonic schizophrenia
    (B) tardive dyskinesia
    (C) akathisia
    (D) pseudoparkinsonism
    (E) Huntington's disorder

89. A reduction in the fluphenazine (Prolixin) dosage would initially lead to

    (A) an increase in abnormal movements
    (B) a decrease in abnormal movements
    (C) a complete cessation of abnormal movements
    (D) no change
    (E) none of the above

90. A medication that would relieve the abnormal movements effectively in a relatively short time is

    (A) benztropine
    (B) vitamin E
    (C) propranolol
    (D) diazepam
    (E) none of the above

91. An appropriate long-term management plan for this person is

    (A) diazepam
    (B) propranolol
    (C) klonopin
    (D) clozapine
    (E) valproic acid

92. A 42-year-old man has the fingernails shown in Figure 8–19. He also has arthritis involving the fingers. What is the most likely associated skin condition?

    (A) pityriasis rosea
    (B) erythema nodosum
    (C) erythema multiforme
    (D) psoriasis
    (E) bullous pemphigoid

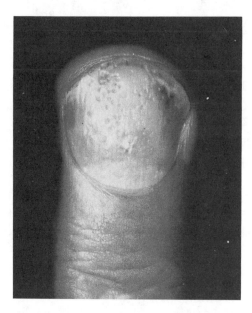

Figure 8–19. Nail with deep, scattered pits and a few larger psoratic papules. *(Reprinted with permission from Zais N. The Nail in Health and Disease, 2nd ed. East Norwalk, CT: Appleton & Lange, 1990.)*

93. An 18-year-old college student presents with severe pain in both legs of sudden onset. Her hematocrit is 26. Her peripheral blood smear is shown in Figure 8–20 (see Color Plate 9). What is the likely diagnosis?

    (A) sickle cell anemia
    (B) iron-deficiency anemia

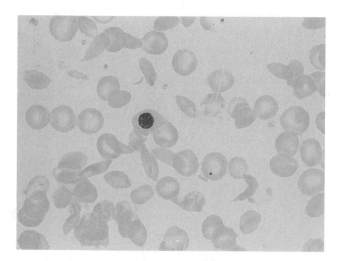

Figure 8–20. Peripheral blood smear of an 18-year-old. *(Reprinted with permission from Hurst JW. Medicine for the Practicing Physician, 4th ed. Stamford, CT: Appleton & Lange, 1996.)*

    (C) alpha-thalassemia major
    (D) beta-thalassemia minor
    (E) anemia of chronic disease

94. A 6-year-old boy has a purpuric and petechial rash over the buttocks and lower extremities. He appears to be well and is afebrile, but has swelling of the right knee. His CBC is normal. The most likely diagnosis is

    (A) idiopathic thrombocytopenic purpura (ITP)
    (B) systemic lupus erythematosus (SLE)
    (C) meningococcemia
    (D) Henoch–Schönlein (anaphylactoid) purpura
    (E) juvenile rheumatoid arthritis

Question 95

A 6-week-old male infant presents with a 5-day history of progressively worsening vomiting. He has not had a stool in 2 days. On physical exam, he is dehydrated. Serum electrolytes are:

(Na$^+$)	(K$^+$)	(Cl$^-$)	(HCO$_3$$^-$1)
136	3.0	88	36

95. Which of the following is the most likely diagnosis?

    (A) congenital adrenal hyperplasia
    (B) gastroesophageal reflux
    (C) pyloric stenosis
    (D) renal tubular acidosis
    (E) gastroenteritis

Question 96

A 27-year-old man is psychiatrically evaluated in jail for making threats to kill himself. He has been arrested for violation of parole, operating a drug house, and selling cocaine. He is enraged with the police for doing this, his fifteenth or "maybe twentieth" arrest since age 15. He feels they are out to get him. He admits to using alcohol and "crack" since age 12; it was easy to obtain since both parents used them. The highest grade achieved was 10th, during which he quit because "both the teachers and principal had it in for him." He was truant most of the time anyway. Currently, he operates his own "chop shop" and talks with pleasure about the "kids" who provide him with cars for the shop and about his dealers who buy parts. "We take care of each other." He admits to hearing voices "occasionally" but denies ever being depressed or manic, except while on crack.

96. Which of the following personality disorders best describes this man?

   (A) histrionic
   (B) narcissistic
   (C) avoidant
   (D) borderline
   (E) antisocial

DIRECTIONS (Questions 97 through 101): For each item, select the indicated best lettered options that is most closely associated with it. Each lettered heading may be selected once, more than once, or not at all.

On the Diagnostic and Statistical Manual of Mental Disorders, 4th edition (DSM-IV) axes, list all the items below that are most appropriate to each axis.

   (A) assessment of functioning
   (B) borderline personality disorder
   (C) dysthymia
   (D) homosexuality
   (E) Huntington's disorder
   (F) loss of job
   (G) mental retardation
   (H) paranoid personality disorder
   (I) poverty
   (J) schizophrenia
   (K) sexually assaulted
   (L) tardive dyskinesia

97. Axis I (select 2)

98. Axis II (select 3)

99. Axis III (select 2)

100. Axis IV (select 3)

101. Axis V (select 1)

DIRECTIONS (Questions 102 through 126): Each of the numbered items or incomplete statements in this section is followed by answers or by completions of the statement. Select the ONE lettered answer or completion that is BEST in each case.

Questions 102 Through 105

A 60-year-old previously healthy woman is scheduled for an elective colon resection for a nonobstructing sigmoid colon carcinoma. The patient began a clear liquid diet 2 days preoperatively. Oral antibiotics were started on the day before surgery, in addition to magnesium citrate. The patient vomited after the first dose of magnesium citrate and was not able to tolerate a second oral dose. At surgery, the patient received a third-generation cephalosporin intravenously on induction of anesthesia. During the colonic anastomosis, there was gastrointestinal spillage.

102. This operative procedure would be classified as

   class I clean
   class II clean-contaminated
   class II clean-contaminated with inadequate bowel preparation and gastrointestinal spillage
   class III contaminated
   class IV dirty

Thirty-six hours after surgery, the patient has a persistent low-grade fever and mild tachypnea. On examination of the chest, there is decreased air entry at the lung bases. The abdominal dressing is clean and dry, and urine output via catheter is clear and adequate in volume.

103. The most likely cause of fever is

   a wound infection
   a urinary tract infection
   pneumonia
   atelectasis
   a pelvic abscess

104. Appropriate evaluation and management should include

(A) empiric antibiotic therapy

(B) blood, urine, and sputum cultures, followed by empiric antibiotic therapy

(C) pulmonary toilet with incentive spirometry and chest physiotherapy

(D) removal of the urinary catheter

(E) CT scan of the abdomen, with percutaneous abscess drainage

By the sixth postoperative day, the patient has normal bowel function and is tolerating a full oral diet. However, she develops a spiking fever pattern and complains of increasing incisional discomfort. On examination, there is a small amount of drainage on the wound dressing, and the incision is erythematous and tender.

105. Appropriate evaluation and management at this point should include

(A) blood, urine, and sputum cultures; chest x-ray and abdominal CT scan

(B) discharging the patient on oral antibiotics

(C) culture of the wound drainage, and initiation of IV antibiotics

(D) opening the incision, culture of the wound drainage, and initiating local wound care

(E) opening the incision, culture of the wound drainage, and initiating IV antibiotics

106. At her first prenatal visit at 8 weeks' gestation, a woman who is pregnant for the second time has a culture of her cervix that is positive for group B *Streptococcus*. Her first child was delivered at 35 weeks after spontaneous rupture of the amniotic membranes and spontaneous onset of labor. During her first labor, she had several recorded temperatures of 101.6°F. Appropriate management is to

(A) prescribe oral amoxicillin for 1 week and repeat the cervical culture in 4 weeks

(B) repeat the cervical culture at 36 weeks' gestation and administer amoxicillin if it is positive

(C) administer IV penicillin when she goes into labor

(D) perform a cesarean section to prevent neonatal infection

(E) do nothing since the attack rate to the infant is very low

107. A 23-year-old woman requests oral contraceptives for contraception. She has no health problems. She requests a low-dose oral contraceptive. The oral contraceptive with the lowest amount of estrogen is

(A) Ovral

(B) Nordette

(C) Micronor

(D) Loestrin 1/20

(E) Modicon

108. The incubation period for an infectious disease is

(A) the interval between exposure to the agent until the onset of symptoms

(B) the interval between exposure to the agent and the time it is maximally infectious to another person

(C) the period between biologic onset and death

(D) the interval between exposure to the agent and disability

(E) the time between infectivity and pathogenicity

109. A child typically reaches 50% of his or her adult height by the age of

(A) 6 months

(B) 12 months

(C) 2 years

(D) 4 years

(E) 6 years

110. During a routine yearly checkup, an 8-year-old boy is found to have 2+ proteinuria on urinalysis. Which of the following would be the most appropriate diagnostic test?

(A) BUN and serum creatinine

(B) urine culture

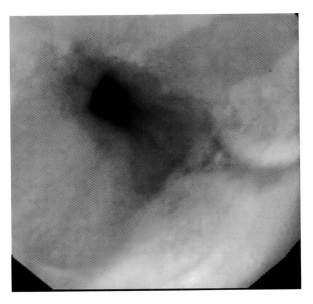

Color plate 1

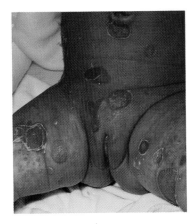

Color plate 2

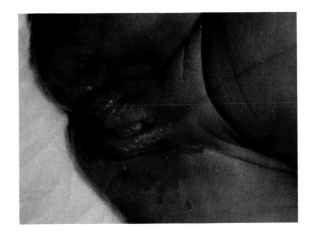

Color plate 3

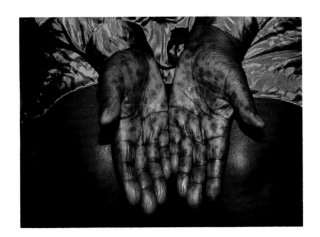

Color plate 4

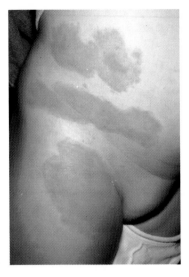

Color plate 5

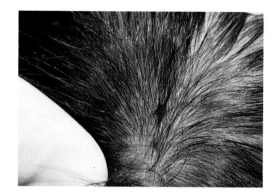

Color plate 6

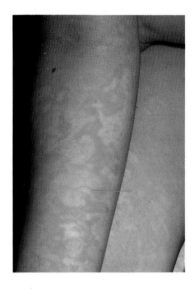

Color plate 7

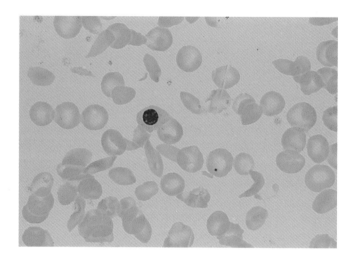

Color plate 8

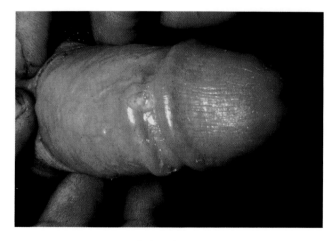

Color plate 9

(C) intravenous pyelogram (IVP)

(D) a repeat urinalysis

(E) renal sonogram

111. A 44-year-old man undergoes evaluation for worsening headaches. His posteroanterior and lateral arteriograms are shown in Figure 8–21. What is the most likely complication?

(A) hypopituitarism

(B) subarachnoid hemorrhage

(C) hypercalcemia

(D) tentorial herniation

(E) chronic meningitis

112. In 1985, the number of beds in mental hospitals throughout the United States was 432,000 as compared with 570,000 in 1995. This shows a considerable increase in the number of mental health patients requiring hospitalization between 1985 and 1995. Assuming full occupancy in both years,

(A) the prevalence of mental illness increased by about one third

(B) sufficient information is not given to calculate either prevalence or incidence

(C) the incidence of mental illness increased by about one third

(D) the incidence of mental illness decreased by about one third

(E) the prevalence of mental illness decreased by about one third

113. A 73-year-old man has been experiencing increasing drowsiness and incoherence. He has a history of arrhythmias and has fallen twice in the past 2 weeks. There are no focal deficits on neurologic examination. A contrast CT scan of the head is shown in Figure 8–22. The treatment of choice is to

(A) give parenteral antibiotics

(B) give antifungal therapy

(C) drill burr holes

(D) observe the patient and repeat the CT scan in 1 month

(E) give fibrinolytic therapy

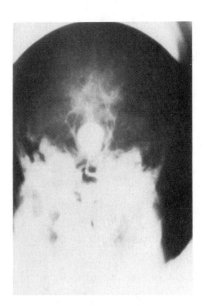
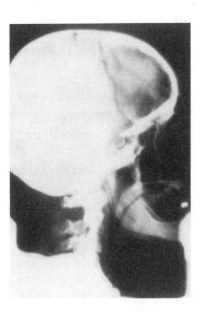

Figure 8–21. Posteroanterior and lateral arteriograms of a 44-year-old man.

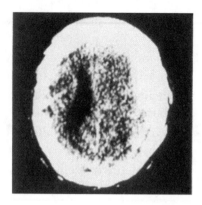

Figure 8–22. Contrast CT scan of a 73-year-old man.

Questions 114 Through 116

An 8-month-old girl is brought to the clinic with a 3-day history of fever, vomiting, and irritability. She has never had a similar problem. On physical exam, her temperature is 40.0°C. She appears moderately dehydrated. She vomits twice during the visit. Her initial workup shows a WBC of 20,000 with 70% neutrophils. Her catheterized urinalysis shows a specific gravity of 1.030, 1+ protein, and trace blood. The microscopic exam reveals 0 to 5 red blood cells per high-power field, numerous white blood cells per high-power field, and moderate bacteria. A urine culture is sent.

114. Which of the following is the most appropriate next step in her management?

    (A) Prescribe trimethoprim–sulfamethoxazole and see her tomorrow in the office.
    (B) Give IM ceftriaxone and see her tomorrow in the office.
    (C) Admit her to the hospital for IV hydration and IV antibiotics.
    (D) Wait for the urine culture and treat her if it is positive.
    (E) Start oral rehydration in the office and prescribe amoxicillin.

115. Her urine culture is positive the next day. Which of the following organisms is most likely to cause her infection?

    (A) *Escherichia coli*
    (B) *Klebsiella*

    (C) nontypeable *Hemophilus influenzae*
    (D) *Pseudomonas aeruginosa*
    (E) *Staphylococcus aureus*

116. You see her in the office 3 weeks later after the infection has been treated. All of her symptoms have resolved and she has a normal physical exam. Which of the following is the most appropriate next step in her management?

    (A) Order a renal ultrasound.
    (B) Order a voiding cystourethrogram.
    (C) Order a renal ultrasound and a voiding cystourethrogram.
    (D) Order a nuclear medicine renal scan.
    (E) No tests are necessary.

DIRECTIONS (Questions 117 through 126): Each set of matching questions in this section consists of a list of 8 to 16 lettered options followed by several numbered items. For each item, select the ONE best lettered option that is most closely associated with it. Each lettered heading may be selected once, more than once, or not at all.

Questions 117 Through 121

Typical side effects are caused by psychiatric medication. In the case reports below, identify the medication that is most likely the cause of the side effect described.

    (A) clozapine
    (B) fluvoxamine
    (C) haloperidol
    (D) imipramine
    (E) lithium carbonate
    (F) lorazepam
    (G) thioridazine
    (H) trazodone

117. A routine blood test showed a WBC of 1.9 K/mm^3 in a man with chronic schizophrenia. Because of this, he was directed to discontinue the medication that had significantly controlled his hallucinations better than any of the many medications he had tried in the past.

118. A young man was successfully medically treated for feelings of discouragement, an early morning awakening sleep disturbance, poor appetite, and sense of hopelessness. Several months after starting this medication, he sought help in the emergency department because of a penile erection that would not subside.

119. A 35-year-old woman with a history of major depression with psychosis appeared in the emergency department. Her eyes were, as she said, "locked up in my head." She had started a drug approximately 2 weeks prior to this episode.

120. A 45-year-old woman with a history of erratic, hostile behavior, pressured speech, flight of ideas, and impulsiveness has had her symptoms controlled with medication. She is seen by her psychiatrist for a routine visit and complains that she might be getting "the flu." She describes symptoms of nausea and diarrhea. As she speaks, the psychiatrist notes that she slurs her words, is tremulous, and is ataxic.

121. A young man with a history of psychotic symptoms has responded well to a low-potency, high-cholinergic drug. He complains to his psychiatrist that he is embarrassed that his semen seems to go "in" rather than "out." He wonders if he is going crazy again.

Questions 122 Through 126

For each of the following patients with a respiratory illness, select the most likely pathogen.

    (A) adenovirus
    (B) *Bordetella pertussis*
    (C) *Chlamydia trachomatis*
    (D) coxsackievirus
    (E) Epstein–Barr virus

    (F) *Hemophilus influenzae*
    (G) herpes simplex 1
    (H) *Moraxella catarrhalis*
    (I) *Mycoplasma pneumoniae*
    (J) parainfluenza virus
    (K) respiratory syncytial virus
    (L) rotavirus
    (M) *Staphylococcus aureus*
    (N) *Streptococcus agalactiae* (group B)
    (O) *Streptococcus pneumoniae*
    (P) *Streptococcus pyogenes* (group A)

122. A 3-month-old infant with wheezing and history of 3 days of cough, congestion, and rhinorrhea

123. A 9-year-old with gradual onset of fever, malaise, and worsening cough over 5 days and rales in the area of the right upper lobe

124. A 3-month-old infant with history of eye drainage at 2 weeks of age who now has insidious onset of staccato cough and is afebrile, with bilateral rales on exam

125. A 6-month-old with history of 2 weeks of congestion and rhinorrhea, who now has worsening paroxysms of coughing

126. A 2-year-old with 2 days of rhinorrhea and cough, now with hoarseness and a barky cough

Answers and Explanations

1–2. (1-C, 2-E) The complications of gastroesophageal reflux disease (GERD) include esophagitis, esophageal ulceration, stricture, and Barrett's esophagus, among others. Though some patients with GERD respond well to medical therapy, such as a proton pump inhibitor, regurgitation and coughing attacks may not improve with medical treatment alone. The results of treatment by antireflux surgery, such as Nissen fundoplication, are generally good under these circumstances and may prevent the progression of the Barrett's. Once present, Barrett's rarely regresses following surgery. Once high-grade dysplasia is found within Barrett's epithelium, up to half of esophagi removed for such a condition demonstrate foci of invasive cancer. Therefore, the recommended treatment for high-grade dysplasia within Barrett's is esophagectomy. *(Greenfield et al, pp 680–694)*

3. (E) External otitis is an infection of the external auditory canal. The primary symptom is ear pain, which is worsened when the pinna is moved. This distinguishes it from otitis media. A foreign body is easily seen in the canal, unless there is secondary infection and drainage. Mastoiditis is a complication of otitis media. Patients have fever, and as the process progresses, displacement of the pinna. Contact dermatitis in the ear is usually due to an earring and would occur on the pinna. *(Rudolph, pp 946–951)*

4. (B) It is true that disease from wild poliovirus has been eliminated from this country. However, approximately eight cases of paralytic polio associated with oral vaccine occur every year. Since this complication does not arise with injectable vaccine, the recommendation was made to change the schedule. Since oral vaccines are more efficient at preventing intestinal infection without disease, and therefore transmission, the decision was made to recommend use of oral vaccines after the first two doses, when vaccine-related paralytic polio is unlikely to occur. *(Fauci et al, pp 1120–1121)*

5. (D) Most cases of travelers' diarrhea are due to *E coli*. *Shigella* and *Salmonella* infections occur in the United States as well. *Vibrio* is obtained from eating undercooked seafood. *Campylobacter* is a common cause of diarrhea in many areas, and is particularly common in children under 5 years and in college-aged people. *(Fauci et al, p 237)*

6–7. (6-B, 7-A) The Mini-Mental State Examination was developed as a screening tool to evaluate cognitive functioning. It is divided into two parts. The first assesses memory, orientation, attention, and calculation. The second part assesses the patient's language capacity. The various elements are assigned value points (eg, one point each for all aspects of orientation—person, time, place). The total possible points is 30. A score of less than 25 suggests impairment, and less than 20 definite cognitive impairment. In the case in question, the woman received an overall score of 26. Using just the Mini-Mental State Exam, no cognitive impairment is suggested. Although depression may be a factor in test performance, the Mini-Mental State Exam, does not screen for depressive disorders. *(Kaplan et al, pp 318–320)*

8. (B) The most likely cause of these physical findings and possibly of the depression suggested by the suicidal behavior is hypothyroidism. If the disorder were Pick's disease or Alzheimer's, one would expect some decreases in cognitive functioning on the Mini-Mental State Exam. In hyperadrenalism and hypoadrenalism, one would see depression, but the physical findings would include hypertension, hirsutism, moon facies, or hypotension and skin pigmentation, respectively. *(Kaplan et al, pp 328–345, pp 361–362)*

9. (D) Hepatitis in pregnancy is caused most often by one of five viruses: hepatitis A, B, C, E, or D. In all forms, hepatocellular damage results in an increase in liver enzymes, such as alanine transaminase (ALT), AST, and alkaline phosphatase. During pregnancy, the normal WBC is elevated, as is the sedimentation rate. Alkaline phosphatase is normally elevated in pregnant patients because of the contribution to total alkaline phosphatase by the placenta. However, in a normal pregnancy, the AST should be normal, whereas in hepatitis, it is usually markedly elevated. Other diseases that may mimic hepatitis during pregnancy, especially in the third trimester, include cholestasis, preeclampsia, and gallstones. The level of elevation of AST is usually the key, being highest in hepatitis. *(Scott et al, pp 439–441)*

10. (D) Prostaglandin inhibition is the key to control of primary dysmenorrhea. Even the dysmenorrhea associated with endometriosis is thought to be secondary to excess prostaglandin formation. Nonsteroidal anti-inflammatory drugs (NSAIDs) such as ibuprofen and others are usually effective in controlling the pain of primary dysmenorrhea (pain with menstruation in the absence of pelvic pathology). Inhibition of ovulation with oral contraceptives, depot medroxyprogesterone acetate, or a gonadotropin-releasing hormone agonist is also effective. Ethinyl estradiol and norethindrone are the most common components of birth control pills; they decrease prostaglandin synthesis by causing atrophy and decidualization of the endometrium. Bromocriptine, clomiphene, and corticosteroids have no discernible effect on ovulation or the production of prostaglandins and are ineffective in relieving primary dysmenorrhea. The presence of pelvic pathology, such as a pelvic mass or nodularity of the uterosacral ligaments suggesting endometriosis, should be evaluated before prescribing medication. *(Speroff et al, pp 523–525)*

11. (D) Treatment needs to be prompt, because death can occur within minutes with a severe anaphylactic reaction. Administration of subcutaneous or IV epinephrine should be given as soon as possible to control symptoms. Beta blockers are relatively contraindicated. Topical steroids are of no benefit, and IV steroids are not effective for the acute event, but may help later recurrence of bronchospasm. Diphenhydramine is appropriate for urticaria, but is second to epinephrine.

12. (E) Type 1 immediate hypersensitivity reactions are characterized by early symptoms such as urticaria, laryngeal edema, bronchospasm, and vasomotor collapse. They result from mast cell or basophil binding by IgE (not IgA) or activated complement fragments C3a or C5a (so-called anaphylatoxins). A persistent delayed rash is not seen with type 1 reactions. The early cutaneous hypersensitivity response of wheal and flare is seen within 15 minutes and resolves in about 90 minutes. Foods, bee stings, drugs, and pollens are examples of inciting agents. Extrinsic (but not intrinsic) asthma is an example of a type 1 allergic reaction. *(Fauci, pp 1860–1866)*

13. (E) Although testing of an animal specimen can give a diagnosis in less than 24 hours, immediate treatment is indicated, because the fox's behavior is clearly abnormal and highly suggestive of rabies. It is appropriate after such an attack to begin preventive treatment immediately for presumptive rabies exposure. The recommended treatment is a five-shot series of immunizations given over 28 days. A dose of rabies-specific immunoglobulin, calculated by weight, is given with the first immunization. One half of the dose is administered in the area of the bite(s), the remainder in the gluteus. Observation of wildlife for rabies is never indicated, since the period in which they may be communicable is unknown. *(Fauci et al, pp 1130–1131)*

14–15. **(14-C, 15-E)** In Figure 8–2, a group of vesicles with early central crusting on a red base can be seen on the shaft of the penis. This is characteristic of genital herpes simplex. Syphilis is usually a painless chancre that develops into an ulcer. Lymphogranuloma venereum is an organism that belongs to the *Chlamydia* group of parasites. The primary genital lesion is a small painless papule that heals spontaneously. *Condyloma acuminatum* is a wart caused by human papillomavirus that may be pinpoint or cauliflower-like. Herpes zoster represents reactivation of the varicella-zoster virus and is not sexually transmitted.

Patients with genital herpes need to be warned that infection can be transmitted even when asymptomatic. Shedding of the organism does *not* stop when the lesions are gone. Patients should refrain from sexual activity while the lesions are present, because condoms are not reliably protective. Patients also need to be told about the risk of having a recurrent episode. Acylovir is the antiviral used to treat herpes. Doxycycline is the treatment of choice for lymphogranuloma venereum. *(Fitzpatrick, pp 914–915)*

16. **(E)** Spontaneous pneumothorax can be seen in otherwise healthy adolescents. It presents very suddenly with chest pain and dyspnea. You would expect to hear wheezing or decreased breath sounds bilaterally if this were an exacerbation of asthma resulting in this much respiratory distress. Pneumonia and empyema would not present over such a short time. He would also be febrile. A foreign body aspiration is unlikely in this age group. *(Kliegman, pp 185–197)*

17. **(E)** Patients with sickle cell disease are at risk for overwhelming infection, especially with encapsulated organisms. This is especially true in infants and young children. The use of prophylactic penicillin has dramatically decreased this risk. It is started as soon as the diagnosis is made. He will need a pneumo-

coccal vaccine, but it is not effective in neonates. It is usually given at age 2 years. Neonates with sickle cell disease are not at any greater risk for iron deficiency than normal infants. These patients are at higher risk for folate deficiency. However, controlled studies have not documented the need for routine folic acid supplementation, so some centers have elected to stop routine supplementation. The only caution in avoiding heat for these patients is that dehydration can exacerbate sickling. When exposed to heat, patients need to be diligent about adequate fluid intake. *(Rudolph, pp 1181, 1203–1207)*

18. **(B)** This is the classic presentation of splenic sequestration, which occurs in these patients in the first few years of life, before the spleen autoinfarcts. Acute chest syndrome, intussusception, and vaso-occlusive crisis are not associated with severe anemia. If this were an aplastic crisis, a very low reticulocyte count would be expected. *(Rudolph, pp 1204–1207)*

19. **(E)** When evaluating a screening program, one must consider several sources of bias. A prognostic (length) bias occurs when disease detected by a screening program is less aggressive than disease detected after symptoms develop. This occurs because less aggressive diseases tend to have a long preclinical phase, increasing the length of time detectable by screening. *(Feinstein, pp 317–318)*

20–22. **(20-B, 21-B, 22-B)** Clinical features of spontaneous esophageal perforation (Boerhaave syndrome) include acute onset of excruciating pain after straining, such as in the case of vomiting. Associated clinical findings may include subcutaneous emphysema, fever, hypotension, tachycardia, and dyspnea. Initial treatment includes resuscitative efforts to stabilize the patient. The diagnostic test of choice is a contrast study of the esophagus. A CT scan is helpful in atypical presentations or to demonstrate related complications. Esophagoscopy is rarely needed to diagnose a perforation. Analysis of the pleural fluid may be suggestive of a perforation, but radiologic studies would be required to make a definitive diagnosis. Time to definitive treatment is the factor that most influences outcome. Poorer survival has been noted in patients in whom a delay in treatment of more than 24 to 48 hours has occurred. *(Sabiston, pp 759–767)*

23–24. (23-D, 24-C) Malignant hypertension is defined by the presence of papilledema and end-organ changes rather than the absolute BP level. Headache may not be the result of his elevated BP, and heart size can be related to factors other than hypertension, such as heart failure and cardiomyopathy. Impairment of renal function provides the best index to prognosis in malignant hypertension. The level of systolic or diastolic BP and size of the heart are features that are readily reversible and do not relate quantitatively to prognosis. A larger heart and more florid retinopathy do not necessarily portend a poorer prognosis, but numerous studies have documented that the worse the renal impairment, the poorer the prognosis. Compliance may play a role in BP control, but is not reliable for predicting prognosis. *(Fauci, p 1393)*

25. (B) Short-acting benzodiazepines especially, such as alprazolam, can produce significant symptoms when abruptly discontinued, a sign of physiologic dependence. Mild symptoms can include anxiety, irritability, sleep disruption, tremor, and nausea; the development of paranoia, depression, delirium, and seizures are serious complications of sudden drug withdrawal. The likelihood of significant withdrawal symptoms increases with dosage, length of treatment, and shorter half-life. *(Kaplan and Sadock, pp 994, 1108; Andreason and Black, p 668)*

26. (C) When individuals perceive their own impulses or traits as unacceptable, it is said that these phenomena are ego dystonic. Such undesirable thoughts or characteristics are experienced as alien to the self, and their presence can create a great deal of subjective distress. The concept of ego dystonic traits is especially important in the consideration of personality disorders. Individuals with an antisocial personality disorder may feel quite comfortable with their own style and thus never seek treatment, even though their so-

ciopathy antagonizes everyone around them. Their antisocial tendencies are thus ego syntonic, that is, acceptable to the self. If the same traits were ego dystonic, however, such individuals would experience a high degree of subjective distress, even if they got along well with others. *(Stoudemire, Human Behavior, pp 70, 71)*

27. (C) The EDD is calculated according to Naegele's Rule by adding 7 days to the first day of the LMP, then subtracting 3 months. For this to be accurate, the woman must have reasonably regular menstrual intervals of 28 to 32 days. The mean duration of pregnancy is 266 days from conception or 280 days from the first day of the last menses if menstrual intervals are about 28 days. *(Scott et al, pp 77–78)*

28. (D) The uterine fundus in pregnancy does not grow beyond the pelvis until after 12 postmenstrual weeks. Subsequently, gestational age can be estimated from fundal height in two ways. At 14, 16, and 18 weeks the uterus is palpable one fourth, one half, and three fourths the distance from the symphysis pubis to the umbilicus. The fundus is palpable at the level of the umbilicus at 20 gestational weeks. *(Scott et al, pp 77–78)*

29–30. (29-E, 30-A) Patients with Alzheimer's disease often have symptoms that may mimic depression (lack of enthusiasm, moodiness) along with their intellectual decline and therefore may score poorly on a depression screening inventory. In early stages, they may be able to perform well on formal mental status testing. CT and MRI scans are not specific for Alzheimer's and may be normal early in the course of the disease. The earliest metabolic changes in Alzheimer's occur in the parietal cortex and can be seen with PET scanning. Tremor is uncommon with Alzheimer's, but is seen with Parkinson's. Pathological features include brain atrophy, neurofibrillary tangles, and granulovacuolar neuronal degeneration. Initial symptoms generally begin after the age of 45 years, with progressive memory loss leading to global dementia. Some familial clustering is reported, but most cases are sporadic. Choline acetyltransferase activity is reduced, not increased, and hallucinations and delusions are common. EEG may be normal or show non-specific slowing. (*Fauci et al, pp 2348–2351*)

31. **(E)** One of the major developmental tasks of adolescence is the acquisition of independence from the parents. Spending time in their own personal space is a part of this. Although prevalent adolescent problems, such as abuse, pregnancy, and drug abuse, can also result in withdrawal from the family, some change in their functioning at school would be expected. If she were hypothyroid, you would expect to see some changes in her physical exam. (*Rudolph, pp 39–42*)

32. **(D)** The patient has the typical CSF findings of bacterial meningitis, with elevated white blood cells and a predominance of neutrophils, elevated protein, and decreased glucose. These values would not be expected in patients with tuberculosis or enteroviral meningitis. Typical bacteria that cause meningitis in this age group are *Streptococcus pneumoniae* and *Neisseria meningititis*. Group B strep is the most common bacterial cause of meningitis in neonates. Group A strep does not commonly cause meningitis. (*Kliegman, pp 878–888*)

33–34. **(33-C, 34-D)** Pyogenic hepatic abscesses may occur following intra-abdominal sepsis, such as diverticulitis. A typical presentation may include fever, abdominal pain, anorexia, and nausea of relatively short duration, along with an elevated WBC and elevation in liver function tests. The most sensitive imaging procedure is the CT scan. An ultrasound is a very useful screening test, especially for suspected biliary tree abnormalities, but may be limited in obese patients or those with non-homogeneous livers. Radionuclide imaging studies are not as useful as CT or ultrasound. The treatment of pyogenic abscesses includes both antibiotics and drainage. Percutaneous drainage of most hepatic abscesses is safe and effective. Surgical drainage is advised for patients exhibiting signs of continued sepsis despite percutaneous drainage and appropri-

ate antibiotics. (*Greenfield et al, pp 958–959; Sabiston, pp 1061–1068*)

35. **(B)** Almost 10% of boys 18 years of age or younger meet the diagnostic criteria for conduct disorder. Although this prevalence rate is significantly higher than in girls, the incidence of the disorder actually is higher in postpubertal girls than in postpubertal boys. Parental alcoholism, sociopathy, neglect, or absence can predispose to the development of conduct disorder in their children. In some children, hyperactivity precedes the emergence of conduct disorder. Various etiologic factors contributing to the development of conduct disorders have been explored. These include attempts to define specific neurologic factors. One such theory states that there is decreased noradrenergic functioning in conduct disorder. The enzyme dopamine beta-hydroxylase, which converts dopamine to norepinephrine, has been found to be in low levels in the plasma of some children with conduct disorder. Additionally, it has been found that attention deficit disorder and conduct disorder often coexist in some children. Other studies indicate the probability of psychosocial etiologic factors, including having parents with serious psychopathology, substance abuse, and alcohol abuse disorders. The number of boys with the disorder is higher and the age of onset is younger (for boys, 10 to 12 years v. 14 to 16 years for girls). (*APA, pp 85–91; Kaplan and Sadock, pp 1205–1208*)

36. **(D)** The concept of the superego was Freud's last addition to the structural theory of individual psychology (the theory that states that the psychic apparatus can be seen as divided into the id, ego, and superego). The id is a collection of primitive instinctual drives. The ego regulates the discharge of those drives either in the avoidance of pain or into agreement with the demands of the real world. The superego, an agency whose contents are sometimes conscious but largely unconscious, acts to ensure that thoughts and actions comply with a personal and social moral code. This set of internalized values and prohibitions is itself part of the superego. When id or ego productions conflict with the

standards of the superego, the individual experiences anxiety or guilt. If the superego is organized along excessively rigid lines, the individual will be prone to an unduly critical style, intense anxiety, and compulsive behavior. When the superego is underdeveloped, an individual is likely to manifest antisocial characteristics. (*Kaplan and Sadock, p 248*)

37. **(G)** Amenorrhea and galactorrhea are usually concurrent findings in women with significantly increased prolactin concentrations. The differential diagnosis of hyperprolactinemia is: thyroid dysfunction resulting in increased hypothalamic thyrotropin-releasing hormone secretion, certain psychotropic and antihypertensive medications, a pituitary tumor, and idiopathic. While it is not certain that this patient has a pituitary adenoma, this is the most likely diagnosis in her situation of anestrogenic amenorrhea and galactorrhea. A serum prolactin concentration exceeding 100 ng/mL (normal is usually less than 20) is associated with a pituitary adenoma in at least 80% of these women. This woman should have a serum prolactin concentration measured, and then a CT scan or MRI of her pituitary if the prolactin concentration is this high. Tumors develop as a result of chronic lactotrope stimulation (or chronic suppression of secretion from the hypothalamus). Treatment is oral bromocriptine (Parlodel) or cabergoline (Dostinex). (*Speroff et al, pp 427–432*)

38. **(I)** Hypertension in a sexually infantile woman with primary amenorrhea is 17α-hydroxylase deficiency until proven otherwise. This is an autosomal recessive disorder in which cortisol, androgen, and estrogen secretion is deficient. The mineralocorticoid pathway is the only steroid biosynthetic pathway that is not impaired. Mineralocorticoid (11-desoxycorticosterone, corticosterone, and aldosterone) secretion is increased because the decreased cortisol causes an increased adrenocorticotropic (ACTH) hormone secretion. Serum pregnenolone and progesterone concentrations will be elevated, while 17-hydroxypregnenolone and 17-hydroxyprogesterone concentrations will be low. Treatment

is glucocorticoid replacement. (*Speroff et al, p 334*)

39. **(C)** Irregular menstrual intervals in women with signs of androgen excess (hirsutism, temporal balding, voice changes, clitoral enlargement, etc) suggest a functional rather than a neoplastic disorder if the problem is chronic and dates from the time of puberty. The absence of a family history, normal blood pressure, and a normal DHEAS level eliminate 21-hydroxylase deficiency. Deficiency of 17α-hydroxylase causes sexual infantilism, not hirsutism. Moderate increases in serum prolactin levels may cause irregular menses, but not hirsutism. Sertoli–Leydig cell tumor is the only other hyperandrogenic disorder listed. Clinical presentation of women with this tumor is usually abrupt onset of amenorrhea and unilateral ovarian enlargement. (*Speroff et al, pp 463–467*)

40. **(J)** Postpartum amenorrhea in a woman with a history of hypertension and hemorrhage is most likely the result of pituitary necrosis and inability to secrete gonadotropins (FSH and leuteinizing hormone). Prolactin secretion is also impaired and lactation is not possible in these women. (*Speroff et al, p 434*)

41. **(L)** Key to making the diagnosis of Turner syndrome (gonadal dysgenesis) is the recognition that 150 cm (4 ft 11 in) is short. Streak gonads (ie, gonadal dysgenesis) should be the first consideration in any woman with primary amenorrhea who is less than 5 feet tall. Other signs of gonadal dysgenesis should be sought: webbed neck, cubitus valgus, heart murmur, shield chest and wide spaced nipples, and others. A karyotype should be obtained to confirm the diagnosis and ensure that there is no Y chromosome. The presence of a Y chromosome requires removal of the gonads because these women have about a 30% chance of developing a gonadal tumor, such as gonadoblastoma. The increased FSH concentration confirms that this woman's amenorrhea is the result of gonadal failure, not hypothalamic–pituitary failure. (*Speroff et al, pp 346–349*)

42. **(K)** Testicular feminization is a disorder in which 46,XY individuals lack androgen receptors or have androgen receptors that do not respond normally to adult male levels of testosterone secretion. This disorder is also known as complete androgen insensitivity. The gonads are testes and are located intra-abdominally or in hernia sacs in the inguinal canals. A cervix and uterus are absent because the testes secreted müllerian duct inhibiting factor during early embryonic life. Because of the risk of a testicular tumor, they should be removed. Orchiectomy can safely be delayed until puberty is complete in subjects with the complete form of testicular feminization. The testes should be removed soon after the diagnosis is made in those with partial forms of androgen insensitivity because variable degrees of masculinization will occur beginning at the time of puberty. These women require estrogen replacement after removal of the gonads to maintain breast development, prevent osteoporosis, and reduce the risk of coronary artery disease associated with estrogen deficiency. *(Speroff et al, pp 339–342)*

43. **(B)** The triad of a pregnancy, endometrial trauma, and endometrial infection in a woman who subsequently becomes amenorrheic is almost pathognomonic of endometrial sclerosis (Asherman syndrome). No treatment is necessary unless the woman wishes to conceive. Treatment consists of lysing the intrauterine adhesions by hysteroscopy, insertion of a foreign body such as an intrauterine device (IUD) into the uterus, and high-dose estrogen therapy for 6 to 12 weeks. The IUD keeps the opposing walls of the endometrium apart, and the estrogen stimulates growth and proliferation of any endometrium still present. *(Speroff et al, pp 418–419)*

44. **(E)** It is always important to remember that the most common cause of amenorrhea in women of reproductive age is pregnancy. Breast soreness, fatigue, and increased urinary frequency are symptoms of pregnancy. A sensitive pregnancy test should be done on all amenorrheic women of reproductive age, even if the possibility of pregnancy is denied. The cyanosis of the vaginal epithelium is Chadwick sign, a sign of pregnancy that appears at about 6 postmenstrual weeks. It is doubtful that post-pill amenorrhea is a frequent disorder. Available evidence demonstrates that conception rates after stopping oral contraceptives are similar to those of women who did not use a contraceptive. If amenorrhea persists for 3 to 6 months or longer after stopping oral contraceptives, it should be evaluated, just as it would under any circumstance. *(Speroff et al, p 445)*

45. **(F)** Premature ovarian failure is suggested by the presence of hot flashes, failure to menstruate after medroxyprogesterone acetate, physical evidence of estrogen deficiency (dry vaginal epithelium and no cervical mucus), and increased FSH concentrations. This disorder affects approximately 1% of women less than 40 years of age. Most have premature menopause secondary to depletion of oocytes. However, approximately 20% of women with premature ovarian failure will have either the gonadotropin-resistant ovary syndrome or autoimmune ovarian failure. In these women, there are a normal number of oocytes for their age and pregnancy is theoretically possible, though extemely unlikely. Chemotherapy, radiation therapy, galactosemia, and overwhelming ovarian infection are other causes of premature ovarian failure. Treatment is hormone replacement with estrogen and progestin. *(Speroff et al, pp 424–425)*

46. **(H)** Abrupt cessation of menses coincident with or followed shortly by signs of masculinization suggest the possibility of a virilizing ovarian tumor, especially if one ovary is enlarged significantly more than the other. The most common virilizing tumor in women of reproductive age is a Sertoli–Leydig cell tumor. The degree of masculinization is variable and seems to depend on the number of testosterone-producing interstitial cells present in the tumor. A pure Sertoli cell tumor will not cause signs of masculinization. It is commonly stated that testosterone concentrations less than 200 ng/dL suggest a functional process, whereas concentrations

greater than 200 ng/dL suggest a tumor. This is a reasonable clinical guide, but with many exceptions. (*Speroff et al, pp 499–501*)

47. **(B)** Abuse of anabolic steroids is most likely to be associated with the development of such manic-like symptoms as euphoria, irritability, and reckless behavior. Depression can result from drug withdrawal, and suicides have occurred. Abuse of anabolic steroids can produce drug dependence. (*Stoudemire*, Clinical Psychiatry, *p 325; Kaplan and Sadock, p 454*)

48. **(E)** Although prior administration of human immunoglobulin containing anti-HAV before or within 2 weeks after exposure is 75 to 85% effective, prior immunization against hepatitis A is even more effective. A two-dose vaccination schedule is 95% effective in preventing disease in adolescents and adults. Consuming untreated water and uncooked food in endemic areas is a risk factor; therefore, relying on bottled water and cooked food is reasonable. However, this will not protect against contact with younger children, who often have subclinical infections and remain significant sources of disease transmission. Pepto-Bismol and ciprofloxacin are preventive treatments for travelers' diarrhea. (*Wallace and Doebbeling, pp 175–178*)

49. **(B)** Diaper dermatitis is a very common problem in infants. This infant's rash is due to bullous impetigo. The classic presentation of this illness is erythema of the skin, followed by the development of bullae that rupture. Allergic dermatitis and irritant dermatitis are most prominent on the convex areas and are intensely red. *Candida* dermatitis is red without bullae and has satellite lesions at the margins. In seborrheic dermatitis, children tend to have the rash on the scalp, neck, and face also. It is scaly and more prominent in the intertriginous areas. (*Hurwitz, pp 27–29*)

50. **(C)** Diaper dermatitis is a very common problem in infants. This infant's rash is due to *Candida*. *Candida* dermatitis is red without bullae and has satellite lesions at the margins. It is common in infants, especially when

they have been on antibiotics. In bullous impetigo, the skin is initially erythematous and then bullae develop. Allergic dermatitis and irritant dermatitis are most prominent on the convex areas and are intensely red. In seborrheic dermatitis, children tend to have the rash on the scalp, neck, and face also. It is scaly and more prominent in the intertriginous areas. (*Hurwitz, pp 27–29*)

51–52. **(51-D, 52-C)** Fibroadenoma represents the most common breast tumor in young women. They are usually well defined, mobile, and firm on exam. Invasive ductal carcinoma is much less frequent in this age group. Ductal carcinoma in situ is usually nonpalpable, but may on occasion present as a mass. Fibrocystic changes can present as a mass, but a well-defined mass identified by sonography is more suggestive of fibroadenoma. Intraductal papillomas have an average size of 3 to 4 mm and are rarely palpable. Excisional biopsy is not necessary for all fibroadenomas, and the patient should be given the option of observation. In patients under the age of 30, observation alone may be sufficient, but a tissue diagnosis, preferably by needle biopsy, should be made in patients over the age of 30. (*Greenfield et al, pp 1374–1376*)

53. **(B)** Syphilis is a sexually transmitted infection caused by the bacterium *Treponema pallidum*. After an average incubation period of 21 days, a painless papule forms and gradually forms a clean ulcer (chancre). The secondary stage begins about 4 to 8 weeks after the appearance of the primary chancre. Malaise, sore throat, fever, and headache are common. The diagnosis can be made by dark-field examination and serologic testing (serologic test for syphilis [STS], Veneral Disease Research Laboratory [VDRL], fluorescent treponemal antibody-absorption test for syphilis [FTA-ABS]). Leprosy may present with hypopigmented macules, plaques, or papules, but fever and headache are not typical symptoms. Chancroid presents with an inflammatory macule that forms a pustule and then ulcerates. Adenopathy may be noted with chancroid, but fevers and

headaches are not typical. The gram-negative organism responsible for chancroid (*Hemophilus ducreyi*) may be obtained by culture. The history of a genital ulcer followed by the rash pictured should raise the suspicion of syphilis as the most likely cause.

54. **(C)** Erythema migrans is the exanthem seen in Lyme disease. It starts as a red macule or papule and then expands to an annular plaque with a raised border. It is seen 3 to 5 weeks after the tick bite at the site of the bite. Patients often have systemic symptoms at the same time. Erythema marginatum is the exanthem in acute rheumatic fever. It is also an annular lesion that usually occurs on the trunk. This patient does not have the other symptoms consistent with rheumatic fever. Contact dermatitis is not annular but intensely erythematous and shaped according to the offending article, such as in a necklace shape if the patient is allergic to a metal necklace. Erythema multiforme classically has target lesions. Tinea corporis is also annular, but has central clearing and is typically not as large as erythema migrans. (*American Academy of Pediatrics, pp 329–330, Hurwitz, pp 388–391*)

55. **(C)** Neonates are exposed to herpes at birth if the mother has a genital infection. Transmission of the infection to the infant is much more likely if the infection is primary. The characteristic lesions are grouped vesicles on an erythematous base. They are likely to occur at a traumatized location such as the scalp if a monitor has been used during delivery. Varicella also is vesicular, but one would expect to see numerous lesions, which usually start on the trunk. Group B *Streptococcus* and *Staphylococcus* can cause cellulitis in the newborn, but the rash would not be vesicular. Exanthems are common with enterovirus but are macular and are present all over the body. (*American Academy of Pediatrics, pp 266–268*)

56. **(A)** Erythema infectiosum (Fifth disease) is caused by parvovirus. This patient has the typical presentation with a prodromal illness, followed by the characteristic "slapped-cheek" rash on the face and the reticular rash

on the extremities. Kawasaki disease is diagnosed clinically. Patients have fever, conjunctivitis, adenopathy, oral changes, and rash and are usually ill. Measles presents with the classic triad of the three Cs—conjunctivitis, coryza, and cough—followed by the rash. Roseola usually occurs in infants. Patients have several days of high fever, followed by a rash on the trunk, which is macular or maculopapular. The rash in scarlet fever is a fine papular rash (sandpaper-like). (*Rudolph et al, pp 669–670, 683–684*)

57. **(C)** The increase in erythrocyte volume requires approximately 500 mg of elemental iron. The fetus and placenta require an additional 300 mg of iron. Given the low rate of absorption of oral iron, a daily intake of 30 to 60 mg of iron is necessary to meet this requirement in a normal pregnancy. Most multivitamins contain approximately 30 mg of iron, and prenatal vitamins about 60 to 65 mg of iron. Anemic women or women with a multiple gestation should receive additional iron supplements beyond those recommended for uncomplicated pregnancies. (*Scott et al, p 94*)

58. **(E)** The primary syphilitic lesion or chancre starts as a papule and over several weeks develops into a small plaque with an erosive surface. It occurs at the site of penetration of the treponemes and is most commonly found on the genitalia. It is not painful. Herpes infection lesions are typically grouped vesicles on an erythematous base. Lesions from trauma and staph infections would be painful. Lesions from condylomata acuminata are soft, flesh-colored, and nodular. (*Jenson et al, pp 1262–1263, 1272*)

59. **(G)** These are the classic history and physical findings seen in Prader–Willi syndrome. Typical features are obesity, almond-shaped eyes, and narrow bifrontal diameter. Patients also have severe neonatal hypotonia, hypoplastic genitalia, small hands and feet, polyphagia, and mental retardation. It is inherited sporadically, and many affected individuals have an abnormality of chromosome 15. (*Rudolph, pp 399*)

60. (D) This child has fetal alcohol syndrome. The facial features shown include narrow palpebral fissures; a short nose with a broad, low bridge; midfacial hypoplasia; and a long philtrum with a narrow vermilion border. Associated anomalies are cleft palate; cardiac malformations (especially atrial and ventricular defects); hearing loss; and joint, skin, and skeletal abnormalities. There are also varying degrees of growth failure and developmental delay. The severity of the defects appears to be proportional to the amount of alcohol consumed during the pregnancy. (*Rudolph, pp 419–420*)

61–64. (61-G, 62-C, 63-F, 64-A) Sinus headache is usually acute in onset, worse on awakening, better on standing, and can worsen on bending over. Often, there is a purulent nasal discharge and pain over the involved sinus. Subarachnoid hemorrhage is often described as "the worst headache of my life" and is very abrupt in onset. Cluster headache predominantly occurs in middle-aged men, and its typical presentation involves intense unilateral headache that is searing, stabbing, and accompanied by ipsilateral lacrimation, nasal stuffiness, and facial flushing. Alcohol is believed to be a precipitant, although alcohol is well tolerated between attacks. Migraine headache is more common in women, and usually begins in childhood or young adult life. Migraine may or may not have an aura, but is unilateral, of pulsating quality, and accompanied by nausea or vomiting, photophobia, or phonophobia. Subdural hematoma is also a subtle condition with earlier head trauma that may be forgotten until the patient displays mental status changes or focal neurologic deficits. A patient with a brain tumor may be asymptomatic other than headache initially, but usually neurologic deficits will be found as the time progresses. Muscle contraction headache is typically worse as the day goes on, bilateral in the frontotemporal area, and described as a tight band around the head. (*Goroll, pp 821–825*)

65–68. (65-B, 66-F, 67-A, 68-G) Diverticulosis is the most common cause of massive rectal bleeding, which is usually bright red and painless. Patients with ulcerative colitis may have diarrhea, abdominal cramps, and weight loss, with a clinical course that may be associated with a severe exacerbation. With severe colitis, there is increased frequency of bloody stools, and signs of systemic toxicity (fever and leukocytosis). Meckel's diverticulum presents as painless rectal bleeding in children. Ischemic colitis usually occurs in the postoperative period after abdominal aortic aneurysm surgery. It is associated with crampy lower abdominal pain, and bloody stools from mucosal sloughing. Endometriosis is not usually associated with rectal bleeding. Bleeding from a gastrointestinal source above the ligament of Treitz (such as a peptic ulcer) will result in melena, which is characterized by tarry, foul-smelling stools. Carcinoma of the colon should be suspected in a patient presenting with rectal bleeding and a history of a change in bowel habits. (*Greenfield et al, pp 1158–1172*)

69. (D) Sinus arrhythmia is a normal variant that is common in pediatric patients. It usually varies with the respiratory cycle, slowing with expiration. On the strip, each normal QRS wave is preceded by a normal p wave. This excludes the diagnosis of atrial premature beats that would have premature p waves that were shaped differently. Patients with sick sinus syndrome usually have episodes of tachycardia and episodes of sinus arrest. In sinoatrial block, the sinoatrial pacemaker is discharging, but occasionally the impulse does not depolarize the atria. The strip shows pauses that approximate the normal P-P interval. This patient does not have a tachycardic rhythm, and patients with supraventricular tachycardia usually have symptoms of palpitations or a sensation of their heart racing. (*Rudolph, pp 1451–1453*)

70. (E) Since this is a normal variant, no further diagnostic testing is necessary. (*Rudolph, p 1451*)

71–72. (71-D, 72-B) A direct blow to the epigastrium compresses the duodenum against the vertebral column, with a shearing injury resulting in an intramural hematoma. With the breakdown of hemoglobin in the hematoma, there is an increase in the oncotic pressure and imbibement of fluid into the hematoma, leading to progressive obstruction. This can contribute to the delay in presentation, which is commonly several days after the initial injury. Bilious vomiting is secondary to obstruction at the junction of the second and third parts of the duodenum. There may be mild hyperamylasemia, related either to the duodenal wall injury or to an associated pancreatic injury. Pancreatitis from blunt abdominal trauma usually presents at the outset with progressive abdominal tenderness and significant elevation of serum amylase. There is often a delay in the diagnosis of small bowel perforation, with the development of tachycardia, fever, and peritonitis on abdominal exam. Gastritis is usually secondary to an acute infectious agent, and cholecystitis occurs in the presence of cholelithiasis. Patients with obstruction from intramural duodenal hematoma are managed with nasogastric decompression and parenteral nutrition. In the majority of cases, the obstruction will resolve in 7 to 10 days. Operative intervention is not usually required. (*Sabiston, pp 314–315; Greenfield et al, pp 345–346*)

73. **(D)** Patients with terminal illnesses have specific needs and present particular problems for in-hospital and outpatient management. Families are often fearful, confused, and unclear as to how to relate to these patients. House officers are not immune to this problem. Analgesics for pain relief are generally more efficacious when administered on a regular schedule, allowing the patient to refuse. The inappropriate use of PRN regimens stems from a prevalent but unsubstantiated fear that patients will become addicted to the medication. In fact, studies have shown that fewer than 1% of patients treated with pain medication become addicted. Patients confronting death are acutely socially sensitive, and miscommunications or evasive discussions are interpreted with the most negative outlook. Patients generally prefer honest information, especially if they have to make decisions about subjecting themselves to often painful procedures and treatments. Checking with the patient on how much in-

formation he or she would like about the illness helps clarify the direction the physician will follow to effectively address the patient's information needs. Studies of groups of terminally ill patients with metastatic carcinoma described group therapy as an exceptionally effective mode of treatment. It offers a close support system based on a common bond and allows the patients to learn from each other how to cope and how to help their loved ones cope with the stresses of terminal illness. (*Cassem, pp 346–369; Kaplan and Sadock, p 67*)

74. **(D)** Established risk factors show a high degree of sensitivity but low specificity for suicidal behavior. Correlates include past suicide attempts, family history of suicidal behavior, a high degree of hopelessness, and decreased serotonergic function. The strength of neurobiologic correlates seems to be directly proportional to the lethality of the suicide attempt and inversely proportional to the likelihood of rescue. Persons who make a suicide gesture tend to be younger, more impulsive, and more characterologically disturbed than persons who have failed in a serious suicide attempt. Risk of suicide in schizophrenia is highest after resolution of acute psychosis, perhaps because of postpsychotic depression. Decreased serotonergic function has been found in depressed persons who have attempted suicide and even further decreased in those who used violent means (eg, guns) in their attempt. (*Andreason and Black, pp 511–520; Kaplan and Sadock, pp 869–871; Tomb, pp 74–78*)

75. **(C)** The recommended amount of folic acid in a folate-replete woman is 400 to 800 μg/day. Most multivitamins contain 400 μg per tablet, and prenatal vitamins usually contain 1000 μg. There is no known toxicity with excess folic acid ingestion. The recommended dietary allowance in nonpregnant women is 180 μg/day, and 280 μg/day in lactating women. (*ACOG, Number 179; Cunningham et al, pp 238–239*)

76. **(E)** Several studies have demonstrated a significant reduction in the rate of fetal anom-

alies with folic acid supplementation. In one study, the malformation rate with folic acid supplementation was reduced from 22.9/1000 to 13.3/1000. In women who previously had an infant with a neural tube defect, consumption of 4 mg of folic acid daily, beginning at least 1 month before conception and continuing through the first 3 months of pregnancy, resulted in a significant reduction in the recurrence of a neural tube defect. Since 1992, the CDC has recommended that all fertile American women take 400 µg folic acid on a regular, continuous basis. None of the other options have been shown to occur. (*Cunningham et al, pp 238–239*)

77. **(B)** In 1976, in the case *Tarasoff* vs. *Regents of University of California*, it was ruled that any physician or therapist who had reason to believe that a patient would kill or injure someone must notify the victim, the victim's relatives or friends, or the legal authorities. The case rose out of the death of a young woman, Tatiana Tarasoff, who was murdered after a patient had told his therapist he would do so. The patient, a student, was being seen at the University Mental Health Clinic. (*Kaplan and Sadock, pp 1308–1309, 1314, 1315*)

78–79. **(78-A, 79-E)** This patient presents with symptoms and signs of a small-bowel obstruction, most probably from intra-abdominal adhesions related to previous abdominal surgery. The diagnosis is strongly suspected on the basis of the clinical presentation. Appropriate initial management should therefore include nasogastric decompression to prevent further distension from swallowed air, and initiation of IV fluid resuscitation *before* obtaining abdominal radiographs. Analgesics may mask physical signs of impending bowel ischemia. A barium enema may be helpful in patients with suspected colonic obstruction, but should not be obtained before resuscitation and plain radiographs. This patient does not have a history of constipation, and therefore enemas and stool softeners are not indicated. This patient has clinical and radiographic signs of a complete small-bowel obstruction. Because of the risk of intestinal

ischemia, surgery is indicated after initial resuscitative maneuvers to correct fluid and electrolyte abnormalities. Continued nonoperative management is appropriate only in patients with partial obstruction who show continued clinical improvement when re-examined. A rectal tube or colonoscopy is not indicated for a small-bowel obstruction, and a "long tube" (Cantor tube) has no additional advantage over standard nasogastric decompression. (*Sabiston, pp 917–919; Niederhuber, pp 300–301*)

80. **(B)** The pincer grasp is attained in the second 6 months of life. Ninety percent of children can do this by age 10 months. The milestone of object constancy (the understanding that an object continues to exist even if the child does not see it) occurs around 9 months. The infant then recognizes the difference between people he knows well and strangers, which leads to the development of stranger anxiety. Ninety percent of infants can stand with support by 10 months. Between 8 and 10 months, babbling becomes more complex, with "mama" and "dada" used nonspecifically. (*Behrman, pp 43–44*)

81. **(E)** Retinal hemorrhages in young children, when seen with other evidence of trauma, especially when the history is not consistent with the physical examination, are pathognomonic of child abuse. Kernig's sign is a sign of meningeal irritation and is seen with meningitis. The rooting reflex is normal in infants. Overlapping cranial sutures can be a normal finding shortly after a vaginal birth. They also can occur when the infant has microcephaly. Neck tenderness could be due to abuse or accidental trauma and of itself does not suggest abuse. (*Rudolph et al, pp 2125–2126*)

82. **(D)** At birth, the average hemoglobin is 17 g/L because of the relatively hypoxic intrauterine environment. After birth, the Pa_{O_2} rises and erythropoiesis decreases. Red cell life span is shorter at this time as well. These two processes lead to the physiologic nadir in hemoglobin that occurs around 2 months of age. Iron deficiency is the most common ane-

mia in childhood but is not typically seen until after 6 to 12 months. Lead toxicity is not seen until children can put objects in their mouths. The patient could have a congenital hemolytic anemia with a *normal* hemoglobin, but this is much less likely. Transfusion is not indicated in this patient unless there are symptoms or signs of cardiac failure. (*Kliegman, pp 803–817*)

83. **(B)** Lung abscesses are localized cavities with pus. They are usually a result of aspiration of infected material from the upper airway and often associated with periodontal disease or poor oral hygiene. The most common pathogens are anaerobes. Penicillin is the drug of choice for most of these anaerobic infections. (*Kelley, pp 1891–1893*)

84. **(D)** The ECG demonstrates T-wave inversions in II, III, and AVF, inferior wall leads. About one third of patients with inferoposterior wall left ventricular infarction have some degree of right ventricular necrosis, and an occasional patient has extensive right ventricular myocardial infarction (MI). The predominant clinical feature of right ventricular MI is severe right ventricular failure with jugular venous distension but no pulmonary vascular congestion, Kussmaul's sign (increased jugular venous distension with inspiration), and often hypotension. The mainstay of treatment is volume expansion. Pressor agents, preload and afterload reducing drugs, and intra-aortic balloon counterpulsation may also be required. (*Fauci, pp 1361–1362*)

85. **(D)** This is a classic case of condyloma (venereal warts). Condyloma acuminatum is caused by the human papillomavirus. Since this is a sexually transmitted disease (STD), women with condyloma should be screened for other STDs, such as gonorrhea, *Chlamydia*, syphilis, and possibly hepatitis B and C. (*Herbst et al, pp 609–612*)

86. **(E)** Each of the listed treatments and others have reported efficacy rates that vary widely. However, excision of the lesions generally has the highest reported efficacy rate, 89 to 93%. Efficacy rates with the other treatments

may be as high as 90+%, but there are also reports of efficacy as low as 22% with podophyllin and 23% with laser therapy. (*Scott et al, pp 483–484; Mishell et al, p 612*)

87. **(C)** Cone biopsy can be performed for diagnostic or therapeutic purposes. Most often, it is employed diagnostically, after the screening modalities (ie, Pap smear and colposcopic biopsy) have identified a lesion without completely identifying the full extent of it. The indications for cone biopsy are: unsatisfactory colposcopy (ie, inability to fully visualize the transformation zone), a more severe lesion found on Pap smear than on colposcopy, dysplasia found on endocervical curettage (ECC), and the need to rule out invasive cancer. In this case, the ECC is positive, and therefore a diagnostic cone biopsy is indicated. (*Mishell et al, pp 822–823*)

88. **(B)** The syndrome of tardive dyskinesia is caused by the use of antipsychotic drugs, usually over a long period of time. Women tend to be more susceptible to it. The use of high-dose and multiple antipsychotic drugs (used concurrently) seem to be factors as well. The type of movements seen in tardive dyskinesia help distinguish it from other disorders. These movements, which can be seen in all parts of the body, tend to be choreiform or tic-like movements. In the hands, they may be seen as jerking movements, opening and closing of all or just one or two fingers. In the trunk and legs, the movement may be twisting, squirming, or random jerking. Like tardive dyskinesia, increased body movement is seen in akathisia and in Huntington's disorder. Restlessness, pacing, and shuffling of the feet, as well as a distressful internal sense of restlessness, discomfort, and need to move, occurs in akathisia. Choreiform and athetoid movements are seen in Huntington's disorder. Family history, severity of disordered movements, and presence of dementia help distinguish this from tardive dyskinesia. In catatonic schizophrenia and pseudoparkinsonism, decreased body movements are present. Seen in a catatonic state are bizarre or inappropriate posturings held for extended periods of time; motor move-

ments are significantly slowed. An exception to this is seen in catatonic excitement, in which movements are agitated and purposeless. In parkinsonism, rigidity, tremor, and bradykinesia are seen. (*Stoudemire, pp 164–165; Kaplan and Sadock, pp 280, 485, 539*)

89. **(A)** Often, when a clinician decreases an antipsychotic, signs of tardive dyskinesia may first appear or increase. The antipsychotic is thought to have masked the signs even as the underlying pathology worsens. (*Kaplan and Sadock, pp 949–953; Stoudemire, pp 164–165; Yudofsky and Hales, pp 517–519*)

90. **(E)** Vitamin E, propranolol, diazepam, and others all have varied effects on the disordered movements of tardive dyskinesia, but none have been entirely effective. Benztropine is not effective for tardive dyskinesia but is used quite effectively for other extrapyramindal effects of the neuroleptics, such as tremors, pseudoparkinsonism, and the dystonias. (*Kaplan and Sadock, pp 960–961; Stoudemire, pp 164–165*)

91. **(D)** Although any of the drugs listed may help ameliorate the signs of tardive dyskinesia, the primary disorder for which the antipsychotic was given (ie, usually schizophrenia) still requires treatment. Clozapine is not believed to be associated with the development of tardive dyskinesia. Newer antipsychotics, such as olanzapine, sertindole, and quetiapine, seem to have little extrapyramidal effects and may offer successful treatment of psychosis without risk of tardive dyskinesia. Ideally, a discontinuation of all antipsychotics would prevent the worsening of the movement disorder. The dire effects of this on the psychotic disorder, however, make it a rare option. (*Kaplan and Sadock, pp 1070, 1077–1079; Stoudemire, pp 164–165*)

92. **(D)** Psoriasis is a chronic skin disease characterized by well-demarcated, erythematous papules and plaques covered by flakes or scales. Common sites of involvement are the scalp, back, extensor surfaces of the knees and elbows, perianal region, and genitalia. Psoriasis is associated with nail dystrophy

(pits, grooves, or crumbling), arthritis (usually monarthric, involving the digits), and acute anterior uveitis (common to the human lymphocyte antigen [HLA]-B27–related diseases). The other skin findings do not have any association with nail pitting. (*Fitzpatrick, pp 46–57*)

93. **(A)** This smear demonstrates sickling of red blood cells. Sickle cell anemia is caused by the homozygous state for the abnormal beta-globin chain gene, resulting in the production of hemoglobin S (Hb S) rather than normal Hb A. During deoxygenation, polymerization of Hb S occurs, resulting in sickled red cells. These cells lead to hemolysis, splenic and hepatic red cell sequestration, and occlusion of microvasculature, the latter being responsible for the pain symptoms. (*Hurst, pp 836–837*)

94. **(D)** Henoch–Schönlein purpura (HSP), the most common vasculitis of childhood, is characterized by petechiae or purpura of the buttocks and lower extremities and occasionally arthritis, nephritis, abdominal pain due to gastrointestinal bleeding, or other fasculitic complications. Remember, HSP is characterized by nonthrombocytopenic purpura. A normal platelet count rules out ITP. SLE, more commonly afflicting females, is not often encountered in children. Children with meningococcemia are acutely ill and febrile. Petechiae are not a feature of juvenile rheumatoid arthritis. (*Behrman et al, pp 677–678*)

95. **(C)** Children with one of the salt-losing forms of congenital adrenal hyperplasia have aldosterone deficiency. In the absence of this hormone, the kidney does not retain sodium normally and there is inappropriate retention of potassium and hydrogen ions, resulting in hyponatremia, hyperkalemia, and metabolic acidosis. The characteristic serum electrolyte aberrations observed in patients with hypertrophic pyloric stenosis include hypokalemia, hypochloremia, and metabolic alkalosis. Children with renal tubular acidosis often present with hyperchloremic metabolic acidosis and hypokalemia. Patients with gastroesophageal reflux usually present with

vomiting over several weeks. Patients with gastroenteritis usually have vomiting and diarrhea. *(Kliegman et al, pp 301–317)*

96. **(E)** The antisocial personality disorder is characterized by an ongoing disregard for and violation of the rights of others. Patterns of these behaviors and attitudes begin in early childhood or adolescence. Persons with such a disorder fail to conform to social norms and are frequently deceitful and manipulative to achieve their aims. They are impulsive and fail to plan ahead. They also tend to be irritable and may get into physical fights as well as assaultive behaviors. *(APA, pp 645–646; Stoudemire,* Clinical Psychiatry, *pp 186–187)*

97–101. **(97-C, J; 98-B, G, H; 99-E, L; 100-F, I, K; 101-A)** In DSM-IV, patients are evaluated along a multiaxial system that identifies both psychiatric and medical disorders, underlying severity of stressors, and a person's level of functioning (social, occupation, and psychological). On Axis I are listed specific clinical conditions being treated (schizophrenia, dysthymia). Axis II is identified as any personality disorder or mental retardation. On Axis III, medical conditions are identified (Huntington's disorder, tardive dyskinesia). Axis IV identifies specific psychosocial stressors and degree of severity (eg, loss of job, poverty). Overall degree of severity would be indicated to complete Axis IV (eg, mild, severe). Axis V is an assessment of functioning with numbers ranging from 1 to 100, with 1 being the lowest and 100 the highest. Homosexuality was listed as an option. Although once considered a disorder, it is now considered an alternative lifestyle. It is possible that some may experience this as a life stressor, in which case it would be listed under Axis IV. *(Kaplan and Sadock, pp 292–299, 682; Stoudemire,* Clinical Psychiatry, *pp 49–62)*

102. **(D)** Surgical procedures are classified into four categories, based on the risk of wound infection. Elective colon surgery with an adequate bowel preparation, and no spillage of gastrointestinal contents, is classified as a clean-contaminated (class II) procedure. In this patient, there was an incomplete, and hence, inadequate bowel prep, with resultant soilage at surgery, converting this to a class III contaminated procedure. *(Niederhuber, pp 161–174)*

103–105. **(103-D, 104-C, 105-D)** Evaluation of postoperative fever should begin with a thorough clinical history and examination of the patient. Empiric cultures and antibiotic therapy are not indicated and are not cost effective. Therapy should be targeted at clearly identified foci. Atelectasis is the most common cause of postoperative fever in the first 24 to 48 hours. It is managed with aggressive pulmonary toilet, chest physiotherapy, ambulation, and adequate pain control. Postoperative wound infection usually presents between the fifth and tenth postoperative days, with fever, increased incisional discomfort, wound erythema, and purulent drainage. Management is directed at opening the wound for adequate drainage and local wound care. Therapy with antibiotics is not usually required if adequate drainage is achieved. A urinary tract infection may develop postoperatively, but usually does not present before the third to fifth postoperative day. There is an increased risk in patients with indwelling urinary catheters for greater than 5 days.

Nosocomial pneumonia is a significant problem in the surgical patient but does not usually present in the first few days after elective surgery. Patients with inadequate pain control, poor pulmonary toilet, and prolonged preoperative hospitalization are at greater risk. Intra-abdominal abscess may develop as a complication after colonic surgery, either as a con-sequence of intraoperative fecal contamination, or as a result of an anastomotic leak. Established pelvic infection does not usually present before the fifth to seventh postoperative day. Management options include percutaneous CT-guided drainage. *(Niederhuber, pp 161–174)*

106. **(C)** As many as 15 to 40% of women have group B *Streptococcus* (GBS) in their lower genital tract. The overall attack rate for early-onset neonatal sepsis is 1 to 2 per 1000 births. In women whose lower genital tracts are

known to be colonized, the attack rate is 1 to 2%. Because of the low attack rate and the high rate of recolonization after antibiotic treatment, antibiotic therapy of the initial positive culture is neither beneficial nor cost effective. For the same reason, a repeat culture and treatment of a positive culture at 36 weeks is not justified. There is no evidence that a cesarean section reduces the probability of neonatal GBS sepsis. The woman who is likely to benefit the most from intrapartum antibiotic prophylaxis is one who has a known positive culture and one or more of the following risk factors:

- Preterm labor (< 37 weeks)
- Preterm, premature rupture of the membranes (< 37 weeks)
- Prolonged rupture of the membranes (> 18 hours)
- Sibling affected by symptomatic GBS infection
- Maternal fever during labor

(Schuchat et al, pp 1–24)

107. **(D)** There are 20 µg of ethinyl estradiol in Loestrin 1/20. Micronor is a progestin-only pill. The others have 30 to 50 µg of ethinyl estradiol. Potency of the hormones in the pill must also be considered in addition to the quantity. In general, a low-dose pill should be the initial choice, provided the woman tolerates it well with minimal side effects. Pregnancy rates and the risk of breakthrough bleeding are not related to the amount of hormones in the oral contraceptive. *(Hatcher et al, pp 223–236)*

108. **(A)** By definition, the incubation period is the time between exposure to the agent and the onset of symptoms. For chronic diseases, this period is usually called the latency period. This period could be as brief as a few seconds for hypersensitivity or toxic reactions or as long as decades for certain chronic diseases. *(Last: Maxcy-Roseau-Last Public Health & Preventive Medicine, p 321)*

109. **(C)** Children usually reach 50% of their expected adult height by the age of 2 years. Additionally, at 2 years of age, children reach approximately 20% of their expected adult weight and 85% of their expected adult head circumference. *(Behrman, pp 21–23)*

110. **(D)** Many healthy children have intermittent proteinuria that can be quite substantial and can be exaggerated by vigorous exercise. In those in whom it is intermittent and not accompanied by hematuria, chronic renal disease is unusual. A child who has proteinuria on a single specimen thus will need repeated urinalyses to establish the intermittent nature of the finding. Careful examination of the sediment to look for red blood cells and casts should also be performed. BP should be determined at each visit. Some clinicians also suggest protein determinations on 12-hour specimens, collected while these children are active and again while they have been resting for 12 hours, thus establishing the link to exercise. If proteinuria remains intermittent, most physicians do not perform invasive procedures such as a biopsy. Proteinuria alone is unlikely to be an indicator of urinary tract infection or structural kidney disease; thus, an IVP and urine culture are unlikely to be helpful. Likewise, with isolated and intermittent proteinuria as the only abnormality, BUN and creatinine levels are highly unlikely to be abnormal. *(Rudolph et al, pp 1338–1339)*

111. **(B)** The arteriograms in Figure 8–18 demonstrate a large aneurysm arising from the basilar artery. Intracranial aneurysms occasionally present with new onset or worsening of headaches or may be asymptomatic and found coincidentally during evaluation of an unrelated disorder. Frequently, they leak or rupture, resulting in a subarachnoid hemorrhage with sudden onset of severe headache and meningeal symptoms and signs (eg, nuchal rigidity, photophobia). Rapid progression to stroke, coma, or death may follow. Intracranial aneurysms are not associated with hypercalcemia, hypopituitarism, or chronic meningitis and rarely cause tentorial herniation without rupturing. Surgical approaches to intracranial aneurysms include excision and ligation. *(Giammarco, pp 131–138)*

112. **(B)** While the calculation of prevalence requires knowledge of the total population from which the cases arose, the calculation of incidence requires the total population at risk at the beginning of the study. In this situation, none of this information is given to permit the calculation of either prevalence or incidence measures. *(Hill, p 241; Colton, p 46)*

113. **(C)** The CT scan shown in Figure 8–19 demonstrates a smooth, biconvex lens–shaped mass in the periphery of the right temporoparietal region. This picture is characteristic of a subdural hematoma that is a result of laceration of veins bridging the subdural space. Unlike an epidural hematoma, which expands quickly and progresses rapidly to coma, a subdural hematoma is initially limited in size by increased intracranial pressure and expands slowly. Symptoms may follow the inciting trauma by several weeks. Altered mental status is often more prominent than focal signs and may progress from confusion to stupor to coma. Treatment consists of evacuation of the clot via burr holes. Antibiotics and antifungal agents have no role, and fibrinolytic therapy or delay in treatment could be harmful. *(Fauci, p 2393)*

114–116. **(114-C, 115-A, 116-C)** The patient appears to have pyelonephritis. Treatment is directed toward treating the most commonly acquired community organism, *E coli*, and ensuring good hydration. Many pediatric textbooks also recommend initial treatment in the hospital for all patients less than one year of age. In this patient, since she is vomiting and has signs of dehydration, initial management with IV fluids and antibiotics is indicated. Aggressive therapy for pyelonephritis is especially critical for younger patients, because their risk for renal scarring is the greatest. Pediatric patients with pyelonephritis are relatively likely to have an anatomic abnormality or vesicoureteral reflux. A renal ultrasound and voiding cystourethrogram are done to check for these. A renal scan could also be used to detect anatomic abnormalities but is more expensive and exposes the patient to radiation, which ultrasound does not. *(Hoberman et al, pp 11–17)*

117. **(A)** Clozapine is a relatively new antipsychotic used in treatment-resistant schizophrenia, as well as in patients who experience severe extrapyramidal side effects of tardive dyskinesia with the standard antipsychotic drugs. Unfortunately, agranulocytosis occurs in 1 to 2% of patients treated with clozapine. Immediate discontinuation of the drug is required, because this condition can be fatal. Weekly monitoring of the WBC has been required since clozapine has been available. Because most cases occur within the first 6 months of clozapine treatment, there is hope that in the future this requirement will be eased. *(Kaplan and Sadock, pp 1070–1071)*

118. **(H)** Trazodone, an antidepressant drug, is used not only for depression, but also for sleep because of its sedating properties. It is associated with the rare occurrence of priapism, a prolonged erection in the absence of sexual stimulation. If not treated early, the condition may develop into an emergent situation. *(Kaplan and Sadock, p 1099)*

119. **(C)** Haloperidol is a butyrophenone antipsychotic drug with a high degree of extrapyramidal effects. The oculogyric syndrome is an example of an extrapyramidal effect called a dystonia. Thioridazine, a piperidine phenothiazine, has some potential to cause extrapyramidal symptoms, but this is significantly less than seen with haloperidol. *(Kaplan and Sadock, p 980)*

120. **(E)** Lithium carbonate is a naturally occurring salt used as a mood stabilizer in the treatment of bipolar disorders. Because of the potential for toxicity, periodic monitoring of blood level is required. Additionally, monitoring is required to confirm a blood level within the therapeutic range, usually 0.6 to 1.2 mEq/L. As serum levels rise above 1.5 mEq/L, symptoms of toxicity emerge in a somewhat predictable manner from early signs such as nausea, vomiting, and diarrhea to more severe signs of coarse tremor, ataxia, lethargy, and coma. Sensitivity to the significance of observable clinical signs provides a means for the clinician to identify toxicity

even though a blood level is not immediately available. *(Kaplan and Sadock, p 1050)*

121. **(G)** Thioridazine causes retrograde ejaculation in men. This is harmless, but nevertheless a cause of embarrassment. *(Kaplan and Sadock, p 1029)*

122–126. **(122-K, 123-I, 124-C, 125-B, 126-J)** The most common cause of lower respiratory infections in infants is respiratory syncytial virus (RSV). It commonly presents during the winter months with rhinorrhea and wheezing. Infants typically are afebrile. Adenovirus can present with wheezing but more typically also includes conjunctivitis and pharyngitis. *Mycoplasma pneumoniae* is the most common cause of pneumonia in school-aged children. The typical course is a gradual onset of fever, cough, and malaise. *Streptococcus pneumoniae* can cause pneumonia in this age group but typically presents more acutely. *Chlamydia trachomatis* is the most common cause for conjunctivitis in the first few months of life. Infants acquire it at birth from their mother. In some infants, it progresses to pneumonitis with the classic "staccato" cough. Adenovirus can cause a respiratory infection as well as conjunctivitis, but the two symptoms occur concurrently. Pertussis presents with an insidious prodrome over several weeks which is difficult to differentiate from other upper respiratory infections except that it lasts longer. The second phase is the paroxysmal phase, with the episodic cough that can be quite severe. Although the pertussis vaccine is in widespread use, the disease is relatively common. The reservoir of infection is typically adults whose immunity has waned. Many pathogens cause respiratory infections in children. In this patient, the course is too long for a typical viral infection, and not acute enough for bacterial pneumonia, such as that caused by group B *Streptococcus*. Croup is a common respiratory infection that occurs in the autumn. The typical course is a few days of cough, rhinorrhea, and low-grade fever, followed by the onset of paroxysms of barky or seal-like cough. It is typically worse at night and resolves in 2 days. The most common cause is parainfluenza virus. *(Kleigman et al, pp 64–80)*

REFERENCES

ACOG Technical Bulletin. *Immunization During Pregnancy.* Number 160. October 1991.

Adrogue HJ, Madias NE. Management of life-threatening acid–base disorders. *New Engl J Med* 1998;338:26–34.

Ameli S, Shah PK. Cardiac tamponade. *Card Clin* 1991;9:665–673.

American Academy of Pediatrics. *Report of the Committee on Infectious Diseases,* 24th ed. Evanston: American Academy of Pediatrics; 1997.

American Psychiatric Association (APA). *Diagnostic and Statistical Manual of Mental Disorders,* 4th ed., revised. Washington, DC: American Psychiatric Association; 1994.

Andreason NC, Black DW. *Introductory Textbook of Psychiatry,* 2nd ed. Washington, DC: American Psychiatric Association; 1995.

Bar-Or O. *Pediatric Sports Medicine for the Practitioner,* 1st ed. New York: Springer-Verlag; 1983.

Bartlett JG, Mundy LM. Community-acquired pneumonia. *N Engl J Med* 1995;333:1618–1624.

Behrman RE, Kliegman RM, Arvin AM. *Nelson Textbook of Pediatrics,* 15th ed. Philadelphia: WB Saunders; 1996.

Berkowitz CD. *Pediatrics: A Primary Care Approach.* Philadelphia: WB Saunders; 1996.

Byrne TN. Spinal cord compression from epidural metastases. *N Engl J Med* 1992;327:614–619.

Centers for Disease Control. *Preventing Lead Poisoning in Young Children.* October 1991.

Champion LAA, Schwartz AD, Luddy RE, Schindler S. The effects of four commonly used drugs on platelet function. *J Pediatr* 1976;89:653–656.

Coffey RL, Zile MR, Luskin AT. Immunologic tests of value in diagnosis. I. Acute phase reactants and autoantibodies. *Postgrad Med* 1981;70:163–178.

Committee on Drugs. Treatment guidelines for lead exposure in children. *Pediatrics* 1995;96:155–160.

Creasy RK, Resnik R. *Maternal–Fetal Medicine: Principles and Practice,* 3rd ed. Philadelphia: WB Saunders; 1994.

Cunningham FG, MacDonald PC, Gant NF, et al. *Williams Obstetrics,* 20th ed. East Stamford, CT: Appleton & Lange; 1997.

Dajani AS, Taubert KA, Wilson W, et al. Prevention of bacterial endocarditis: recommendations by the American Heart Association. *JAMA* 1997; 277:1794–1801.

DeArce MA, Kearns A. The fragile X syndrome: the patients and their chromosomes. *J Med Genet* 1984;21:84–91.

Diabetes Control and Complications Trial Research Group. The effect of intensive treatment of diabetes on the development and progression of long-term complications in insulin-dependent diabetes mellitus. *N Engl J Med* 1993;329:977–986.

DiSaia PJ, Creasman WT. *Clinical Gynecologic Oncology.* St. Louis: Mosby; 1997.

Dixon AC, Parrillo JE. Managing the cardiovascular effects of sepsis and shock. *J Crit Illness* 1991;6: 1197–1214.

Ellenhorn MJ. *Ellenhorn's Medical Toxicology: Diagnosis and Treatment of Human Poisoning,* 2nd ed. Baltomore: Williams & Wilkins; 1997.

Fauci A, Braunwald E, Isselbacher KJ, et al. *Harrison's Principles of Internal Medicine,* 14th ed. New York: McGraw-Hill International Book Co; 1998.

Feigin RD, Cherry JD. *Textbook of Pediatric Infectious Diseases,* 3rd ed. Philadelphia: WB Saunders; 1992.

Feinstein AR, *Clinical Epidemiology the Architecture of Clinical Research.* Philadelphia: WB Saunders; 1985.

Fink JN, Fauci A. Immunological aspects of cardiovascular disease. *JAMA* 1982;248:2716–2721.

Fitzpatrick TB, Johnson RA, Polano MK, Suurmond DS. *Color Atlas and Synopsis of Clinical Dermatology,* 2nd ed. New York: McGraw-Hill; 1994.

Gartner LM. Neonatal jaundice. *Pediatr Rev* 1994; 15:422–432.

Giammarco R, Edmeads J, Dodick D. *Critical Decisions in Headache Management.* Hamilton, Ontario: BC Decker, Inc; 1998.

Goroll AH, Lawrence AM, Mulley AG. *Primary Care Medicine,* 3rd ed. Philadelphia: JB Lippincott; 1995.

Greenfield LJ, Mulholland M, Oldham KT, Zelenock GB, and Lillemoe KD, eds. *Surgery: Scientific Principles and Practice.* Philadelphia: Lippincott-Raven; 1997.

Guyer B, Martin J, MacDorman M, Anderson R, Strobino D. Annual Summary of Vital Statistics-1996. *Pediatrics* 1997;100:905–918.

Hales RE, Frances AJ, eds. *Psychiatry Update: American Psychiatric Association Annual Review,* vol. 6. Washington, DC: American Psychiatry Press; 1987.

Hatcher RA, Trussell J, Stewart F, et al. *Contraceptive Technology,* 16th ed. rev. New York: Irvington Publishers; 1994.

Hill BA. *Principles of Medical Statistics,* 8th ed. Oxford University Press; 1966.

Hogan DE. The emergency department approach to diarrhea. *Emerg Clin North Am* 1996;14:673–692.

Hurst JW. *Medicine for the Practicing Physician.* Stamford, CT: Appleton & Lange; 1996.

Hurwitz S. *Clinical Pediatric Dermatology: A Textbook of Skin Disorders of Childhood and Adolescence.* Philadelphia: WB Saunders; 1981.

Joint National Committee on Prevention, Detection, Evaluation and Treatment of High Blood Pressure. The sixth report. *Arch Intern Med* 1997; 157:2413–2446.

Kaplan HI, Sadock BJ. *Synopsis of Psychiatry: Behavioral Sciences Clinical Psychiatry,* 8th ed. Baltimore: Williams & Wilkins; 1998.

Kelley WN. *Textbook of Internal Medicine,* 2nd ed. New York: JB Lippincott; 1992.

Kliegman RM. *Practical Strategies in Pediatric Diagnosis and Therapy.* Philadelphia: WB Saunders; 1996.

Koehler JE. Bartonella infections. *Adv Pediatr Infect Dis* 1996;11:1–27.

LaDou I. *Occupational Medicine,* 2nd ed. Stamford, CT: Appleton & Lange; 1997.

Laine L, Suchower L, Connors A, Neil G. Twice-daily, 10-day triple therapy with omeprazole, amoxicillin, and clarithromycin for *Helicobacter pylori* eradication in duodenal ulcer disease: results of three multicenter, double-blind, United States trials. *Am J Gastroenterol* 1998;93:2106–2112.

Last JM, ed. *Maxcy-Rosenau-Last Public Health & Preventive Medicine,* 13th ed. East Norwalk, CT: Appleton & Lange; 1992.

Last JM. *Public Health and Human Ecology,* 2nd ed. Stamford, CT: Appleton & Lange; 1997.

Light RW. Parapneumonic effusions and empyema: current management strategies. *J Crit Illness* 1995;10:832–842.

McAnarney ER, Kreipe RE, Orr DP, et al. *Textbook of Adolescent Medicine.* Philadelphia: WB Saunders; 1992.

The Medical Letter on Drugs and Therapeutics: Drugs for Treatment of Acute Otitis Media in Children. New Rochelle; Medical Letter, Inc; 1994;36:19–21.

Mishell DR Jr., Stenchever MA, Droegemueller W, Herbst AL. *Comprehensive Gynecology,* 3rd ed. St. Louis: Mosby; 1997.

MMWR Morbidity and Mortality Weekly Report. Recommendations and Reports. *1998 Guidelines for Treatment of Sexually Transmitted Diseases.* Volume 47, No. RR-01. January 23, 1998. U.S. Department of Health and Human Services.

Niederhuber JE. *Fundamentals of Surgery.* Stamford, CT: Appleton & Lange; 1998.

Norman ME. Vitamin D in bone disease. *Pediatr Clin North Am* 1982;29:947–971.

Oski FA, DeAngelis CD, Feigin RD, et al. *Principles and Practice of Pediatrics,* 2nd ed. Philadelphia: JB Lippincott; 1994.

Rankin AC, Brooks R, Ruskin JN et al. Adenosine and the treatment of supraventricular tachycardia. *Am J Med* 1992; 92:655–664.

Relman DA, Schmidt TM, MacDermott RP et al. Identification of the uncultured bacillus of Whipple's disease. *N Engl J Med* 1992;327:293–301.

Rock JA, Thompson JD. *TeLinde's Operative Gynecology.* 8th ed. Philadelphia: Lippincott-Raven; 1997.

Rowe MI, O'Neill JA, Grosfeld JL, et al. *Essentials of Pediatric Surgery.* St. Louis: Mosby; 1995.

Rudolph AM, Hoffman JIE, Rudolph CD. *Pediatrics,* 20th ed. Stamford, CT: Appleton & Lange; 1996.

Sabiston DC, ed. *Textbook of Surgery,* 15th ed. Philadelphia: WB Saunders; 1997.

Schuchat A, Whitney C, Zangwill K. Prevention of perinatal group B streptococcal disease: a public health perspective. *Morbid Mortal Wkly Rep* 1996; 45(No. RR-7):1–24.

Schumacher HR, ed. *Primer on the Rheumatic Diseases,* 10th ed. Atlanta: Arthritis Foundation; 1993.

Schwartz SI, Shires GT, and Spencer FC, eds. *Principles of Surgery.* New York: McGraw-Hill; 1994.

Scott JR, DiSaia PJ, Hammond CB, Spellacy WN, eds. *Danforth's Obstetrics and Gynecology,* 7th ed. Philadelphia: JB Lippincott; 1994.

Second Report of the National Cholesterol Education Program Expert Panel on Detection, Evaluation and Treatment of High Blood Cholesterol in Adults. NIH Publication No. 93-3095; 1993.

Speroff L, Glass RH, Kase NG. *Clinical Gynecologic Endocrinology and Infertility,* 5th ed. Baltimore: Williams & Wilkins; 1994.

Stoudemire A, ed. *Clinical Psychiatry for Medical Students,* 2nd ed. Philadelphia: JB Lippincott; 1994.

Stoudemire A, ed. *Human Behavior: An Introduction for Medical Students.* Philadelphia: JB Lippincott; 1990.

Sweet RL, Gibbs RS. *Infectious Diseases of the Female Genital Tract,* 3rd ed. Baltimore: Williams & Wilkins; 1995.

Tancredi LR. Emergency psychiatry and crisis intervention: some legal and ethical issues. *Psychiatry Ann* 1982;12:799–806.

Tecklenburg FW, Wright MS. Minor head trauma in the pediatric patient. *Pediatr Emerg Care* 1991;7:40–47.

Tomb DA. *Psychiatry,* 5th ed. Baltimore: Williams & Wilkins; 1995.

Traugott L, Alpers A. In their own hands. *Arch Pediatr Adolesc Med* 1997;151:922–927.

U.S. Preventive Services Task Force. *Guide to Clinical Preventive Services,* 2nd ed. Baltimore: Williams & Wilkins; 1996.

Wedding D. *Behavior and Medicine,* 2nd ed. St. Louis: Mosby; 1995.

Yamada T, Alpers D, Owyang C, et al. *Textbook of Gastroenterology.* Philadelphia: JB Lippincott; 1991.

Yen SSC, Jaffe RB. *Reproductive Endocrinology: Physiology, Pathophysiology and Clinical Management,* 3rd ed. Philadelphia: WB Saunders; 1991.

Zais N. *The Nail in Health and Disease,* 2nd ed. East Norwalk, CT: Appleton & Lange; 1990.

Zenz C. *Occupational Medicine,* 3rd ed. Editors. Dickerson BO, Horvath EP. St. Louis: Mosby; 1994.

Zinner MJ. *Maingot's Abdominal Operations,* 10th ed., vols. I and II. Stamford, CT: Appleton & Lange; 1997.

Subspecialty List:
Chapter 8—Practice Test 2

83. Infectious diseases
84. Cardiovascular system diseases
92. Skin diseases
93. Hematology
111. Vascular
113. Vascular

SURGERY

1. Digestive system diseases
2. Digestive system diseases
20. Digestive system diseases
21. Digestive system diseases
22. Digestive system diseases
33. Infectious diseases
34. Infectious diseases
51. Oncology
52. Oncology
65. Digestive system diseases
66. Digestive system diseases
67. Digestive system diseases
68. Digestive system diseases
71. Trauma
72. Trauma
78. Digestive system diseases
79. Digestive system diseases
102. Digestive system diseases
103. Digestive system diseases
104. Digestive system diseases
105. Digestive system diseases

PSYCHIATRY

6. Assessment
7. Assessment
8. Assessment
25. Intervention
26. Personality theory
35. Child psychiatry/Assessment
36. Personality theory
47. Disease control
73. Oncology
74. Psychopathology
77. Intervention/Legal
88. Assessment
89. Intervention
90. Intervention
91. Intervention
96. Psychopathology
97. Assessment
98. Assessment
99. Assessment
100. Assessment
101. Assessment
117. Intervention
118. Intervention
119. Intervention
120. Intervention
121. Intervention

PREVENTIVE MEDICINE

4. Disease control
13. Disease control
19. Biostatistics
48. Assessment
108. Epidemiology
112. Biostatistics

Practice Test 2

NAME _____
  Last   First   Middle

ADDRESS _____
  Street

_____
  City   State   Zip

<table>
<tr><td>S</td><td></td><td>0 1 2 3 4 5 6 7 8 9</td></tr>
<tr><td>O</td><td>N</td><td>0 1 2 3 4 5 6 7 8 9</td></tr>
<tr><td></td><td>U</td><td>0 1 2 3 4 5 6 7 8 9</td></tr>
<tr><td>C</td><td>M</td><td>0 1 2 3 4 5 6 7 8 9</td></tr>
<tr><td></td><td>B</td><td>0 1 2 3 4 5 6 7 8 9</td></tr>
<tr><td>S</td><td>E</td><td>0 1 2 3 4 5 6 7 8 9</td></tr>
<tr><td></td><td></td><td>0 1 2 3 4 5 6 7 8 9</td></tr>
<tr><td>E</td><td>R</td><td>0 1 2 3 4 5 6 7 8 9</td></tr>
<tr><td>C</td><td></td><td>0 1 2 3 4 5 6 7 8 9</td></tr>
</table>

DIRECTIONS   Mark your social security number from top to bottom
in the appropriate boxes on the right.
Use No. 2 lead pencil only.
Mark one and only one answer for each item.
Make each mark black enough to obliterate the letter
within the parentheses.
Erase clearly any answer you wish to change.

1. (A) (B) (C) (D) (E)
2. (A) (B) (C) (D) (E)
3. (A) (B) (C) (D) (E)
4. (A) (B) (C) (D) (E)
5. (A) (B) (C) (D) (E)
6. (A) (B) (C) (D) (E)
7. (A) (B) (C) (D) (E)
8. (A) (B) (C) (D) (E)
9. (A) (B) (C) (D) (E)
10. (A) (B) (C) (D) (E)
11. (A) (B) (C) (D) (E)
12. (A) (B) (C) (D) (E)
13. (A) (B) (C) (D) (E)
14. (A) (B) (C) (D) (E)
15. (A) (B) (C) (D) (E)
16. (A) (B) (C) (D) (E)
17. (A) (B) (C) (D) (E)
18. (A) (B) (C) (D) (E)
19. (A) (B) (C) (D) (E)
20. (A) (B) (C) (D) (E)
21. (A) (B) (C) (D) (E)
22. (A) (B) (C) (D) (E)

23. (A) (B) (C) (D) (E)
24. (A) (B) (C) (D) (E)
25. (A) (B) (C) (D) (E)
26. (A) (B) (C) (D) (E)
27. (A) (B) (C) (D) (E)
28. (A) (B) (C) (D) (E)
29. (A) (B) (C) (D) (E)
30. (A) (B) (C) (D) (E)
31. (A) (B) (C) (D) (E)
32. (A) (B) (C) (D) (E)
33. (A) (B) (C) (D) (E)
34. (A) (B) (C) (D) (E)
35. (A) (B) (C) (D) (E)
36. (A) (B) (C) (D) (E)
37. (A) (B) (C) (D) (E) (F) (G)
    (H) (I) (J) (K) (L) (M) (N)
38. (A) (B) (C) (D) (E) (F) (G)
    (H) (I) (J) (K) (L) (M) (N)
39. (A) (B) (C) (D) (E) (F) (G)
    (H) (I) (J) (K) (L) (M) (N)
40. (A) (B) (C) (D) (E) (F) (G)
    (H) (I) (J) (K) (L) (M) (N)

41. (A) (B) (C) (D) (E) (F) (G)
    (H) (I) (J) (K) (L) (M) (N)
42. (A) (B) (C) (D) (E) (F) (G)
    (H) (I) (J) (K) (L) (M) (N)
43. (A) (B) (C) (D) (E) (F) (G)
    (H) (I) (J) (K) (L) (M) (N)
44. (A) (B) (C) (D) (E) (F) (G)
    (H) (I) (J) (K) (L) (M) (N)
45. (A) (B) (C) (D) (E) (F) (G)
    (H) (I) (J) (K) (L) (M) (N)
46. (A) (B) (C) (D) (E) (F) (G)
    (H) (I) (J) (K) (L) (M) (N)
47. (A) (B) (C) (D) (E)
48. (A) (B) (C) (D) (E)
49. (A) (B) (C) (D) (E)
50. (A) (B) (C) (D) (E)
51. (A) (B) (C) (D) (E)
52. (A) (B) (C) (D) (E)
53. (A) (B) (C) (D) (E)
54. (A) (B) (C) (D) (E)
55. (A) (B) (C) (D) (E)
56. (A) (B) (C) (D) (E)

57. (A) (B) (C) (D) (E)
58. (A) (B) (C) (D) (E)
59. (A) (B) (C) (D) (E)
    (F) (G) (H)
60. (A) (B) (C) (D) (E)
    (F) (G) (H)
61. (A) (B) (C) (D) (E) (F) (G)
62. (A) (B) (C) (D) (E) (F) (G)
63. (A) (B) (C) (D) (E) (F) (G)
64. (A) (B) (C) (D) (E) (F) (G)
65. (A) (B) (C) (D) (E) (F) (G)
66. (A) (B) (C) (D) (E) (F) (G)
67. (A) (B) (C) (D) (E) (F) (G)
68. (A) (B) (C) (D) (E) (F) (G)
69. (A) (B) (C) (D) (E)
70. (A) (B) (C) (D) (E)
71. (A) (B) (C) (D) (E)
72. (A) (B) (C) (D) (E)
73. (A) (B) (C) (D) (E)
74. (A) (B) (C) (D) (E)
75. (A) (B) (C) (D) (E)
76. (A) (B) (C) (D) (E)

77. (A) (B) (C) (D) (E)

78. (A) (B) (C) (D) (E)

79. (A) (B) (C) (D) (E)

80. (A) (B) (C) (D) (E)

81. (A) (B) (C) (D) (E)

82. (A) (B) (C) (D) (E)

83. (A) (B) (C) (D) (E)

84. (A) (B) (C) (D) (E)

85. (A) (B) (C) (D) (E)

86. (A) (B) (C) (D) (E)

87. (A) (B) (C) (D) (E)

88. (A) (B) (C) (D) (E)

89. (A) (B) (C) (D) (E)

90. (A) (B) (C) (D) (E)

91. (A) (B) (C) (D) (E)

92. (A) (B) (C) (D) (E)

93. (A) (B) (C) (D) (E)

94. (A) (B) (C) (D) (E)

95. (A) (B) (C) (D) (E)

96. (A) (B) (C) (D) (E)

97. (A) (B) (C) (D) (E) (F)
    (G) (H) (I) (J) (K) (L)

98. (A) (B) (C) (D) (E) (F)
    (G) (H) (I) (J) (K) (L)

99. (A) (B) (C) (D) (E) (F)
    (G) (H) (I) (J) (K) (L)

100. (A) (B) (C) (D) (E) (F)
     (G) (H) (I) (J) (K) (L)

101. (A) (B) (C) (D) (E) (F)
     (G) (H) (I) (J) (K) (L)

102. (A) (B) (C) (D) (E)

103. (A) (B) (C) (D) (E)

104. (A) (B) (C) (D) (E)

105. (A) (B) (C) (D) (E)

106. (A) (B) (C) (D) (E)

107. (A) (B) (C) (D) (E)

108. (A) (B) (C) (D) (E)

109. (A) (B) (C) (D) (E)

110. (A) (B) (C) (D) (E)

111. (A) (B) (C) (D) (E)

112. (A) (B) (C) (D) (E)

113. (A) (B) (C) (D) (E)

114. (A) (B) (C) (D) (E)

115. (A) (B) (C) (D) (E)

116. (A) (B) (C) (D) (E)

117. (A) (B) (C) (D) (E)
     (F) (G) (H)

118. (A) (B) (C) (D) (E)
     (F) (G) (H)

119. (A) (B) (C) (D) (E)
     (F) (G) (H)

120. (A) (B) (C) (D) (E)
     (F) (G) (H)

121. (A) (B) (C) (D) (E)
     (F) (G) (H)

122. (A) (B) (C) (D) (E) (F)
     (G) (H) (I) (J) (K) (L)
     (M) (N) (O) (P)

123. (A) (B) (C) (D) (E) (F)
     (G) (H) (I) (J) (K) (L)
     (M) (N) (O) (P)

124. (A) (B) (C) (D) (E) (F)
     (G) (H) (I) (J) (K) (L)
     (M) (N) (O) (P)

125. (A) (B) (C) (D) (E) (F)
     (G) (H) (I) (J) (K) (L)
     (M) (N) (O) (P)

126. (A) (B) (C) (D) (E) (F)
     (G) (H) (I) (J) (K) (L)
     (M) (N) (O) (P)

ISBN   0-8385-0341-1

90000

9 780838 503416